W9-AGI-413

PRAISE FOR *A LIBERATED MIND*

"In all my years studying personal growth, Acceptance and Commitment Therapy is one of the most useful tools I've ever come across, and in this book, Dr. Hayes describes it with more depth and clarity than ever before."

—Mark Manson, *New York Times*–bestselling author of *The Subtle Art of Not Giving a F*ck*

"In our crisis-ridden society psychological flexibility is more needed than ever. Transcending shallow and ineffective behavioral approaches, Dr. Steven Hayes here presents a methodology, a skill-set, for emotional liberation that enables us to pivot from self-limitation to self-awareness and self-affirmative action."

—Gabor Maté, MD, author of *When the Body Says No: Exploring the Stress-Disease Connection*

"We can spend our lives avoiding the thoughts and feelings that cause us pain. But Steve Hayes has become a leader in his field by understanding that things that cause us pain are things about which we care. By learning to use psychological flexibility we can turn toward the difficult places to live with richness and meaning. Compassionate, helpful, and authoritative, *A Liberated Mind* shows us a powerful way to a fulfilling life."

—Susan David, PhD, author of *Emotional Agility*

"The key to evolving consciousness is cultivating a flexible mind—open, present, empowered and aligned with deep values—and Steven Hayes does a brilliant job showing us how. This book is organized around developing six psychological skills that clinical research shows, beyond all other factors, promote flexibility and translate into a happier and healthier life. As you read this illuminating book, you'll see how these skills are learnable, that you can start right now, and how when woven together, they offer a path to inner freedom."

—Tara Brach, PhD, author of *Radical Acceptance* and *True Refuge*

"*A Liberated Mind* provides an outstanding introduction to a psychological approach that has changed many lives by turning us toward focusing on our values. The ideas and advice presented here help us truly understand what matters so that we can live with greater freedom, courage, and joy."

—Kelly McGonigal, PhD, author of *The Willpower Instinct* and *The Upside of Stress*

"Steven Hayes possesses an extraordinary trifecta of skills: A brilliant theoretical and research psychologist, he's also a compassionate clinician and a wonderfully engaging writer. *A Liberated Mind* is packed with jewels of insight and information that could change the way we deal with suffering as individuals and as a society. A compelling, revelatory read."

—Martha Beck, PhD, author of *Finding Your Own North Star*

"Dr. Steven C. Hayes is one of the greatest thinkers, psychological theorists, and clinicians alive. He has contributed an enormous amount to the field of psychology and is well-known for being the creator of ACT (Acceptance and Commitment Therapy), a treatment that has now become the first-line approach for many psychological problems. The book, *A Liberated Mind: How to Pivot Toward What Matters*, tells a very personal story about the origin and development of this treatment. Written for a very broad audience, Dr. Hayes is able to clearly translate the science and clinical complexity of this treatment into concrete guiding principles for people's lives. These principles not only apply to psychological suffering, but also to physical illnesses, relationships, corporations, societies, and cultures. The book is honest, compassionate, and profoundly insightful. It will transform your life by liberating your mind."

—Stefan G. Hofmann, PhD, professor of psychology at Boston University

"In this highly accessible book, Steven Hayes identifies pathways to connecting with our deepest values and pursuing what really matters. Filled with compassion, wisdom, and down-to-earth methods for change, *A Liberated Mind* is a refreshing 'how to' manual for overcoming the obstacles, judgments, habits, and prejudices that so often stand in the way of a life worth living."

—Richard M. Ryan, professor at the Institute for Positive Psychology and Education, Australian Catholic University, and co-developer of Self-Determination Theory

"Many of our inborn behavioral tendencies were wonderfully well adapted to the world they evolved in fifty thousand years ago. But disaster ensues when our primitive and automatic impulses inflexibly control us, rather than us flexibly controlling them. Hayes combines a scientist's precision with a poet's sensitivity in freeing us to be more loving and fully human. This is a great self-help book for people who would never dream of reading a self-help book."

—Allen Frances, professor emeritus and former chair at the Duke Department of Psychiatry, chair of the DSM-IV Task Force, and author of *Saving Normal*

"Steve Hayes is a brilliant thinker and doer, and nowhere is this more evident than in this book. It weaves together research and a lifetime of practical experience into an accessible, personal, and positive guide to thinking about our lives in a fundamentally more helpful way."

—Kelly D. Brownell, PhD, director of World Food Policy Center and Robert L. Flowers Professor of Public Policy at Duke University

"Steven C. Hayes is today's B. F. Skinner—a great intellect, equally passionate about basic knowledge and practical applications. In *A Liberated Mind*, you can get to know him as a person and apply his wisdom to your own life."

—David Sloan Wilson, president at The Evolution Institute and author of *This View of Life: Completing the Darwinian Revolution*

"Based on a broad and deep knowledge of cutting-edge psychological science and a wide-ranging appreciation of philosophical and religious wisdoms, one of the leading psychologists in the world, Steven C. Hayes, provides an antidote to the conundrum of human struggle and despair. Everyone experiencing anxiety, depression, or pain in their life and striving for emotional well-being should be aware of the surprising revelations in this well-written and easy-to-read book."

—David H. Barlow, professor of psychology and psychiatry emeritus, founder and director emeritus at the Center for Anxiety and Related Disorders, Boston University

A LIBERATED MIND

How to Pivot Toward What Matters

STEVEN C. HAYES, PhD

AVERY
an imprint of Penguin Random House LLC
New York

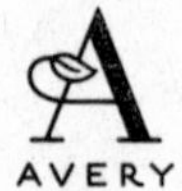

an imprint of Penguin Random House LLC
penguinrandomhouse.com

Most Avery books are available at special quantity discounts for bulk purchase for sales promotions, premiums, fund-raising, and educational needs. Special books or book excerpts also can be created to fit specific needs. For details, write SpecialMarkets@penguinrandomhouse.com.

Library of Congress Cataloging-in-Publication Data

Names: Hayes, Steven C., author.
Title: A liberated mind : how to pivot toward what matters / Steven C. Hayes, PhD.
Description: New York : Avery, 2019. | Includes bibliographical references and index.
Identifiers: LCCN 2019004734 | ISBN 9780735214002 (hardback) |
ISBN 9780735214026 (ebook)
Subjects: LCSH: Self-help techniques. | BISAC: PSYCHOLOGY / Mental Health. |
MEDICAL / Psychiatry / General.
Classification: LCC BF632 .H299 2019 | DDC 158.1—dc23
LC record available at https://lccn.loc.gov/2019004734
p. cm.

International edition: ISBN 9780593085875

Printed in the United States of America
10 9 8 7 6 5 4 3 2 1

Book design by Lorie Pagnozzi

Neither the publisher nor the author is engaged in rendering professional advice or services to the individual reader. The ideas, procedures, and suggestions contained in this book are not intended as a substitute for consulting with your physician. All matters regarding your health require medical supervision. Neither the author nor the publisher shall be liable or responsible for any loss or damage allegedly arising from any information or suggestion in this book.

This book is dedicated to the memory of
John Cloud: reporter, rascal, raconteur, friend.
You believed in me and in this book, which
has lifted me up every single day I've worked on it.
The world asks reporters to do such hard things,
without understanding the cost.
Be at peace, my friend. Be at peace.

CONTENTS

Part Three

ACKNOWLEDGMENTS

I began to think about this book shortly after my first self-help book, *Get Out of Your Mind and Into Your Life*, became popular in 2006. I drafted a crude proposal but it was odd and it languished. I'm a geek by training and personality, and even among psychologists it is a bit of a joke that I can be incomprehensible. It was not until Linda Loewenthal reached out a few years later and became my agent that the project began to move. Linda brought that needed mixture of support, pushing, wisdom, skill, patience, and caring that by 2011 had turned the project into something real. Her trust in me, and her unwaveringly honest feedback over the years, lifted me up and pushed me forward.

The late John Cloud, the *Time* magazine reporter who plucked me out of obscurity in 2006 when he wrote the story that launched the success of *Get Out of Your Mind*, helped produce the first well-crafted proposal and sample chapter drafts. I have dedicated this book to him because in an alternate universe, he and I would have written the entire volume together as I had originally hoped. He was a brilliant writer and a deep soul, and I so hope the spirit of John is reflected in this book.

Spencer Smith, a professional writer and co-author of *Get Out of Your Mind*, also helped with the proposal. Spencer is what my Jewish relatives would call a mensch—he is an honorable, kind, reliable, ethical straight shooter. I am blessed to call him a friend and colleague.

Emily Loose was my development editor for this book. Amazingly able, wise, and persistent, she deliberately allowed the ideas in the book to enter into her life so she could bring her gut feel to the development process. I was honored, moved, and impressed by that approach—she is simply the best.

Caroline Sutton at Penguin/Avery gave very helpful input on the text at critical points of the development processes.

All of my adult children (Camille, Charlie, and Esther) were sounding boards and gave specific input, from Esther's drawings to Camille's title ideas.

My wife, Jacque, stood by me for the many years and endless rewrites it took to get these words produced. Trips, interviews, writing binges, research—all shifted obligations onto her shoulders. I can't ever repay that debt, but it brings tears to my eyes to acknowledge and remember it. Jacque also provided key input regarding the new ideas in this book as they were vetted one at a time in long discussions that delayed our sleep. She especially pushed me to look more closely at social context and privilege issues, which are critical to the arc of this work. Thank you, my love.

My doctoral graduate students of the last few years helped with discussions of nuances of ACT theory, including Brandon Sanford, Fred Chin, Cory Stanton, and Patrick Smith. Almost all of the forty-eight doctoral students of mine who already have their PhDs are in the backstory of specific parts of this book. I mentioned just a few of them in the text and endnotes but they are there anyway, in ways that only they and I will know specifically but that the reader will benefit from. Thank you, gang. (No, this does not mean you can tell people the secret behavioral handshake.)

I was helped in considering various titling options by Greg Stikeleather and Till Gross. Hank Robb and Inge Skeans kindly helped with proofing and calling out confusing sentences.

The section on lying in Chapter Four was originally written for a book that Guy Ritchie and I were considering writing, to go along with a film he was working on regarding the impact of the ego. The book project did not move forward (I hope someday the film will appear—it is a powerful piece), but it was Guy who first made me aware of the deep connection between the conceptualized self and lying, and the clarity of his vision made a lasting impact. I would like to thank him for his insights.

I would also like to acknowledge the clients who have changed ACT work with their very lives. Some of their stories are in this book, anonymized, but others are here indirectly because of the ways their pain and courage informed the work. For example, a substantial portion of the metaphors used to explain ACT came from clients, not me or any other professional. We will all be forgotten, but maybe, just maybe, your courage has put things into the culture that will reverberate for a long time. 'Tis a consummation devoutly to be wished.

I want to give a deep bow of appreciation to the entire contextual behavioral science community. It is an amazing group of clinicians, teachers, basic researchers, philosophers, applied researchers, policy experts, evolutionists, behaviorists, cognitivists, prevention scientists, nurses, physicians, coaches, psychologists, and social workers (I could go on like that for a while) spread across the globe. I've told some of their individual stories in this book, but the reader should know that behind every name in every endnote relevant to ACT, RFT, and CBS is a committed human being. I know many of them, perhaps the majority of them, and they deeply care about working together to create a psychology more worthy of the challenge of the human condition. I have tried to give their ideas and aspirations voice in this book. I may have instigated this work, but I am only a co-founder or co-developer because by the time it came together in book form in 1999, it needed the able hands of Kirk Strosahl and Kelly Wilson, and to be refined for research and practice it needed hundreds of caring professionals and researchers. That continues to be even truer as it has entered the world community. We are all better human beings when we are groups, and my colleagues have lifted me up with their values, vision, and friendship every step of this journey.

As I will repeat in the very end of this book, life is a choice between love and fear. Those human beings who have loved me—friends, family, and colleagues—have helped me choose love. There is no better gift. Thank you.

Steven C. Hayes, Reno, Nevada

AUTHOR'S NOTE

This book is fairly heavily referenced, but in order not to distract the reader almost all of the documentation is in the endnotes. If you see me writing about a study, stating facts, or suggesting that books are available and so on, and you want to follow up, check in the back. The endnotes are "blind," meaning there is no indication in the text that I've provided references, comments, or resources, but I've tried to do so whenever I detected a possible need, so look there first whenever you need further information. In order not to slow down the volume by mentioning names of people the normal reader will not have a reason to learn, I sometimes cite and credit people in the endnotes rather than the text, even using words like "my colleagues" or "my team" to speak of people in my lab tradition or the contextual behavioral science community writ large. To normal academic readers that will at times seem self-focused, but it is in the service of the reader and seems to be necessary in books of this kind. All I can do is to beg for tolerance of that decision and ask people to look in the endnotes.

I also mention my website with some regularity (http://www.stevenchayes.com) for tests you can take or lists of resources you can access and the like, but that too can get tiresome, so in the final edit I cut that down a fair amount. In some of those cases I wrote an endnote instead.

There is also a lot of useful information about this work on the website for the Association for Contextual Behavioral Science (ACBS), which is the group most focused on the development of the work I write about in this book: http://www.contextualscience.org. Some of the information on that site requires that you log in as a member in order to see it, but public members are welcome and it is inexpensive.

Finally, vast resources are also available for free online, such as an ACT YouTube channel, ACT-based TED talks (you can see my two TEDx talks at http://bit.ly/StevesFirstTED and http://bit.ly/StevesSecondTED), Facebook groups, an ACT discussion list for the public (in Yahoo Groups—https://groups.yahoo.com/neo/groups/ACT_for_the_Public/info), and so on—a careful online search will turn up such things.

A LIBERATED MIND

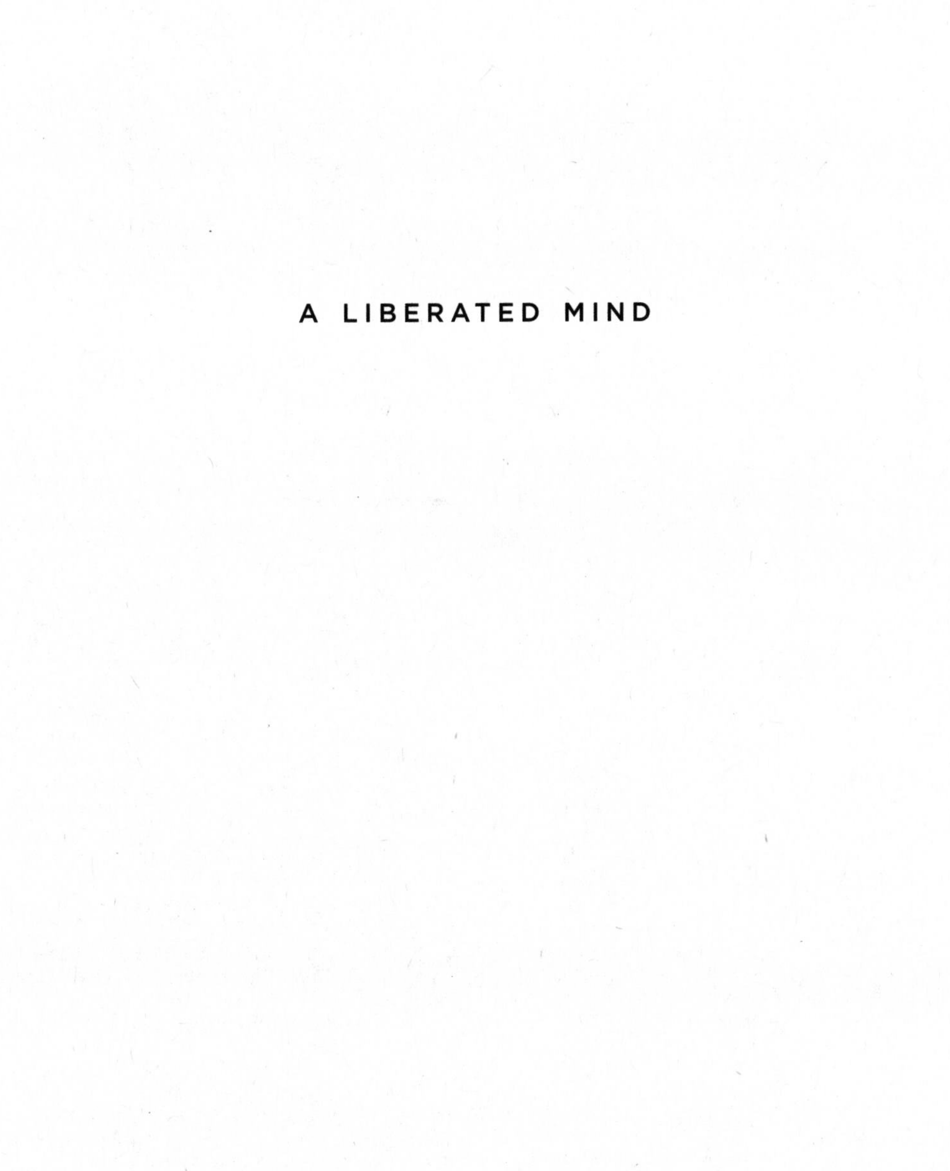

Part One

Chapter One

THE NEED TO PIVOT

Life should be getting easier, but it's not. It's a paradox of the modern world. At the very moment that science and technology are providing us previously unimagined longevity, health, and social interaction, too many of us struggle to live meaningful, peaceful lives full of love and contribution.

There is no question that we've made incredible progress over the last fifty years. That computer in your pocket called your phone is 120 million times more powerful than the guidance computer for Apollo 11—the first rocket to land people on the moon. Progress in health technology has been similar. Leukemia killed 86 percent of the children who contracted it fifty years ago—now it kills less than half that. In the last twenty-five years, child mortality, maternal mortality, and deaths from malaria all declined 40 to 50 percent. If physical health and safety were the issue and you could pick only the moment to be born in the world but not to whom, you could not do better than to choose today.

Behavioral science is another matter. Yes, we are living longer. But it is hard to make the case that we are living happier, more successful lives.

We have more accurate information than ever about illnesses that are largely due to lifestyle. Yet despite billions of dollars spent on research, our healthcare systems are staggering under the dramatically rising rates of obesity, diabetes, and chronic pain. Mental illness is rapidly becoming much *more* of a problem, not less. In 1990, depression was the fourth leading cause of disability and disease worldwide after respiratory infections, diarrheal illnesses, and prenatal conditions. In 2000, it was the third leading cause. By 2010, it ranked second. In 2017 the World Health Organization (WHO) rated it number one. Approximately forty million Americans over age eighteen have been diagnosed as having an anxiety disorder, and almost 10 percent of Americans report "frequent mental distress." We don't feel as though we have adequate time. We don't take care of ourselves the way we'd like. Our health suffers. Many of us are putting one foot in front of the other while lacking a real sense of purpose and vitality. Every day, someone who seems to have a good life decides to eat a bottle of pills rather than continue one more day.

How can this be?

I believe it is because we have not risen to the challenges of being human in the modern world. Some of the very things we have been doing over the last hundred years to foster human prosperity have created our conundrum. Take the case of innovations in technology. Each step forward—radio to TV to the Internet to the smartphone—has created greater mental and social challenges, and our culture and minds haven't adjusted rapidly enough in effective and empowering ways.

As a result of our technology, we are all exposed to a constant diet of horror, drama, and judgment. In addition, many of us are left feeling overwhelmed and threatened by the rapid pace of change. A concrete example: only a few decades ago children ran and played freely in ways that could bring child endangerment complaints today. This increased protectiveness is not due to the world actually becoming more dangerous; research suggests it has not. Our impression that the world is less safe results more from exposure to uncommon events through the media. No matter how calm we feel, we can turn on our computers and see a tragedy unfold, complete with images of those who died just minutes ago. The twenty-four-hour news cycle shreds our veil of safety with constant videos of capricious violence.

When the external world changes at this speed, our internal world needs to change too. That sounds logical, but it is hard to know what steps to take.

The good news is that behavioral science has developed a plausible answer to how we can do better. Over the last thirty-five years, my colleagues and I have studied a small set of skills that say more about how human lives will unfold than any other single set of mental and behavioral processes previously known to science. That is not an exaggeration. In over one thousand studies, we've found that these skills help determine why some people thrive after life challenges and some don't, or why some people experience many positive emotions (joy, gratitude, compassion, curiosity) and others very few. They predict who is going to develop a mental health problem such as anxiety, depression, trauma, or substance abuse, and how severe or long-lasting the problem will be. These skills predict who will be effective at work, who will have healthy relationships, who will succeed in dieting or exercise, who will rise to the challenges of physical disease, how people will do in athletic competition, and how they will perform in many other areas of human endeavor.

This set of skills combines to give us *psychological flexibility*. Psychological flexibility is the ability to feel and think with openness, to attend voluntarily to your experience of the present moment, and to move your life in directions that are important to you, building habits that allow you to live life in accordance with your values and aspirations. It's about learning not to turn away from what is painful, instead turning *toward* your suffering in order to live a life full of meaning and purpose.

Wait, turning *toward* your suffering?

That's right. Psychological flexibility allows us to turn toward our discomfort and disquiet in a way that is open, curious, and kind. It's about looking in a nonjudgmental and compassionate way at the places in ourselves and in our lives where we hurt, because the things that have the power to cause us the most pain are often the things we care about most deeply. Our deepest yearnings and most powerful motivations lie hidden inside our most unhealthy defense systems. Our impulse is usually either to try to deny our pain, by suppression or self-medication, or to get caught up in dwelling on it through rumination and worry, allowing it to take charge of our lives. Psychological flexibility empowers us to accept our pain and live life as we desire, *with* our pain when there is pain.

I believe psychological flexibility is a means of achieving human liberation; it is the counterweight that people need to rise to the increasing challenges of the modern world. And hundreds of studies show that the skills that allow us to develop psychological flexibility can be learned, to a degree even through books such as this one. I know these are big claims, but if I do my job, by the end of this book you will understand why the skills that build flexibility are so powerful and how you can begin developing them in yourself.

It's perhaps not surprising that the core message of turning toward our pain echoes other approaches, such as the mindfulness literature developed out of spiritual traditions, or the emphasis on exposure in cognitive behavioral therapy. But the new science of psychological flexibility is not aping old themes—by repeatedly asking *why* these methods work, it has arrived at a deeper understanding of the importance of flexibility skills and how to establish them. This understanding was produced by a scientific community that followed a new path of research, resulting in a new and more integrated set of methods for living happier and healthier lives.

Our own natural tendencies and life experiences have provided a deep wisdom inside us that naturally guides us toward the manner of living that science is showing is the healthy way to rise to life's challenges. You would think that having the wisdom within would steer us on a healthy course, and it might except for one thing: the organ between our ears. Our minds are constantly tempting us to head in the wrong direction.

Every one of us engages in behaviors that, deep down, we know don't serve our best interests. The examples are endless: the diet that goes awry when you binge on a pint of Ben and Jerry's after a long day at work; those extra drinks you have at the party even though you know you won't feel your best the next day; the looming deadline that you keep procrastinating about; or the time you picked a fight with your spouse for no real reason. Each of these alone is innocuous enough. But the same psychological mechanisms that drive these behaviors can lead us to very dark places when left unchecked. For too many of us, the occasional binge becomes habitual. That extra drink at the party turns into substance dependence. Procrastinating on a deadline unfolds into life dreams that are not pursued. Picking fights with the people you love becomes a method for avoiding the intimacy you so desperately crave.

Why do we do these things?

The simple answer is that our minds get in our way. We fall into patterns of *psychological rigidity*, where we try to run from or fight off the mental challenges we face, and we disappear into rumination, worry, distraction, self-stimulation, work without end, or other forms of mindlessness, all in the attempt to evade the pain we're feeling.

Psychological rigidity is at its core an attempt to avoid negative thoughts and feelings caused by difficult experiences, both when they occur and in our memory of them. Let's say you fail a test. A frightening thought may flicker by: "I'm a failure." Before you know it, that thought is pushed off into a corner and told to stay there, and you have decided to self-soothe by going out to have some drinks with friends. That is fine so far as it goes, but if the cycle repeats itself and you then begin avoiding preparing for the next test, you are paving a route to pathology by suppression and unhealthy forms of self-soothing.

Suppose instead you try to reassure yourself that you are smart and able. Doing so makes enormous sense, superficially speaking. Surely it is helpful to think positive thoughts, right? It is logical, yes, but it may not be wise. If you're thinking positive thoughts explicitly to avoid or contradict negative thoughts . . . well, that's another form of psychological rigidity and now the positive thoughts will remind you of the very thoughts you hoped to avoid. A recent study showed that positive affirmations like "I'm a good person!" work great as long as we don't really need them. When we do need them, like when we start feeling bad about ourselves, such affirmations make us both feel and do worse!

It's a cruel joke.

The punch line is that if the purpose of any coping strategy is to avoid feeling a challenging emotion or thinking an upsetting thought, to wipe out a painful memory or look away from a difficult sensation, the long-term outcome will almost always be poor.

Psychological rigidity predicts anxiety, depression, substance abuse, trauma, eating disorders, and almost every other psychological and behavioral problem. It undermines a person's ability to learn new things, enjoy his or her job, be intimate with others, or rise to the challenges of physical disease. Mental rigidity even plays a role in areas we wouldn't necessarily expect. For example, suppose you examine rates of trauma in people who were in New York near Ground Zero during the 9/11 attacks. Who do you suppose developed more trauma afterward? Those who were more horrified, such as by seeing people jump to their death, or those more determined *not* to be horrified by the same experience? The research was done and we know the answer. It's the latter.

But mental rigidity doesn't only expose us to greater incidence of psychological disorders and behavioral problems; it does two final terrible things that truly make it monstrous. First, although you begin on a path of rigidity to avoid pain, soon enough you have to avoid joy as well. Studies have shown that anxious people who are rigid and avoidant start out intolerant of anxiety, but they end up intolerant of happiness too! Joy makes them nervous. If you are happy today, you might be disappointed tomorrow. Better to be numb.

Second, rigidity makes it more difficult to learn from your emotions. If you are a chronic emotional avoider, it can lead to alexithymia—the inability to know what you are feeling at all. This is part of the most hidden and most horrible cost of psychological rigidity: as you fight, and run, and hide from your insides, you become distant from your own history, your own motivation, and your own caring. Studies show that if you do not understand your emotions well simply because your family never discussed them, then you can improve your emotional understanding by intentionally learning more about them, and the outcomes are not bad. But if you don't know what you feel because you're avoiding your feelings, horrible outcomes follow in a vast range of areas. I'll give you an example: people who have been abused by others are more likely to be abused again, but that effect is not direct—it's particularly likely to happen to those who respond to the initial abuse by becoming distant from their own feelings. Once that lack of feeling settles in, victims of abuse have a hard time reading who is safe and who isn't, and the last people who should ever have to face abuse again are the very ones revisited by it. It is unfair, cruel, and yet predictable.

Why are we so given to psychological rigidity? Even if a wiser part of our minds knows what is good for us, a domineering problem-solving part does *not*. I call this aspect of our minds the Dictator Within, because it is constantly suggesting "solutions" for our psychological pain, even though our own experience, if we listen carefully, whispers that these solutions are toxic. As with many political dictators, this voice within our minds can cause great harm. It can lead us to buy into a damaging story about our pain and how to deal with it. It weaves its advice into tales about our childhoods, about our abilities and who we are, or about the injustices of the world and how others behave. It seduces us into acting on these stories even though there is a part of us, deep inside, that knows better. We are being conned by ourselves.

Think about how often we run from the things we fear in our daily lives and how much needless suffering it causes. You've been feeling down recently and you know that somehow this is connected to the fact that you haven't been working out enough, but going for a jog or a hike or getting to the gym just seems like more than you can bear, so you turn on the TV instead. You have a deadline at work on a project you aren't in the mood to deal with so you procrastinate, which only compounds the problem. You're totally stressed out because you spend sixty hours a week in the office. You know you need time off, but you don't take it because you're trapped in the idea that if you don't go in on the weekend or carry work home, something catastrophic is going to happen. The Dictator convinces us that engaging in these mentally rigid avoidant behaviors makes good sense.

Running from our pain, or trying to deny it, seems logical. Because we don't like feeling pain, it seems appropriate to treat difficult thoughts, feelings, and memories as "the problem" and to view elimination of them as "the solution." We bring all of our problem-solving tools to the task. Unfortunately, too often this leads to following rigid problem-solving formulations or rules such as "get rid of it" or "figure it out" or "just fix your problem."

We are paying a psychological price because what is really wrong within is treating life as a problem to be solved rather than a process to be lived. In the external world, acting to eliminate pain is a vital survival instinct. Responding to *get your hand off the hot stove* or to *eat because you haven't eaten all day* is important to our successful functioning, and anyone who ignores such commands will pay a high price. But in the internal world of thoughts or feelings, it's a different story. A memory or emotion is not like a hot stove or a lack of food. What makes logical sense for action in the outside world does not necessarily make psychological sense in the world of thoughts and feelings.

Take the example of a painful memory, such as that of a major betrayal or trauma. Difficult emotions tempt us to try to protect ourselves against ever having to experience that suffering again, to attempt to make the emotions *just stop*. But in order to get rid of something deliberately, we have to focus on it. If we are working to get rid of something, we need to check to see if it's gone. When we do that with internal events laid down by our own history, such as memories, we have now reminded ourselves of the events connected with these memories yet again. When we do this with echoes of the past, we increase their centrality and build out the history we have with them.

If we instead distract or self-soothe in order to deal with the pain—say, by reading a good book or listening to a favorite piece of music—these otherwise enjoyable activities can actually over time become *related* to what we are avoiding and can even open a back door into them. After just a few times, that soothing book or piece of music might remind you of the memory you are avoiding or trigger a revisiting of the trauma you hoped would recede.

Meanwhile we often attempt to fuel our motivation to change with mental threats about the dire things that will happen if we do not, which also often only makes painful or traumatic memories *more* powerful and central. Those threats produce emotional reactions—which sometimes are kin to the reactions we are trying to evade, thus *increasing* the pain we feel. We end up in a kind of demonic feedback loop. Trying to combat anxiety, for example, can lead to increased anxiety *about* our anxiety. Similarly, when we disappear into rumination, we convince ourselves we are figuring out how to solve our problems, but we become so focused on them that they increasingly control our lives. We turn our insides into virtual war zones in a frantic but losing attempt to find peace of mind by eliminating and subtracting offending experiences.

I am not telling you anything you do not know, at least intuitively. Most of us have noticed that our minds can lead us to strange places. But most of us don't yet understand that when we have a painful memory or a frightening feeling, doing things to escape them can increase their importance. If we are afraid of being rejected by others, we see signs of imminent rejection everywhere. We know that buying into that fear will not liberate us, but the possibility of rejection is so fear-inducing that it seems like a violation of basic logic not to focus on it. If we are browbeating ourselves about supposed weaknesses, we are likely to feel even less able, and we are more likely to fail.

Liberating ourselves from the trap of rigidity is made harder by the messages we're barraged with by the culture at large. Many businesses thrive on this messaging. Are you worried about your appearance? A beauty product will remove the worry. Unhappy? The right beer will cheer you up. Look at the themes of virtually all the major self-help books and programs—it's more of the same: manage your anxiety, feel good, control your thoughts, and life will be better.

Most self-help books also ask people to do one or another form of self-soothing or self-correction. Somehow, we are supposed to relax, focus on the positive, or have different thoughts. In the conventional conception, our names for mental conditions hang the hook of blame on emotions and thoughts. We have "anxiety disorders" or "thought disorders." An array of pills and therapy approaches promise the elimination of difficult thoughts and feelings (for example, notice that term *anti-* in *antidepressants*). And yet as the adoption of this entire model has spread around the world, misery and disability have increased, not decreased.

Piled on top of this encouragement to avoid or eradicate our pain is the new addictive invitation that social media constantly offers us to compare ourselves to others and to distract ourselves. No matter how successful we are, we can reach into our pockets and find a social-comparison tool called a smartphone that will dutifully show us that others are seemingly doing far better.

The fields of psychology and psychiatry have also inadvertently contributed to the problem. Ideas that are not evidence-based proliferate, such as Freud's Oedipus complex (you are sexually attracted to your parents, which creates a hidden conflict, giving rise to anxiety), while evidence-based ones lie dormant.

But even the major science-based efforts have not given the public the tools they need. They have also promoted a compelling but flawed understanding of how we ought to cope with our negative emotions and thoughts. In the midtwentieth century, psychological strength would often have been defined largely as emotional avoidance. One of the most famous scenes from the award-winning drama *Mad Men* shows the lead character—successful ad man Don Draper—visiting a young colleague in the hospital after she has given birth to an unwanted baby in 1960. Peggy Olson has denied that she was pregnant—even to herself—and becomes depressed to the point of psychosis after she delivers. In the psych ward, Draper leans in toward Olson and tells her to snap out of it. "Do whatever they say," he says of her doctors. "Get out of here . . . This never happened. *It will shock you how much it never happened.*" In the next scene, he's pouring himself a long shot of whiskey at his office.

Sure, that's just television. But the cultural rule delivered in that scene—that you can and must learn to change your thoughts at will, and only if and when you do so will you reduce or eliminate uncomfortable emotions—has been deeply ingrained in our minds. One of the most important approaches to psychotherapy is partially responsible.

Working separately in the 1960s, University of Pennsylvania psychiatrist Aaron Beck and New York City psychologist Albert Ellis (1913–2007) wrote papers arguing that many damaging emotions were caused by faulty cognitions: "black-and-white thinking," for instance—seeing complicated relationships or life events as simply awful without considering the more nuanced possibilities. They argued that people look at a difficult discussion with a boss or a fight with an old friend—typical things in life—and see them in an unrealistic, irrational, or distorted way.

The solution suggested came to be called *cognitive behavioral therapy* (CBT). CBT is a whole package of therapeutic approaches that includes many very well-supported behavior change methods, and CBT is now evolving in ways I support. But a central tenet of traditional CBT that is problematic came to dominate the popular understanding of the approach—we need to change negative or distorted thoughts and convert them to positive and rational ones. This "cognitive restructuring" was supposedly the route to mental health because it was flawed habits of thinking—not Freud's "neuroses," not nightmares, not repressed memories—that most controlled our emotions and shaped our behavior.

The idea permeated our culture. When Phillip McGraw (stage name Dr. Phil) gives advice, for instance, much of it flows from a cognitive behavioral perspective. "Are you actively creating a toxic environment for yourself?" he has asked on his website. "Or are the messages that you send yourself characterized by a rational and productive optimism?"

The research I describe in this book has led to a fundamental reappraisal of the notion that we should challenge and restructure our thoughts. Research shows that this part of the CBT approach is not what is powerful about it, and it often doesn't work as well as learning to accept that we are having unpleasant emotions and thoughts and then working to reduce their role in our lives instead of trying to get rid of them.

On a parallel track, psychiatry has promoted the idea that we need to treat a host of psychological conditions as if they are the face of a hidden disease. That implies they will eventually be shown to have known causes, mechanisms of development, and responses to treatment. Yet after spending several decades and many billions of dollars on research in this pursuit, in how many cases have mere conditions turned into mental diseases with a known cause?

The answer may shock you. Not one. The truth about mental health is that the causes of all of the mental conditions you hear about are unknown, and the idea that "hidden diseases" lurk behind human suffering is an out-and-out failure.

Meanwhile the idea that psychological conditions should be treated as hidden diseases has taken a troubling toll. It is a soothing idea because it contains a real truth: suffering is not your fault. But when people buy into it, they often begin to feel that they must be on medication for life because of what they "have" hidden inside.

Consider just the ten-year period from 1998 to 2007 (the most recent decade with solid numbers) and people in the United States who sought out treatment for psychological struggles. In that time, the number of people using only psychological change methods fell nearly 50 percent, while the number of those using psychological approaches along with medications fell about 30 percent. What shot up? People using only medications to address their difficulties. By the end of that decade, more than 60 percent of people with psychological conditions were using only medication; it has only gotten worse since.

That would be fine if science supported that approach, but it doesn't. Medications can be helpful if they are used to leverage psychosocial methods, with lower doses and shorter durations, but as prescriptions have skyrocketed and medication-only has become the norm, the incidence of mental health problems has risen. What's more, when people are falsely convinced that they have a "mental disease," they tend to be more pessimistic that they can do anything on their own to improve their condition, such as through behavior change. Friends and family feel less hopeful for them as well.

This book will reveal how powerfully we can transform our lives by seeking not to eradicate our difficult thoughts and emotions or numb them away but to cultivate psychological flexibility, which allows us to accept them for what they are and not let them rule our lives. It will show that trying to eliminate or completely restructure our thoughts is unnecessary and even futile. Our nervous system does not contain a delete button, and thought and memory processes are too complex to make them neat and tidy. It will also reveal how flawed the cultural message is that people *have* something that makes their lives difficult. It is what we *do* that matters, and that gives us the means to live in a way that is richly meaningful to us, despite even quite difficult challenges.

Getting Out of the Trap

I once had a dog who would walk in circles while scratching the rug to prepare a place to lie down. Sometimes this ritual would go on for many minutes. The rug did not change with the scratching . . . but eventually my poor pooch would flop down virtually in exhaustion and sleep.

Metaphorically we walk in circles—watching silly TV shows, surfing the net, posting to our Facebook page—while waiting for a sense of wholeness, or peace of mind, or purpose to arrive. The rug-scratches of distraction, avoidance, and indulgence are not changing anything of importance. We need a place we can be *comfortable*, in the original etymological sense of that word: with (*com*) strength (*fort*, like "build a fort," from the Latin *fortis*). Living with our strength in the world requires far more of us than distraction, avoidance, and indulgence. If you want to find peace of mind and purpose, you will have to let go of finding a way out and instead pivot toward finding a way in. I am acutely aware that this is easier said than done.

I learned about the power of pivoting the hard way. I am a panic-disordered person in recovery. Through years of struggle, I saw anxiety and panic gradually take away my peace of mind. A shrill voice in my head demanded that I run, or hide, or fight against anxiety, gradually driving me into an unlivable place in which my experience was my enemy. Learning to accept my anxiety started me on the path to recovery, and to the discoveries and methods of building psychological flexibility presented in this book.

My first panic attack occurred in a meeting of the psychology department faculty in the fall of 1978. The full professors were fighting—again. As a young assistant professor, I dearly wanted to yell for them to please stop! I raised my hand and asked for attention to make my appeal, but they were too busy fighting. After a minute or so I lowered my hand, not because I no longer wanted to speak, but because I thought I was going to pass out. My heart was racing so fast I couldn't count the beats. Something in that awful fighting had triggered an anxiety attack the likes of which I'd never felt before. I would see what the trigger was only years later, after I developed a therapy approach to help face monsters of this kind—Acceptance and Commitment Therapy (ACT . . . it's said as the word *act*, not as initials). In this initial panic experience, I was too caught up with my anxiety to get any mental distance from it. Whatever I was going to say to my colleagues was lost in the urgent command to flee. But I was seated across the room from the door with an obstacle course of chairs and bodies blocking my way out. Extracting myself was impossible.

As I was desperately trying to come up with a plan for escape, the room suddenly quieted and I realized my colleagues had seen me raise my hand. They were all now looking at me, expecting me to speak. I opened my mouth but no sound came out. My eyes darted helplessly around the room, taking in the horrifying sight of so many others looking, looking, and looking at me. I struggled to breathe. After what seemed like ages but was probably only ten or fifteen seconds, the perplexed group went back to their fighting as I was left still clutching my chair, opening and closing my mouth like a fish out of water, having never uttered a sound.

I was humiliated and terrified. I had felt strong and unexpected anxiety before, but never to the point where I could not function. When the nightmarish meeting ended, I slunk out of the room on unsteady feet, sure that my colleagues were wondering what was wrong with me. My mind was already plotting courses of action that seemed logical, but that we now know exacerbate panic disorder. I was frantically asking myself: How can I control this? How can I keep this from happening again? I soon began to take many small steps to avoid and control the situations, places, or actions that could be a problem if anxiety suddenly removed my ability to function. As I took those steps I initially felt relieved—and I began my journey into the hell of panic disorder.

The situation was a kind of "monkey trap." In some parts of Africa, natives drill small holes in gourds that are then filled with banana chips and tied to trees. The holes are just big enough for a monkey to insert its hand, but when it grabs the banana chip the fist that results is too big to pull out through the hole. The monkey is trapped.

You would think the monkey would just let go of the chip, but it doesn't. It hoots and hollers and struggles and fights—all the while clinging to the chip—until the natives come back to claim their prize.

I was clinging to the "prize" of an anxiety-free life, or at least one with far, far lower levels of anxiety. It seemed reasonable to do so. Who in their right mind would give up on such a thing? Wouldn't that mean giving up on the possibility of a healthy life? Instead, like the monkeys in the banana trap, I hooted and hollered and struggled and fought, but all to no avail. I was caught in the anxiety trap.

It was only when I abandoned the attempt to control anxiety that I began discovering how to heal. It was only when I gave up on that false vision—when I dropped that mental banana chip—that my mind was free to stop frantically making my anxiety worse.

Eventually, I would turn toward my anxiety with an attitude of self-kindness and dispassionate curiosity, and then turn toward my own yearning to love and to make a difference, even though these were precisely the areas in my life where I felt the most vulnerable. This taught me that if we want to change the impact of the difficult parts of our history, we need to learn how to carry those parts with us lightly, with self-kindness—and without giving them any more attention than they deserve. My panic gradually retreated. At the very moment that I stopped running and turned toward my pain and suffering, life possibilities began to open up, whether or not I was feeling anxious.

My own experience led me to search for answers about why our minds are so enthralled to the Dictator Within and its powerful impulse to problem-solve our pain away. I also wanted to find scientifically proven ways to learn to make the pivot toward acceptance and then build habits of healthier living. Through decades of research, we've learned that people are better able to understand the "how" of pivoting when they understand certain key discoveries we've made about how our minds work. When you see how the Dictator does what it does, you are closer to adopting a new mode of mind—a liberated mind—that will help in almost every area of human life.

We've learned that the tendency toward psychological rigidity evolved right alongside human language and cognition. These prodigious mental talents that allow us to use elegant forms of symbolic thought to solve problems, to perform scientific experiments, to create great literature, or to invent new technology, also give rise to the voice in our minds of the Dictator Within. Our symbolic thinking talents invest our thoughts with a reality comparable to that of the external world. We can craft memories so vivid that recalling them provokes much the same emotions or brain responses we felt when the events occurred. The messages we tell ourselves, through the voice of the Dictator, are not heard simply as things we're thinking but as hard truths. When they are threatening, we react to them in the same instinctive ways we combat threats out in the world. Our thoughts can be as frightening as a lion charging at us on the ancient savannah, and we apply the same fight-or-flight impulse to trying to run away from them, hide from them, or slay them.

The manner in which our thinking processes evolved also accounts for how automatically our minds are triggered to launch into negativity. Our thoughts are embedded in dense networks of permanently stored thought patterns, and at any moment, a given thought, such as *He doesn't seem happy to see me*, can trigger a whole cascade of negative thinking, such as about moments of disappointment in our childhood that come rushing back to us. We can't press a stop or delete button, and our efforts to do so only tend to intensify the power of our negative thoughts.

As I will introduce here in Part One, ACT research not only illuminated how our symbolic thinking talents lead to these difficult consequences but also discovered methods for freeing us from their negative effects. We discovered that psychological flexibility involves six skills, and building each of these involves its own specific kind of pivot away from rigid mental processes. So the big pivot fostered by ACT is really six specific pivots, which combine to enable us to live with more psychological flexibility.

Central to understanding why the pivots are so powerful is that each of the rigid ways in which our minds trap us in unhealthy patterns of thinking and behaving contains a healthy yearning hidden deep within it. We are doing the wrong things, but for the right reasons—because we want our lives to have important qualities. The flexibility pivots allow us to redirect that hidden yearning toward a more open and flexible way of being that can actually satisfy the yearning. We can then continue to develop our flexibility skills so that we are able to stay on the course of living according to our values and aspirations.

Here is a brief introduction to each of the skills and the yearning each pivot redirects.

1. **Defusion.**

   Requires pivoting from cognitive fusion to defusion; redirects the yearning for coherence and understanding.

   Cognitive fusion means buying into what your thoughts tell you (taking them literally, word for word) and letting what they say overdetermine what you do. This trick of mind happens because we are programmed to notice the world only as structured by thought—we see the terrible this or the awful that—but we miss the fact that we are thinking. In our attempts to have the world make sense, we judge our experiences and then buy into the judgment instead of realizing it *is* a judgment to begin with. The flip side of fusion is seeing thoughts as they actually are—ongoing attempts at meaning-making—and then choosing to give them power only to the degree that they genuinely serve us. This flexibility skill involves just noticing the act of thinking, without diving in. Our made-up word for "just noticing" is *defusion*. With this ability to distance from our thoughts, we can begin to free ourselves from our negative thought networks.

2. Self.

Requires pivoting from allegiance to a conceptualized sense of self, or our ego, to a perspective-taking self; redirects the yearning for belonging and connection.

In the simplest sense, what I mean when I'm talking about your *conceptualized self* is your *ego*—your stories about who you are and who others are in relation to you. Inside our stories, we note what is special about us (our special skills; our special needs), and we hope this will earn us a place in the group. We all have these stories, and, held lightly, they can even be helpful. However, when we hold tightly to them it becomes difficult to be honest with ourselves or to make room for other thoughts, feelings, or behaviors that would benefit others and ourselves but that don't fit the story. In this event, the conceptualized self leads us to defend these stories as if our life depends on it, which creates alienation, not true connection. The alternative is to connect more deeply with a *perspective-taking self*—a sense of observing, witnessing, or purely being aware. This sense of self allows us to see that we are more than the stories we tell ourselves, more than what our mind says. We also see that we are connected in consciousness to all of humanity—we belong not because we are special, but because we are human. Some people think of this as a transcendent or a spiritual sense of self.

3. Acceptance.

Requires pivoting from experiential avoidance to acceptance; redirects the yearning to feel.

Experiential avoidance is the process by which we run from or attempt to control our personal experiences (thoughts, feelings, sensations) and the external events that give rise to them, all the way from going to a party to trying to cope with the death of a loved one. We do this because our mind tells us it's an easy way to avoid pain, and we will be able to feel freely only when we feel GOOD. But avoidance typically only compounds our difficulties and restricts our capacity to feel at all. *Acceptance* is the full embrace of our personal experience in an empowered, not in a victimized, state. It's choosing to feel with openness and curiosity, so that you can live the kind of life you want to live while inviting your feelings to come along for the ride. As a result of the Acceptance pivot, the focus moves from feeling GOOD, to FEELING good.

4. Presence.

Requires pivoting from rigid attention driven by past and future to flexible attention in the now; redirects the yearning for orientation.

Processes of *rigid attention* show up as ruminating about the past, or worrying about the future, or mindlessly disappearing into our current experience the way teenagers disappear into video games. As we struggle with life's challenges, we often fear becoming lost, and we tend to look to the past and future to become oriented. But instead we find ourselves in a mental fog of what was or what will be, when there is really only what *is*. *Flexible attention in the now*, or being present, means choosing to pay attention to experiences here and now that are helpful or meaningful—and if they are not, then choosing to move on to other useful events in the now, rather than being caught in mindless attraction or revulsion.

5. Values.

Requires pivoting from socially compliant goals to chosen values; redirects the yearning for self-direction and purpose.

People often attempt to achieve goals because they feel that they *have to*. Otherwise people we care about, or whose views we care about, would be displeased, or they will be disappointed in themselves. Research shows that such *socially compliant goals* give rise to motivation that is weak and ineffective. We may try to drive our own behavior with such external goals, but we also secretly resent them because they undermine our own process of unfolding. The yearning for self-direction and purpose cannot be fully met by goal achievement since that is always either in the future (I haven't met my goal yet) or the past (I met my goal).

Values are chosen qualities of being and doing, such as being a caring parent, being a dependable friend, being socially aware, or being loyal, honest, and courageous. Living in accordance with our values is never finished; it is a lifelong journey. And it provides a way to create enduring sources of motivation based on meaning. Ultimately what your values are is up to you—they are a matter between you and the person in the mirror.

6. Action.

Requires pivoting from avoidant persistence to committed action; redirects the yearning to be competent.

We are always building larger patterns of action, known as habits. When we think about building habits, we tend to focus on perfect outcomes, such as quitting smoking entirely hard-stop. In fact, habit building is a moment-by-moment process. If we try to change our habits in one fell swoop, our efforts tend to lead to procrastination and inaction, impulsivity, or avoidant persistence and workaholism. The Action pivot focuses us instead on the process of competently and continuously building habits in small steps linked to the construction of larger habits of loving, caring, participating, creating, or any other chosen value.

The six pivots can be more simply summarized with this cheat sheet:

1. **See our thoughts with enough distance that we can choose what we do next, regardless of our mind's chatter.**

2. **Notice the story we've constructed of our selves and gain perspective about who we are.**

3. **Allow ourselves to feel even when the feelings are painful or create a sense of vulnerability.**

4. **Direct attention in an intentional way rather than by mere habit, noticing what is present here and now, inside us and out.**

5. **Choose the qualities of being and doing that we want to evolve *toward*.**

6. **Create habits that support these choices.**

I've dubbed the initial moves to embrace these practices "pivots" because the word *pivot* in English comes from an old French word that referred to the pin in a hinge. Pivots in hinges take the energy that is headed in one direction and immediately redirect it in another. When we pivot, we take the energy inside an inflexible process and channel it toward a flexible one. If we learn to feel feelings as they are—with openness, curiosity, and self-compassion—*pain can be a powerful ally in living.* Take for example, the pain of personal betrayal that can lead to a process of experiential avoidance: with acceptance skills we can channel that painful energy of wanting to feel loved and cared for back toward its original purpose—creating the very relationships for which we yearn.

Pain and purpose are two sides of the same thing. A person struggling with depression is very likely a person yearning to feel fully. A socially anxious person is very likely a person yearning to connect with others. You hurt where you care, and you care where you hurt.

Think of making these pivots as learning the moves to a dance, like following steps laid out on the floor. As with dance steps, the pivots combine to form a seamless whole, and without each, the dance will not flow smoothly. As you practice the skills, you develop increasing flexibility. And just as it is easier to swing your partner around if your partner is always in fluid motion, rather than stopping after each move, by continuously developing your flexibility skills, you become increasingly able to take the energy of your existing thoughts and feelings, even the negative ones, and swing them into energy for growth. Ironically, when we pivot we can actually begin to satisfy the deeper yearnings that lie inside our logical but mistaken strategies.

Relatively speaking, these flexibility practices account for the lion's share of psychological health. Learning them leads to more effective patterns of living and behaving, of being and doing. Said in another way, the flexibility skills not only help contend with specific life problems, such as depression, chronic pain, and substance abuse, they allow all of us to live healthier and more meaningful lives. They promote prosperity.

Making the pivots may seem daunting, but ACT research has shown that we can learn these six skills through quite simple methods and can turn them into living habits. I will introduce a host of research studies that have shown how to make the pivots and build the skills and have proven the remarkable positive effects of the practices on growth and life enhancement.

For a taste of the findings, take the example of one recent study. Researchers randomly assigned several hundred people who were recovering from a completed course of cancer treatment with its horrors of chemo and surgery to receive either usual aftercare (such as following up with the needed lifestyle changes in diet and exercise to avoid a relapse) or eleven short ACT-based phone calls about how to use flexibility skills to rise to the challenge of cancer recovery. Finding out you have a serious, life-threatening illness can be traumatic. But over the next six to twelve months, compared to the usual care group, the ACT participants not only showed lower anxiety and depression and better compliance with their new medical regimen (e.g., they started following a better diet and exercising—key steps to avoid relapse), they showed notably higher levels of quality of life, especially in terms of physical well-being, as well as higher levels of acceptance and posttraumatic growth.

In some ways, that last result is the most exciting because it is a clear indication of what it means to respond to life's challenges with flexibility. Yes, cancer is a shock, but if you survive, life is giving you a chance to learn and to change. That is what *posttraumatic growth* means. Over the next six or twelve months, those in the ACT group showed more appreciation of life, more spiritual growth, more of an embrace of new possibilities, and more focus on relationships with others. They *grew*, and they turned their recovery from cancer into an asset—a source of personal strength.

In another study, my colleagues and I looked at one population many researchers had avoided because of its complexity: poly-drug users. These are the addicts who often show up in rehab facilities and say, "Oh, I take everything. I'll take a bunch of Gas-X if someone tells me you get high when you use it" (by the way, you don't). To make it even more challenging, we chose to examine those whose addiction patterns included opioids such as heroin and who were already being treated with methadone (which is a legal, long-acting opioid) but were failing.

We randomized well over a hundred participants into three groups: one that would simply continue taking methadone; one that would take methadone but also learn ACT; and one that would continue on methadone but be exposed to a program that facilitated the use of a twelve-step program like AA or NA. After six months, the ACT participants were taking far fewer opiates (as measured by their urine) compared to the group that just stayed on methadone. The twelve-step facilitation group showed an initial change but by the end of the follow-up they were not better than those on methadone alone. Since that study, dozens of studies on substance use have confirmed that people can stop smoking, reduce excessive marijuana use, get through detox, or succeed in alcohol addiction treatment more quickly using ACT. The methods work because urges become less dominant; values become more important; unpleasant sensations less entangling. It becomes possible to choose what you do.

The science of psychological flexibility now spans well over a thousand studies, which have tested it in almost every area of human functioning. In clinical research this breadth is called a *transdiagnostic*, meaning that targeting psychological flexibility works across a wide range of traditional mental health categories (anxiety, depression, substance abuse, eating disorders, and so on). It turns out even that is not broad enough. ACT is transdiagnostic on steroids. The same flexibility processes also help us step up to the challenge of physical disease, or manage our relationships better, or reduce stress, or organize our business well, or play competitive sports. Psychological flexibility measures can predict whether you can manage your diabetes, or the number of assists and points the professional hockey team makes while players are on the ice. Specific psychological flexibility measures predict whether you will develop trauma when bad things happen, or whether you will be an effective parent.

In Part One I tell the story of the discoveries that led to the development of ACT methods. Part Two introduces important additional findings about why flexibility skills are so powerful and shares a wealth of methods developed to help people make the initial pivots and then continue to develop the skills. In both parts, I share the stories of people who have transformed their lives. Part Three introduces findings about how helpful the ACT skills are in coping with a host of specific challenges, such as facing substance abuse, dealing with cancer, managing chronic pain, letting go of depression, quitting smoking, losing weight, sleeping better, learning better, and being more engaged and fulfilled in one's work.

People's problems and difficulties are not fixed by the snap of fingers; fundamental change takes time for most people. Our lives are never smooth and our growth is never "finished." But a change in *direction* does not take much time at all. Like pivoting on the ball of your foot as you turn a corner, the core of the process of creating a more psychologically flexible life can take just an instant—especially when you know how to undo the trick our minds are playing on us. Learning how to pivot in that way need not take years, or even months. In the over 250 randomized controlled trials of ACT currently available, dozens were based on only a handful of hours dedicated to creating a new life direction.

An example—one of many—is a study I conducted with my graduate students that examined the impact of a single day of ACT training targeting shame and self-stigma for overweight and obese people already in other weight-loss programs (e.g., Weight Watchers). We found that our training reduced shame and improved both psychological flexibility and quality of life. We did not target weight loss specifically, so it was a real surprise that when overweight people learned to pivot with their self-shaming and blaming, they naturally lost more weight over the next three months as well. Weight loss came along for free once people stopped beating themselves up for being heavy and instead learned to sit with their emotions and thoughts. In a related study, we showed that the level of psychological flexibility overweight people exhibit correlates directly with their ability to lose weight, engage in exercise, and stop binging.

My deeply hopeful message is that dramatic change is possible, and it is not very far away. How far away? How much effort will be needed? Well, let me ask you this: If you are walking in one direction and you pivoted on the ball of your foot in another direction, how far away was that? How much effort did it take?

You might be tempted to answer my question by saying it takes virtually no time and no effort to do it, but that is true only after a fashion.

Have you ever watched a baby learn to walk? If you have, you know that walking takes time and effort to learn. Research shows that infants learning to walk take about 2,400 steps an hour—enough to cross seven football fields!—and they fall, on average, seventeen times. Do the math: this means that if a baby walked even half of its waking hours, it would cover forty-six football fields and fall a hundred times in a single day. No wonder parents of toddlers are tired! Even with all this enormous practice, toddlers initially can change direction only by a series of short rocking steps, adjusting direction a little each time. That is why we call them "toddlers." Eventually, a new skill will be learned and normal children and adults can pivot smoothly on the ball of the foot, shifting from one direction and carrying momentum into another direction. Pivoting while walking is both effortless and a skill that took effort and practice to learn.

The good news is that mental pivots are actually a *lot* simpler to learn than walking. With guidance, you will not need to fall down anywhere near as often as you did as a toddler.

If I'm right, and psychological flexibility is a key missing ingredient in addressing the modern world in a healthy way, it means we are not very far from creating more loving and empowered environments at home, at work, in our communities, and in our hearts. There are no money-back guarantees, of course, but it has been shown again and again that once you learn the key set of pivotal psychological skills, beginning a healthy process of change is about as far away as saying the word *begin*.

Chapter Two

THE DICTATOR WITHIN

I began to develop ACT in earnest after I hit bottom with my struggle against anxiety in the middle of one dreadful night. Many people with anxiety disorders, as well as many of those who've experienced addiction, depression, and so many other entrapping psychological conditions, will recognize parts of the experience. I share the story not only because it demonstrates how the psychological rigidity of avoidance can become so crippling, but also because that night I made several important steps toward recovery. In fact, I made three of the six pivots, though I didn't come to think of them as such until I'd done a good deal of later reflection and research focused on what had happened to me that night. The story illuminates what the experience of pivoting is like; how rapidly we can make pivots—often making more than one at once—and how they can lead to the conviction to pursue a new course in our lives. My experience that night led me to the conviction that we in psychology needed to discover methods by which people could learn to make pivots without hitting bottom and that would allow them to truly free themselves to live healthy, fulfilling lives.

The studies that my team and I conducted in the several years following this dreadful but transformational night confirmed the core hypothesis at the heart of ACT: that changing our relationship to our thoughts and emotions, rather than trying to change their content, is the key to healing and realizing our true potential. Had I not experienced the set of realizations I had that night, I don't think that I would have come to understand that as fully, or as quickly. I was firmly in the grip of the monkey trap.

When We Run from Our Experience

My anxiety had been growing steadily. The rancor in my department that had triggered my first panic attack had broken out into a full-fledged civil war, with my colleagues fighting in a way of which only wild animals and full professors are capable. Adding to the strain, the divorce that had been set in motion shortly before my first panic attack was now becoming final. Despite outward appearances of getting on with my life and work, panic had gradually become the central focus of my life.

I tried to gain control over the attacks using all the methods I could think of, not realizing that all of them were based on the same flawed premise—they were all in one way or another attempts to escape, avoid, or diminish anxiety. The goal was to be achieved by any means necessary: situational, chemical, cognitive, emotional, or behavioral. The specific tactics I told myself to use included:

* **Try to expose yourself to frightening situations because that is supposed to make the fear subside.**
* **Learn and practice relaxation techniques.**
* **Try to think more rationally.**
* **Sit near the door so you can get out easily.**
* **Don't rush before going into a meeting—your heart rate might go up.**
* **Always have an excuse to leave, just in case you need it.**
* **Check your heart rate subtly just to make sure it's OK.**

* **Have a beer.**
* **Joke.**
* **Overprepare.**
* **Avoid giving talks—let graduate students do them.**
* **Take tranquilizers.**
* **Have a friend in sight when you're talking.**
* **Distract yourself with soothing music.**

Many of these efforts were harmless enough over the short term—there was nothing wrong with me joking, relaxing, or kicking back with a beer. Some could even have been helpful—in a different set of circumstances, like trying to think more rationally or exposing myself to anxiety-provoking situations. The problem was that the foundational message my mind was sending me was toxic: anxiety is my opponent and I have to defeat it. I have to watch out for it, manage it, and suppress it. My anxiety itself became my chief source of anxiety.

As I came to consider anxiety my mortal enemy, my panic attacks increased in intensity and frequency. One day in a lab meeting I had an attack so strong that I abruptly fled, offering no explanation. An attack on a flight to a conference made me move my seat, so that my friends would not see what was happening . . . and then move it again. I had an attack in a department store so strong I could not remember how to find the escalator. I sat down behind the bedspread display and wept quietly. I scheduled films in class rather than lectures, but even then, the panic could come on so strongly I could barely thread the film into the machine. Soon, no place was safe. By the time two years had gone by, 80 to 90 percent of my waking hours were focused on trying not to panic. On the outside I smiled and laughed and looked normal, even if I might have seemed a bit withdrawn or spacey. Inside I was constantly scanning the mental horizon for signs of the next attack.

I was like a person living with a baby tiger who had bitten my foot when hungry, and my response was to try to placate it by throwing it chunks of steak. That worked fine in the short term, but every day that went by, the tiger got bigger and stronger and needed more meat to be satisfied. The meat I was feeding it was chunks of my freedom; chunks of my life. As the tiger grew, my attention throughout the day was more focused on planning what to do if an attack showed up. It was exhausting. Eventually, my own home provided no respite, and sleep no refuge. I began waking in the middle of the night in a full-blown state of panic, a striking testament to how automatic our rigid and avoidant thinking processes are. I didn't even need to be awake, experiencing an external trigger of some kind, in order for the vicious mental cycle to be activated.

I had fallen completely under the iron grip of the Dictator Within. The voice in my head was telling me more and more urgently either to avoid my anxiety or to somehow overpower it. We all know this self-judging, bullying voice within our minds. One could think of it as our internal advisor, judge, or critic. When we learn to tame it, it can be very useful. But if we allow it free rein it deserves the name Dictator because it can become that powerful. Just like a real dictator, the voice can tell us many positive things: it can boost our confidence, saying "nicely done," and it can reassure us that things that have gone wrong are not our fault. It can tell us that we are intelligent and hardworking. It can just as easily turn against us, however, telling us that we are bad, or weak, or stupid. It can tell us we are hopeless, or that life is not worth living.

Whether the voice is positive or negative is not as important as whether it dominates us. In the name of positivity, for example, it can sell us on delusions of grandeur—convincing us that we are so special that we are secretly envied or assuring us that we are smarter than other people and are unequivocally right while others are just flat-out wrong. On the flip side, in the name of supposedly constructive criticism it can steep us in self-loathing, rip our lives into shreds of shame, or put life on indefinite hold.

What is so potentially dangerous about the power this voice can have over us is that we lose contact with the fact that we are even listening to a voice. It is almost constantly weaving a story about who we are, about how we compare to others, what others are thinking of us, and what we must do to ensure that we are OK, that we're coping with whatever challenges are confronting us.

The dictation is so constant and seamless that we disappear into the voice; we identify with it, or "fuse" with it. If we were pushed to say where that voice comes from, it would be natural for us to consider the Dictator to be *our* voice, *our* thoughts, or even our *true self.* That is why we call this voice the *ego*—which is just Latin for *I*. But it is really the *story* of I. It becomes so entangling that we take its dictates literally.

I had done that in spades during my multiyear descent into panic disorder. The voice had generated thoughts like *I need to get a grip, I'm such a loser, Why can't I solve this problem?,* or *I'm a psychologist, for God's sake; I need to fix it!* In hindsight, I can see the "I, I, I" in every single one of those thoughts. My "story of I" had become entangling, and overwhelming.

Virtually all of my patients have told me of similar corrosive messages from their internal Dictator. Cognitive behavioral therapists have assembled virtual butterfly collections of such automatic negative thinking patterns, putting them into questionnaires that can be used to assess maladaptive thought patterns. For example, one of the earliest and best-known measures is the Automatic Thoughts Questionnaire (ATQ), created in 1980 by two psychologist friends and colleagues—Steve Hollon and Phil Kendall. The ATQ measures how frequently people think thoughts like *I've let people down, My life is a mess, I can't stand this anymore,* or *I'm so weak.* Such thoughts correlate with many different kinds of poor mental and physical outcomes, but especially depression and anxiety.

I saw the effects clearly in my clinical practice. For example, an obsessive-compulsive client of mine could lay out in incredible detail all of the ways it might be possible for her to contaminate others. Her worries dominated her mind, and every area of her functioning deteriorated.

Given the negative effects of these thoughts, it is no wonder that cognitive therapists were so focused on changing them. Obviously, ruminative thoughts about contamination were the problem, right? And if they were, then obviously they needed to be changed, right?

This conclusion is logical, but I found that focusing on changing my thoughts as I wrestled with my anxiety only empowered my Dictator Within. The more determined I became that I needed to get over panic, or through it, or around it, the more I had panic attacks. What made the notion that I had to be at war with my anxiety especially insidious was that over a period of minutes or hours my efforts appeared to work. My anxiety quieted down for a while. But over days, months, and years my condition only worsened. Then I had the experience that led me to steer a new course.

Turning Toward Our Experience

On a cold winter night in 1981, I woke up to a stabbing pain in my left arm and I felt my heart racing and skipping beats wildly. I got out of bed and sat cross-legged on the floor, gripping the thick gold and brown shag carpeting, trying to come to terms with what was happening to me. A heavy weight seemed to sit on my chest. And I realized with a perverse and deep satisfaction that I was having a heart attack. This was not yet another anxiety attack; this was not in my sick mind. This was real. This was physical. *You are having a heart attack,* I thought. *You need to call an ambulance.*

I remember thinking how bizarre it was that I should be having a heart attack, telling myself, *This should not be happening to a thirty-three-year-old man.* My father, Charles, had had a heart attack at age forty-three, but he was an overweight alcoholic who smoked like a chimney. A loving but sad man, he had washed out of a promising career in professional baseball to become a salesman (he even sold brushes door to door for a time) and could not accept that fateful turn of events. I didn't smoke cigarettes and didn't drink too much. I was not carrying life failures around with me like a sack of rotting meat whose odor could only be covered by gin and tonics. I was about to be recommended for tenure at a major state university.

Yet the signs were unmistakable; I put two fingers to my neck to check my pulse. *At least 140 beats per minute*, I told myself. My sense of righteous satisfaction swelled. This. Was. Real.

The voice in my head now became urgent. *You need to go to the emergency room. This is not a joke. Call an ambulance. You can't drive in this condition.* I paused, but the voice became more urgent still. *Do it. Do it NOW.*

I reached for the phone to make the call, but my hand was shaking so badly I knocked it to the floor. And then, oddly, as it lay there, I began to feel strangely disconnected from my body, as though I were standing aside looking over at myself. Time seemed to decelerate as though I were now watching a film in slow motion. My mind claimed I was facing death, but I seemed to be viewing myself dispassionately from a place far removed from that drama. I watched a hand extend out for the now-beeping phone on the floor and was surprised to see that hand then hesitate and retreat slowly back to my lap. The hand did it again—it reached out quickly and came back slowly. And again.

How curious. Look at that, I thought.

I began to imagine what would happen if I did make that call. I saw the drama of being rushed to the hospital and into the ER unfold as though in a film trailer. But it was the final scene that horrified me as I suddenly realized what this "movie" was actually going to be about. *Oh, no*, I pleaded internally, hoping for a reprieve. *Please, God, not that.*

In my imagination, a smug young doctor in a white coat casually sauntered over to the gurney, and as he came close, I could see his expression of disdain. My stomach sank, and a cold shudder ran through my body. I knew what he was going to say.

"Dr. Hayes . . . you are not having a heart attack," he intoned over a growing smirk. "You"—he paused and then breathed in for effect—"are having a panic attack."

I knew he was right. I was not going to make that call. There would be no medical drama that night. I had just descended another level down into panic disorder hell; my mind had actually convinced my body to mimic a heart attack.

There was something wrong with me that no one and nothing could save. I had tried everything I could think of to conquer my anxiety, and it just kept getting stronger and stronger. No. Way. Out.

A long, strange, breathy scream of hopelessness erupted unbidden from deep within me. I'd heard that scream come out of my mouth only once before when, working my way through college at a factory job, I was caught in an enormous machine that made aluminum foil and was nearly crushed to death. I felt that same entrapment now. This was not just any scream. This was a scream of despair—of unavoidable death.

Something indeed *was* going to die that day. But it wasn't my physical self. Rather, it was my identification with the voice in my head; the incessant, judgmental voice that had turned my life into a living hell.

That long scream was not hopeful. It was not a plan. The scream meant just one thing. Enough is enough. I. Was. Done.

I sat in silence for several minutes. No plans. No solutions. No counterarguments. Just "No! No more!"

And then something happened. As I hit bottom, a door opened up. I saw that I had a powerful alternative that lay 180 degrees in the other direction.

I suddenly had a clear sense of the Dictator Within almost as a foreign entity—and one that *I* had let become my ruler; *I* had let the voice take the place of the part of me that is aware and can choose. The experience was like disappearing into a movie, only to realize that you are sitting in a chair, watching it. I had disappeared for years on end into my own mind and its dictates. Suddenly I was seeing my situation not from the vantage of the "story of I"; the "I" who was watching was beyond those ego-based stories, good, bad, or indifferent. The "I" that was watching had no edges that could be consciously felt—it was just awareness; awareness from the perspective of here and now. In a profound sense, I was awareness itself.

That was my first pivot, from my conceptualized self, as defined by the Dictator, to a perspective-taking self. I saw with sudden clarity that the stories my analytical mind told me about myself were not me: the stories were rather the product of a set of thought processes that were *in* me. Those processes were tools I could use if I chose to, but I did not have to listen to them and certainly was not defined by them.

From that new perspective, making the pivot to defuse from my thoughts—from taking my thoughts literally to watching the process of my thinking *as a process*—was only a hair's width away. I realized that what the voice was telling me did not necessarily have any more "weight" than any of the other thoughts that raced through my mind. I did not have to buy into them. Thoughts flit in and out of our awareness automatically all the time, like "I'm getting hungry, maybe I'll get some ice cream," or "I hope the laundry is done." Some thoughts that are off-base also pop into our minds, like thinking someone is staring at us who isn't even paying us attention. Memories suddenly resurface for no apparent reason.

While we tend to think of our thought processes as logical, many of them are anything but. Thoughts are constantly being generated automatically and mindlessly. We cannot pick which ones pop up, but we can pick and choose which of them to focus on or to use to guide our behavior. Doing so takes skill, of course, but our ACT work has shown that this is a learnable skill.

A helpful way to think about defusion is to imagine that you are sitting in a chair watching a movie. You're quite engaged in the film, but then you notice down in the corner of the screen a tiny little window showing a parallel film. This other film is about the screenplay writer as he or she creates the lines of dialogue in the main film. It's a film about authoring a movie, not the story being authored. When you hear dialogue in the main movie you can focus on that drama, but you can also turn your eyes to that small authoring film within the film and watch the writer doing the work. You can get a sense of the wheels turning in the mind of the writer as one line follows another in an attempt to construct an engrossing and consistent story that people will watch and find credible.

Seeing your thought processes that way is the critical shift from cognitive fusion to defusion; it is shifting from looking at the world structured by thought (the "main movie" or story), to looking with a sense of dispassionate curiosity at the process of thinking itself.

It's extremely liberating to calmly watch this second film. Instantly, whether the main story is true or false becomes far less important than whether it is *useful*. The author is neither your friend nor your enemy. It's just a part of you, creating lines of thought.

Once I was able to see my thoughts this way, I quickly made the pivot from avoidance to acceptance. I suddenly understood that in convincing me that my anxiety was my blood enemy, the Dictator was telling me to run and hide *from myself*, and to fight *with myself*. According to the voice, I had to repudiate the experiences I was having because having them was unacceptable—they were signs of weakness, maybe even of imminent collapse. I realized in that moment that the storyline I had been drawn into was that it was not OK to be me.

I also realized that I was so much freer to choose my actions than my mind supposed. Infinitely more. I could sense it; see it. If the voice was not me, and my thoughts were just thoughts, I could do *anything* in the presence of whatever thought presented itself. I could even turn 180 degrees and *get with* anxiety. I could choose to feel it instead of fighting it or running from it.

I mentally drew a line in the sand. The "No! No more!" message that was in the scream took on a new meaning—no more running from my anxiety. I was going to feel it, fully and without defense. Period. End of story. Sue me if you do not like it.

I've come to think of this pivot to accepting the difficult experiences we've been trying to avoid as *turning toward the dinosaur.* When I was a child, I had constant nightmares about dinosaurs. In my dreams, they would come to my house. I would hide, but they would look through the windows with their huge eyes and find me. Inevitably, I would bolt from the house and run. No matter how hard I tried, I could never get away. It felt as though I were running in slow motion. I struggled and struggled, but even enormous effort was not enough to get away. I headed down this street and that, but the direction taken did not matter. No matter what I did or what turn I made, they would finally catch me—and in the very instant that they did and I met my doom, I would wake up.

One night, in yet another futile sprint race with a creature from the Jurassic, it occurred to me I could accelerate that process. I suddenly turned and ran right toward the dinosaur, on purpose. I leapt into its huge mouth full of enormous teeth—and . . . I woke up! I didn't always remember that solution, but many nights I did. Gradually, the nightmares stopped. It seemed dinosaurs did not like my new game.

This night I turned and ran *toward* that inner dinosaur again. I'd realized the dinosaur was my own thought processes and the emotions they produced. I'd seen every inch of its huge mouth and counted every one of its enormous teeth, and I leapt into its mouth anyway. And then just as in my childhood dreams, I woke up. Only this time the awakening was more profound. I had made a life choice.

This whole process of pivoting from one life direction to another took far less time than it just took for you to read about it. In real time, I suspect these pivots took just seconds. I turned that rising sense of freedom and liberation into a kind of personal declaration of independence. "I don't know who you are," I said to the Dictator out loud, in my empty room at two in the morning. "Apparently, you can make me hurt; you can make me suffer. But there is one thing you cannot do"—and now the words came more forcefully—"*you—cannot—make—me—turn—from—my—own—experience.*

"*You . . . can't . . . do it!*"

As the echo of my declaration died away, the sense of time being suspended faded, and I was once again fully behind my own physical eyes. Looking down, I noticed that my hands were clenched, and I loosened them. I felt a sense of extension, as if an inner part of me were touching the world around me with new fingers. It was quite a different set of sensory fingers than were braced against the carpet a while earlier. I was not trying to keep my balance or to find the footing to force anxiety to go away. Instead, I was simply being.

It was as if a filter between myself and my own experience had been removed, like removing sunglasses you'd accidentally left on inside or taking out earplugs and finding gentle music in the background. I felt grounded and alive. I had a sense of gaining an ability to see the world more clearly as it is. *Never again*, I mentally promised myself as I stood up, realizing from my aching knees and a dried tear track on my face that I'd been on the floor a very long time. "I will not run from me."

I would not always know *how* to keep that promise—in small ways I would violate it almost daily and in larger ways, occasionally—but in the several decades since that night I would not for a single moment forget it, nor waver in my commitment to it. The promise was unconditional: no more running away from my thoughts, feelings, memories, and sensations. My experiences and I would succeed or fail together—as a collective, as a kind of family—all of us together.

At the time, I did not have much idea of what experiences I was avoiding, deep down. I would start here, with anxiety, and see what unfolded. It was only later that I would find sadness and shame and other emotions that were hiding in plain sight, underneath the panic. But that journey began with a commitment to myself: whatever happened, I would take all of me—the "strong" parts and the scared parts—and move forward with my life

Rising, I already sensed that the insights I'd had would carry forward not only to helping me change my relationship to my own anxiety, but also to finding better methods of working with my clients through new avenues of intervention and research. It was not long—just days—before I knew I had to understand what had just happened to me in a scientific sense. How did it work?

Spiritual writings, motivational blogs, and self-help books make plentiful reference to such turnaround stories. I'm hardly unique. If you talk to a friend who has overcome an addiction, or an anxiety disorder, or a compulsion, very often they have a story of hitting bottom and then finding the resources within to take a new direction. What was different in my case is that I channeled this moment into research.

A New Research Journey

My team of five doctoral students in clinical psychology soon developed a scientific research program designed to find the answers. I realized that to do so we would have to try to move beyond serious limitations in each of the psychological approaches that had come to dominate the field, one after the other, during the twentieth century. That included not just Freud and the psychoanalysts, but humanism, behaviorism, and the approach that was becoming dominant at the time, cognitive behavioral therapy (CBT). Some of these prior approaches were not based on solid experimental scientific research (e.g., psychoanalysis and humanism). Some were focused too much on the content of our thoughts rather than their impact on our lives (e.g., Freud in analyzing memories and dreams; CBT in its focus on irrational thinking and the disputation of problematic thoughts); some cared about the processes by which our thoughts had their impact, but the underlying theory of those processes was inadequate.

None of the schools of research and therapy had grappled well with a set of questions I now perceived as vital. How does the voice of the Dictator Within develop in our minds? Why are our thought processes so automatic, and why are the messages of the Dictator so incessant? I wanted to understand why negative thought patterns can be set in motion by the slightest triggers, even while we're not fully conscious, as I had found with my panic attack coming upon me while I slept. In addition, why do we find these negative thoughts so compelling? Why do they continue to hold such power over us even after we've told ourselves rationally they're not good for us? Why isn't the effort to think them away through the rational sorts of argumentation that traditional CBT instructs more powerful?

I could see that answering these questions would require a better understanding of human language and cognition. I expected we would not be able to find ways to help people consciously distance themselves from the voice, not needing to hit bottom as I had, without understanding how our thoughts take on so much power over us. I also suspected that with the answers we could achieve myriad positive goals, not only helping people break free from the monkey traps of thought that imprison them in so many unhealthy conditions, but also training children with deficiencies in thinking and emotional skills how to reason or how to connect with others in a healthy way.

No approach to psychology had provided good answers to all of these questions about human cognition. That was what I and my research team set out to try to do. We wanted a robust evidence-based, scientific understanding that told us how to predict and influence what people did with their thoughts.

We certainly haven't come up with all the answers, but we *have* found explanations that have allowed us to develop methods for helping people to defuse from the voice of the Dictator and make the crucial turn toward acceptance, and then to develop habits of committed action that allow them to live healthier and more fulfilling lives. These discoveries have indeed also provided the field with new ways to help children develop language and cognition skills, along with many other positive outcomes, such as improving performance in sports, succeeding in dieting, or helping a whole African community rise to the challenge of the Ebola epidemic. Our discoveries began with understanding the need to make the first three pivots, and finding ways for people to do so. Those discoveries led the way to finding methods to help people make the last three pivots.

In the chapters that follow, I will introduce the discoveries in this same sequence, explaining the science and beginning to introduce the simple methods we developed for making the pivots and continuing to develop your psychological flexibility. The methods will then be introduced more fully in the Part Two chapters, and I will show you how you can apply them to whatever challenges you or your loved ones are struggling with.

Understanding why the ACT practices are so powerful and why I felt developing such a different approach to psychological well-being was needed really requires knowing more about the limitations of the major prior therapeutic approaches, and the flaws in popular cultural assumptions about the causes of psychological challenges. Appreciating those limits is also important because not only have the prior traditions exerted a powerful influence over current therapeutic practice, but many of their notions about how we can heal ourselves have entered our broad culture. And while some of the insights and practices of these traditions continue to be highly valuable, some of them were off-base in ways that are counterproductive in the daily enterprise of pursuing a more fulfilling, purposeful life. So before introducing more about ACT, a quick excursion through the story of the prior traditions and one or two of our currently popular approaches is in order.

Chapter Three

FINDING A WAY FORWARD

Several mainstream traditions of psychology and psychiatry have powerfully influenced how people think about the human mind and our behavior, despite being scientifically flawed. Some of the notions that have been popularized are known to be incorrect, and at times even counterproductive. Others have just never been proven through systematic research. Understanding how those approaches have fallen short is important to appreciating the power of the ACT findings and methods.

Here is what the world should expect from an intervention approach in psychology and psychiatry: it should contain a broadly useful set of strategies for producing important life changes that work, and we should know why they do. Wide-ranging effectiveness indicates that an approach is tapping into fundamental aspects of human emotion, cognition, biology, and motivation. Broad and consistent usefulness focuses us on the big picture—not tiny details. We are all a bit fed up with the ingredient-by-ingredient findings of research in some areas, like nutrition science—dairy fat will kill you; no, wait, it's good for you; well, OK, sometimes it's good and sometimes it's bad. The last thing people need from psychologists is more elaborate and contradictory advice about what is good for living life well.

It's also important to understand *why* methods work so that you don't inadvertently misuse them. For instance, people who use a "time out" disciplinary approach with kids need to know that it is premised on the power of withdrawing positive reinforcement. Otherwise, you might put your eleven-year-old in time out, not think to take away the smartphone he has in his pocket, and find that little Junior *loved* the distraction-free chance to play Minecraft, giving him positive reinforcement for his bad behavior rather than withholding it.

To be useful, the "why" explanations have to be clear and specific (we will call that *precision*), but still apply to a lot of conditions (we will call that *scope*). To be consistent over time they also shouldn't contradict important things we know in other areas of science, such as research on genetics or the brain (we will call that *depth*). In psychology these explanations also have to tell us how to make specific changes in the way we're approaching life so that we will reach our goals (we will call those *change processes*).

The bottom line is this. Consumers of psychological change advice should demand *broadly useful methods of change that work, and that do so through change processes that have precision, scope, and depth.*

That's it and that's all. Put a period at the end of that sentence. Consumers deserve that from the behavioral scientists they help support with their tax dollars.

ACT and its underlying processes meet that test reasonably well. You'll be able to judge that yourself from the introduction of the ACT science and methods to come. ACT arguably applies to more types of problems and situations, and has consistently provided more good "why" explanations than any other widely used change approach in applied psychology. I know how that sounds and I feel a little frightened to say it so boldly—but I stand by it because I believe it is correct.

Few methods of behavior change have even really tried to answer the "why" questions. Most of what you think of as "psychology" has not shown much of an interest in them. That is probably because answering the "why" questions is so hard, and it's never really done. ACT researchers themselves keep searching for more answers. But those we've found thus far have led to powerful results. The other psychological traditions have not yet produced both "how" and "why" answers that are as consistent, or as widely useful.

A Fifteen-Minute History of Psychotherapeutic Intervention

The field was dominated in the first half of the last century by psychoanalysis and psychodynamic theory. It exerts vast influence to this day. So influential have Sigmund Freud's ideas been that he is among the most cited scholars in the world, not just in psychology but in *any* scientific area. He was a careful clinical observer and some of his insights have been validated, but others have no basis in science and are rather fantastical speculations. Freud's focus was on the hidden, or repressed, motivations behind problematic behavior. In particular, he famously argued that awakening sexual impulses might engender deep conflicts and fears, which then lead to pathological behavior as a way to avoid those conflicts and fears, which he called *defense mechanisms*. His arguments were eloquently written and persuasive, but Freud and his followers initially produced little in the way of experimental support.

It took many decades before psychoanalysts got around to the hard business of trying to verify that their methods actually work, and when they did they found that many were in fact relatively unhelpful. To this day, the explanations of *why* they work when they do is often vague and empirically inconsistent. Many of the specifics of Freud's arguments have been repudiated or gradually ignored by psychology. His theory had wide scope (seemingly applying to everyone), but it was imprecise and did not provide enough good evidence for specific change processes.

Take the famous case of Little Hans, which Freud published in 1928. You can immediately sense how hard it would be to prove the "why" claims Freud made in his assessment of it. Hans was a little boy who wanted to stay home instead of going to school. Hans feared horse-drawn carts and said they were a reason he did not want to leave the house, but Freud saw deep symbolism and unconscious motives in Hans's fear. He believed that Hans had a hidden sexual impulse toward his mother, which had engendered a fear of being castrated by his father should his father find out. Staying home allowed Hans to partially fulfill his secret desire to be with her, or, Freud theorized, perhaps his desire to have sex with his mother, while also meeting the primary purpose of avoiding his deeper fear and sense of conflict. Freud's evidence consisted of such things as a comment Hans made to his mother about his penis while she gave him a bath, or the possibility that horses' blinders reminded the little boy of his father's big glasses, while the animals' big teeth reminded the little boy unconsciously of what his father might want to do with him if he knew about his secret desires.

About here one's eyes begin to roll.

Freud was trying to find valid principles, but he did not devise experimental tests of his theories, and he overlooked factors in his patients' behavior that we now realize were probably quite important. For example, in the case of Little Hans, the boy had seen a horse-drawn cart fall over amid the cries and screams of riders, but Freud did not take account of how that experience may have naturally led to the boy's fear of horses, quite apart from Dad's big, scary glasses.

To be fair, some of Freud's ideas are now relatively well supported scientifically, through subsequent work done by other researchers. There is much to like about the concept of defense mechanisms, for example. We do indeed appear to reject facts about ourselves that are too painful to admit, regardless of the strength of the evidence, a defense mechanism Freud called *denial*. We do generate feelings and actions that go in the exact opposite direction of our true feelings if those are too hard to admit, a defense mechanism called *reaction formation*. Addressing these unhealthy avoidance tendencies is a major function of ACT methods.

However, the idea that a conflict between urges and restrictions placed on them underlies abnormal behavior (such as Little Han's "Oedipal" urges and his fear of castration by his father) is largely unfounded. What's more, Freud's approach encouraged as a primary method of therapy a deep interrogation of our feelings and thoughts in order to discover our hidden motivations and desires. No evidence supports that as a change process with precision, scope, and depth. Thoroughly exploring thoughts and feelings can be helpful in therapy, but without good guidance by solid, scientifically validated principles, it is easy to get lost in such explorations and make little progress with becoming happier and healthier.

There are rich modern versions of the psychoanalytic tradition that have begun to enter the world of evidence-based therapy, but they have done so by leaving fantastical speculation behind. Most of the new methods have emphasized the importance of examining present thoughts and emotions or interpersonal relationships (sometimes including the therapeutic relationship itself), and learning to appreciate the intentions and mental states of others. Some of this work has begun the scientific journey of developing evidence-based change processes. I personally find a lot to draw from in these modern forms of psychoanalysis, especially ideas about the need to understand the psychological world of others, and to see ourselves in a social context. But a deep dive into the search for unconscious conflicts, which is the part of the Freudian approach the public most took away from the explanations of psychoanalysis, is not likely to be helpful.

Humanistic and Existential Therapy

The humanistic tradition emerged partly in opposition to the fantastical qualities of psychoanalytic theory, and it became quite popular in the middle part of the last century. It focuses on how people experience the world, how we conceptualize ourselves and relate to others, and how we create a life of meaning. The central issues attended to are important: empathy, authenticity, and a sense of self.

I became interested in psychology because of humanists like Abraham Maslow (famous for discovering the importance of *peak experiences*), and I loved people like Fritz Perls (Gestalt therapy), Viktor Frankl (a concentration camp survivor who focused on the creation of meaning and developed a method called *logotherapy*), and Carl Rogers. Still do. I love how they want to focus on human potential and not just human problems. I love their appreciation of the whole person and their interest in the whole of human experience.

The problem is that while humanists from the beginning said research was important, they had a hard time agreeing on how to do it. Maslow argued that traditional scientific methods simply could not capture the essence of human experience. Rogers argued that research was needed to avoid self-deception, but he also argued that "the growth of knowledge in the social sciences contains within itself a powerful tendency toward social control [and the] weakening or destruction of the existential person." In other words, he worried that if scientific principles were directly linked to deliberate behavior change they might be used in ways that undermine human freedom, and human freedom was so important that knowledge about how to change behavior is a potential threat.

No doubt that is true. Advertisers and tobacco companies have clearly done research that would fit such a description. Casinos, the pharmaceutical industry, the food industry, and video game companies have done the same. The list is actually not short. But stand back from that claim, and you can see why such an attitude meant that humanists could never quite prove that their methods were broadly effective, nor could they adequately answer the hard "why" questions. This attitude gave humanists and existentialists little room to work on an adequate science of change. As a result, the public has to take many humanistic ideas on faith, and that is a high cost.

ACT is sometimes covered in books on humanistic therapy, and I like that. We've drawn on some of the best ideas inside this tradition, and we've found a way to overcome Maslow's and Rogers's worries about how to verify them scientifically.

Behavior Therapy: The First Wave

Most clinical psychologists would mark the beginning of a more scientific approach to psychological intervention with the rise of behavior therapy and behavior modification in the 1960s. This is not totally fair—the traditions of psychoanalysis and the humanistic approach did have *some* scientific basis. But well-controlled studies that tested behavior change methods were innovations brought to the table by behavior therapists.

I am old enough to have witnessed the rise of behavior therapy firsthand. I originally embraced this approach in college in part because B. F. Skinner and other behaviorists who had made important discoveries about how behavior can be learned and modified had presented a compelling picture of a better world. Skinner's utopian novel *Walden Two* laid out a future world in which the environments we live in would foster human cooperation, better child rearing, healthier environments, and more satisfying workplaces. I was so struck by the idea that I enrolled at the behavioral stronghold of West Virginia University in 1972 to do my doctoral training.

The core of the behaviorists' work was in showing how behaviors would become more or less likely to occur based on the consequences that followed them. The relationships between setting, actions, and outcomes are what behaviorists call *contingencies*. If a pigeon inside a box is given food after it pecks at a small colored plastic disk, it will likely peck that disk more and more often. That's an example of the principle of *reinforcement*, which many parenting methods today draw on, such as the previously mentioned "time out" technique. Other wings of the behavior therapy movement relied more on principles drawn from the Russian physiologist Ivan Pavlov. His classical conditioning principles explain how animals can come to associate a previously neutral event, such as the ringing of a bell, with, say, the presentation of food immediately following it, so that the animal learns to salivate at the bell tone.

These principles were applied to work with humans by the early behavior therapists, who, for example, worked to pair relaxation with gradual exposure to frightening events, hoping that the pairing would reduce anxiety and allow more natural behavior. That was the core of a powerful new psychotherapy technique called *systematic desensitization*, in which people with phobias imagined gradually more and more anxiety-provoking images while staying relaxed through the use of methods of muscular relaxation. In its heyday desensitization was the most studied psychotherapy method on the planet. It often worked (and still does), but it is rarely used today because it ultimately failed the "why" test.

Research showed that the relaxation part of the treatment did not matter—exposure alone helped, even if the exposure was just in the person's imagination, by being asked to envision a source of fear. Nowadays psychologists use exposure extensively (in one's imagination, through virtual reality, or in real life) but generally without relaxation and the other trappings of desensitization. We still are not entirely sure why *that* works either, but the developer of desensitization, the late South African psychiatrist Joseph Wolpe, deserves enormous credit for having tried very seriously to find answers.

I've called this era of behaviorism the First Wave of the behavioral and cognitive therapies. Principles developed through work with nonhuman animals were tested systematically with human clients, and a number of powerful methods of behavior modification were created that to this day are on the lists of evidence-based procedures. What was and is great about behavioral psychology is its focus on principles of change that have high precision, scope, and depth. But the behaviorists of the day could not adequately explain the complexity of human thought and its role in our behavior. It wasn't that they were closed to analyzing human thought processes and emotion. Contrary to popular perception, when they referred to "behavior" they meant *all* human actions, including thinking and feeling. But they didn't have a good model of how the human mind works. Their explanation of how principles like reinforcement or classical conditioning could produce the complexity of our thinking, feeling, or caring just did not work well enough. Said in another way, the behaviorists I knew had heart, but they could not really explain our heads.

The behaviorists knew this was a problem, or at least Skinner did. In 1957 he wrote a book titled *Verbal Behavior* in which he tried to explain how we develop language through behavioral principles. It was brilliant, and I was initially charmed by it, but I soon began to worry that his explanations were far too limited. That feeling only grew after I got my degree and started trying to do research using his ideas. Very early in my academic career I concluded they were largely wrong. Skinner could explain only some of the earliest stages of language development, and his ideas about human cognition were gradually relegated primarily to work in early language training, especially with children with severe developmental delays.

Most people wrote off behaviorism in part because of its failure to explain human cognition. But they also did so because of the notion that Skinner and other behaviorists were pursuing dangerous efforts toward thought and behavior control. It was not true, but Skinner inadvertently fueled speculation that behaviorists were pursuing totalitarian control methods by writing a book titled *Beyond Freedom and Dignity*, in which, with a totally deaf ear to how his words would sound, he complained that we should not let flowery expressions like *freedom* and *dignity* get in the way of discovering how we can learn to change behavior. As a result, reporters writing about behavior modification at the time regularly associated it with terms like *mind control*, *brainwashing*, or even *psychosurgery*, though behavior therapy never had anything to do with such efforts. It was painful to watch this happen.

I spent many hours with Skinner and the other early behavior therapists and I found that far from being coldhearted manipulators, they were warm, caring, and inspirational. These folks wanted to use the insights they'd discovered in the laboratory in all sorts of positive ways—to reduce energy consumption (that would eventually be the topic of my dissertation), to make workplace settings more humane, to help parents raise their kids, or to help patients learn to use their kidney dialysis machines at home. But their theory and methods simply weren't up to the breadth of this challenge, and the culture began to pass them by.

Traditional Cognitive Behavioral Therapy (CBT): The Second Wave

Behavior therapy was not even a decade old when Aaron Beck, Albert Ellis, and others led the way in developing CBT. The central focus of this Second Wave of behaviorism was to correct the failure to account for the role our thoughts play in governing our behavior. CBT did not jettison behavioral methods—it incorporated virtually all of the earlier behavioral practices, such as the gradual exposure to sources of fear in order to cure phobias. But many practices aimed at changing the content of people's thoughts were added—and these new methods became the real heart and soul of CBT.

The core of the theory was that maladaptive thoughts lead to maladaptive emotions, which in turn drive abnormal behavior. In trying to change people's maladaptive thoughts, the pioneers of CBT asked clients what they were thinking and then, based on various theoretical ideas, challenged the thoughts they believed to be pathology-promoting. The basic method was to get patients to consider their thoughts and emotions rationally, examine the evidence for and against them, and then deliberately adopt a view that was consistent with evidence about the situation and thus was relatively accurate.

The fundamental argument behind CBT was logical and clear, which was part of its attraction. It also had the benefit of familiarity. The basic notion had been part of cultural wisdom for ages. Your grandmother could probably tell you about some of your cognitive errors—"You are making too big a deal about it, dear. It doesn't *always* turn out badly." But I was again skeptical. Very.

While behavior therapy was based on thousands of careful experimental studies of learning processes drawn from the animal lab that had high precision and scope, the CBT conception of how the mind works was based primarily on talking to clients and having them fill out questionnaires. There was, in fact, no tight definition of what a "thought" even was! Laboratory science still had no means of explaining human cognition adequately, and the CBT community did not know how to fill that gap.

CBT methods do produce good outcomes, which is why I trained in early CBT methods and employed them in my work with clients. What CBT added to behavior therapy was helpful in leading people to see how thoughts can dominate our behavior. For example, one of the practices of CBT was to have patients keep a thought record, which helped clients become aware of their thoughts and their impact. One of my earliest clients initially denied he had thoughts that led to his anger. He also denied he was angry, even when the veins stuck out of his neck in rage. I pushed him to keep a thought record, tracking the internal and external situation before the thought appeared, and what happened afterward. He came back the next session a changed man. "I have them!" he declared. "I caught them! It was amazing. Right before I got angry I was thinking, 'This is not fair'!"

I also saw, however, that sometimes the cognitive change that CBT argued was critical actually came *after* changes in mood or behavior, not before. How we felt and what we did, it seemed, might sometimes drive maladaptive thinking rather than the other way around, which CBT could not readily explain. It was when it came to the "why" questions that Second Wave CBT really began to falter, which most researchers in CBT nowadays concede at least to a degree.

I decided I would try to determine whether mainstream CBT explanations were accurate.

Moving On from Traditional CBT

During my panic struggle times through the earliest days of ACT I focused my research group on rigorously assessing CBT methods. My students and I conducted eight studies on the cognitive model of CBT, examining whether the answers it gave to the "why" questions were correct. In every case, our results said "no."

Let me describe my favorite of these studies, done for his master's thesis by Irwin Rosenfarb, who went on to a long academic career. An important CBT study had shown that children who were afraid of the dark could stay in the dark a lot longer after watching a short video that tried to teach them to think differently about their fear. The video was very simple: it asked the children to say positive things to themselves when in the dark, such as "I'm a brave boy and I can stay in the dark!" The researchers concluded that the children could now stay in the dark longer because they were talking to themselves in a more affirming and rational way.

We thought that explanation might be wrong. Maybe the children just stayed in the dark a lot longer because they would look like a failure in the eyes of the experimenter if they promptly left a dark room after being told to say, "I'm a brave boy and I can stay in the dark!" In other words, maybe the video set a kind of social standard against which the children knew they might be measured, much as when a parent says to a child, "I expect you to read for the next hour. No getting on the computer!"

To test that idea, we had to trick the children into thinking no one could know what video they watched. In our version of the study, the fearful children sat in a room alone and watched the video—just as had been done in the classic study. They were tested before and after for how long they could stay in the room, again just as in the original. To set up the deception, though, we told all of the kids that we had many different shows that they could watch to help them with their fear. A panel with lots of buttons supposedly controlled the different TV channels and all were told that after we left the room they could press any button, and the show they picked would appear.

The children were randomized to one of two conditions (*conditions* is the way researchers refer to the specific setup for each group in an experiment, and *randomized* just means their condition was assigned by chance, sort of like flipping a coin). In one condition, before leaving the room we asked the children to point to the button they would soon press "so we will know what you are watching." This is like the classic study, except in ours they supposedly had lots of channel options. In the deception condition we told them *not* to show us what button they would press "so we won't know which one you are watching." In fact, of course, the same show popped up for all kids once they pushed a button, regardless of which channel they'd picked, so we *did* know what they were watching, but the children thought we didn't.

The result? The group who thought the experimenter knew what they were watching stayed in the dark a lot longer—exactly as in the original study. But those in the other group, the ones whom we deceived into thinking no one knew what they were watching, did *not* stay in the room any longer. The advice had no effect. Nada. Not even the tiniest trend.

Our new answer to the "why" question about the results of that initial CBT study was that it was not what you knew that mattered, it was who knew you knew it. The cognitive model said it was the *content* of thoughts that matters, not the social context you have them in. The conclusions about the "why" question in this classic study were simply wrong.

I had also seen in my work with patients, and in trying to overcome my anxiety, that traditional CBT often didn't work, especially the cognitive change methods. It was torturous to me to be using CBT methods in my practice when they did not work for me in trying to cope with my growing anxiety disorder. But they were the best methods we had in psychology at the time. I found myself over and over again telling my patients to practice doing what failed me when dealing with the exact same issues. I felt like a total fraud.

Now, all these years later, a wealth of additional research has revealed that CBT generally does not work in the way that was originally postulated, or at least not consistently. Very large and carefully done studies have shown that disputing and trying to change thoughts doesn't add much to CBT outcomes. In fact, cognitive thought change methods can even *subtract* from the impact of the behavioral methods, such as encouraging depressed people to become more active, that are still part of CBT! We now know that CBT has good effects mostly due to its behavioral components. In many areas, compelling proof of its "why" answers have eluded traditional CBT. It does not yet meet the standard of change processes with precision, scope, and depth, even if its outcomes are still the gold standard.

The Third Wave

Researchers and therapists are still struggling to accept the ramifications of these findings about CBT's limits, but a major transition is under way in which many CBT researchers are moving CBT itself broadly in an ACT direction, a transition that has begun in recent years to move at light speed. I have called the period of transformation we've been through during the last fifteen years or so the Third Wave of cognitive and behavioral therapies.

The central shift is from a focus on *what* you think and feel to *how do you relate to* what you think and feel. Specifically, the new emphasis is on learning to step back from what you are thinking, notice it, and open up to what you are experiencing. These steps keep us from doing the damage to ourselves that efforts to avoid or control our thoughts or feelings inflict, allowing us to focus our energies on taking the positive actions that can alleviate our suffering.

It's important to say that in championing this change and developing the ACT methods, I drew on key sources in First and Second Wave behavioral and cognitive therapy. One was a new form of exposure therapy developed by David Barlow. He was (and still is) one of the premiere anxiety researchers on the planet. I was fortunate that he was my mentor and supervisor at Brown University during my clinical psychology internship as I completed my doctorate. Shortly after I left Brown, he had begun innovative work on treating anxiety disorders. Instead of having patients gradually put themselves into the *situations* they were afraid of—such as, for those who were afraid of heights, taking steps up a ladder and, ultimately, riding in a glass elevator up a skyscraper—Dave was asking clients to experience progressively more intense internal *sensations* of fear without putting them in those situations. For example, he would take people with panic problems and spin them around in a chair to get them dizzy, or make them hyperventilate by breathing very rapidly until they felt like passing out. Or he would have them run until their hearts pounded. The idea was that if you could get used to progressively more intense sensations that you avoided, you would be less sensitive to them and less likely to overreact to them, in the same way that a person with a height phobia could get used to progressively higher heights.

At the time, David thought these methods worked by actually reducing the fear of panicky sensations. That "why" guess turned out to be largely wrong. I thought the answer might be slightly different. His results suggested to me that it was *not fear itself or its associated sensations and thoughts that cause our problems, but our relationship to these experiences that does the damage.* That was the implicit message, after all, in, say, asking a person to hyperventilate. To do that task they had to be open to the sensations that would come—but that very willingness means that it is not the content of the sensations per se that is the problem. No matter how many times you hyperventilate, doing so will still produce very odd and even aversive sensations that are caused by excess oxygen and low levels of CO_2 in your blood. Exposure in that case implicitly suggested to patients that it is the *function* of sensations that's the problem—in other words, what they cause us to do, such as running from them. I thought that finding other ways to deliberately develop a new relationship with unpleasant sensations, as well as emotions and thoughts, might be the key to a better approach to intervention.

I had written some thoughts in that regard years before. My first undergraduate psychology paper was on the possibility of using exposure not just to focus on the situation but also to focus on openness to emotion. David's work clicked into that old interest and helped me link it to a search for principles of change. If what is important is how we relate to sensations, learning to experience them without trying to expunge them, could the same thing apply to all experiences, including thoughts and emotions? My personal experience with turning toward my anxiety seemed to suggest this was the key.

Humanistic methods, mindfulness practices, and the Human Potential Movement also pointed to the importance of accepting negative thoughts and feelings. As a child of the 1960s and 1970s growing up in California, I had dabbled in various methods for putting our minds on a leash—distancing ourselves from the Dictator Within—such as contemplative practice, body awareness, chanting, yoga, psychedelic drugs, and mindfulness training. I was exposed to zen during my college years in Los Angeles by the late Joshu Sasaki Roshi. I lived for a time in an Eastern religious commune in Northern California directed by a swami named Kriyananda. I also took part in college in encounter groups and sensitivity training sessions—long and fairly unstructured gatherings in which a facilitator guided group members to express their emotional reactions, especially those that arose in reaction to other group members. The idea was that if we were open enough to our emotions and thoughts, no matter how unpleasant, and could express them freely, our actions would be liberated and more coherent.

A few years into my job as a professor I participated in and was moved deeply by Erhard Seminars Training (est), a large-group awareness training that was a logical extension of humanistic practices, examining ways that emotions and thoughts can be given power by how we relate to them. I decided to try est because my graduate advisor, John Cone, changed so obviously after he experienced "the training" that I could not deny there might be value in it. There was no written tradition in est, but the workshops were incredible. The focus was on how the mind overwhelmed experience and how awareness itself provided a foundation to experience life in a more open way. Many of these ideas ended up in ACT.

None of these methods (encounter groups, est, religious chants, and so on) had been scientifically developed, however, and they could be misused. Encounter groups, for example, could become abusive, providing cover for cruel lashing out at members under the auspices of honest communication. I had seen things like that happen. Some humanistic gurus were notorious for using their position of power to sexually harass trainees. Mindfulness traditions suffered the same thing.

I was shocked and disappointed when Kriyananda was first accused of violating his vows of chastity with multiple female members of the commune (I say "first" because after nearly losing the commune he'd built, he created another wave of similar troubles much later on in his career). Even the venerable zen master Joshu Sasaki Roshi gained a similar reputation. There is no way my night on the carpet could have happened without est, but the excessive commercialism and weak empirical support for large-group awareness training more generally convinced me that its best ideas needed to be brought into an open process of scientific investigation and refinement. I valued mindfulness methods but thought they too needed to follow that path.

I and many other researchers have since conducted solid scientific studies of the fruit-nut-seed mix of ideas that were floating around in the 1960s and 1970s. Some of them turned out to be worthwhile and as a result, they are now part of the picture in Third Wave CBT methods, such as ACT.

Brains and Genes

I've been summarizing what has happened in the development of psychology, but you notice I've not yet even mentioned biology. I need to, both because most of us are aware of some important advances in the biological understanding of human action, and because some harmful notions about how our biology determines our psychology have been popularized.

When I was in training in the 1970s, many researchers studying the role of genes in behavior believed that one day we would know that there are handfuls of genes responsible for many psychological conditions, such as major depression and schizophrenia, and that a great deal of human behavior would be easily explained by genes. Meanwhile, the field of neuroscience was rapidly developing and the idea was taking hold that understanding the structure of our brains would reveal the ways they determine how we think, feel, and act. Most behavioral psychologists, though, believed that behavior and psychological conditions were as influenced by life experience as by genetic and neurobiological factors, and that each impacted the other in a system. Said another way, psychology is biological but cannot be reduced to biochemistry or neurobiology without losing what is important.

The biological community at large didn't put much stock in that idea. I gave a talk in 1993 to the behavioral genetics lab at the University of California, San Diego, and when I stated my view that learning strongly impacted how genes and the brain operate, the students literally laughed in my face.

Today the idea is hardly laughable. Instead, the dream that simple genetic causes of mental health conditions would be discovered is dead. Research has proven that we in behavioral psychology were largely right.

A huge blow to the expectation that a clean line between specific genes and behavior could be drawn followed the 2003 mapping of the complete human genome. As clear relationships between genes and particular traits and conditions were sought, and hundreds of thousands of people's specific genomes were mapped and scoured, simple correlations between genes and conditions proved more and more elusive. The idea that there are genes "for" depression or "for" being an upbeat person was soundly repudiated. Not only are scores of genes implicated in any given condition, but even so, they account for only a few percentage points of the likelihood of developing a condition.

We've also learned that the body has evolved a vast array of "epigenetic" processes—meaning ones that affect the activation of genes and are influenced by our life experiences. Geneticists have long agreed that experiences cannot change genes, and that is still technically correct. But we now know that experiences do significantly determine which genes are allowed to operate in your body. And some of this epigenetic "coding" that is imprinted in our biology can be inherited. The general agreement of geneticists of the last century needs to be modified.

If your grandparent experienced abuse as a child, you may have inherited some of the epigenetic effects of that experience. Studies have shown that the grandchildren of people who went through the Holocaust, or who were abused as children, or who nearly starved in Holland during World War II, have bodies that are more genetically vigilant for stress and trauma, because their epigenome is different.

Let me share an example of a genetic discovery to demonstrate how complicated the influences of experience on genetic function are. Researchers were very excited when in 2003 they learned that variation in a gene related to the flow of the chemical serotonin in the brain was associated with depression and other maladies. After the initial "Eureka!," a *flood* of research followed. It was soon revealed that the variation in the gene seemed to be important primarily if you were maltreated as a child. Then more studies showed that several other factors influenced the degree that the variation mattered, including one's gender, ethnicity, and amount of social support. It began to appear that the gene created a greater sensitivity to experiences and became especially relevant when adversity struck and social support was lacking. Based on these factors, the same genetic condition that predicted *more* depression in some circumstances predicted *less* depression in others!

The notion that has made its way into the mainstream culture that those of us who struggle with psychological well-being were just dealt a bad genetic hand is grossly inaccurate. And the idea of a "bad genetic hand" can lead to a lack of commitment to do what you can to improve your well-being.

ACT research has shown that developing psychological flexibility can have powerful effects on the functioning of our genes. For example, an epigenetic process called *methylation* interferes with your body's ability to read your genes. Harmful methylation can result from trauma, but learning the flexibility skills can undo part of the damage, and recent evidence shows that it does so by changing methylation. Flexibility processes literally alter how genes work.

You can say it this way: if you learn to be less reactive to stress through the cultivation of flexibility pivots, the body starts turning off those reaction systems, including genetic expression switches that may have been originally thrown not by you but by your parents and grandparents.

How cool is that?

What about how our brain controls our psychological health? It can also be significantly altered by learning the skills. If you have chronic pain and you go through a course of ACT, the brain starts not sending as much pain information to parts of the brain involved in decision making. It's not exactly right to say you hurt less as a result—it is more that hurt is just less central to your thought processes.

High experiential avoiders have brains that are busy watching out for possible negative events, as you plan and talk to yourself about what to do with these events if you detect them. As psychological flexibility increases, your brain quiets. You are spending less time in defensive scanning and planning, and that allows for more focus on what you want to be attending to, like work tasks or listening thoughtfully to a friend. Attentional control increases and the parts of the brain that regulate attention grow in strength.

Yes, it is correct to say that your brain determines your behavior. But it is equally correct to say that your behavior changes your brain. To say one without the other is like saying, "I can only pick up fifty pounds because my muscles are weak," without noting that they are weak because you never exercise.

An enormous body of research illuminates why the ACT skills lead to helpful brain changes and changes in gene expression. We now know that if you change your mind and behavior in a healthy way, helpful changes in your body will come along for the ride, down to almost every single cell you have. I will review some of that evidence later in the book. For now, suffice it to say that psychology is no longer the weakling in the study of life; it is now right at the center of the most important advances in understanding how our biology works.

Launching ACT Research

As I sought to discover better methods for helping people improve their psychological health and pursue the course of life they aspired to, I knew that understanding the distinctive complexity of human thought was at least as important as research in genetics and neuroscience. I realized that in order to learn how to help people adopt a new relationship with their thoughts and emotions, I had to understand how we develop the voice of the Dictator in our minds. That was crucial because of the enormous power "the voice" has over us. I wanted to understand why it is so compelling to us: why we have such a hard time ignoring the bad advice it often gives. I knew it was also important to figure out why our thought processes can be so automatic and impervious to change. Perhaps, I hoped, my research partners and I could find ways to neutralize the power of the Dictator and free people to act in healthy ways in response to difficult experiences, thoughts, and emotions.

I will introduce our findings about human thought in the next two chapters because they are powerful in explaining why ACT and other Third Wave methods are so effective. We've found that a bit of understanding about them really helps people embrace the methods. I also think you'll find them fascinating. We've learned remarkable things about human language and symbolic thought. We know much more today about how the human mind works. But the most important thing about these findings is that they've led to clear guidance about how we can live more purposeful and rewarding lives.

Chapter Four

WHY OUR THOUGHTS ARE SO AUTOMATIC AND CONVINCING

How does the Dictator Within get its power over us?

That is not an abstract intellectual question. Understanding how human thought works is fundamental to our freedom and prosperity. Our minds play tricks on us, but once we know how the tricks work, we can't be fully fooled so easily.

In the classic film *The Wizard of Oz*, the Wizard is initially a fearsome disembodied head that looms over Dorothy, her dog, and her three companions. When the Wizard commands in a booming voice, "Bring me the broomstick of the Wicked Witch of the West!" they cower in fear and proceed to risk their lives to follow the command. Once the little dog Toto has pulled back the curtain on the Wizard, however, his command, "Pay no attention to that man behind the curtain!" impresses them not at all. They've seen though the trick, and the power of illusion has disappeared. "You humbug!" Dorothy cries. "You're a very bad man." The old man comes out from behind the curtain and pleads his case: "Oh, no, my dear. I'm a very good man. I'm just a very bad wizard."

Early on in the development of ACT, my research team became convinced that if we were going to liberate people from negative thought patterns, we needed to pull the curtain back on the mind's inner workings, so that people could begin to see the Dictator for what it is and release themselves from following its commands automatically. Much as in the movie, we don't need to do that because we have very bad minds—to the contrary, what we have are very good minds, just very bad Dictators. Once we stop letting our thoughts automatically control our behavior, we can make far better use of our own cognitive talents.

Scholars and researchers have long believed that the way we formulate and express our thoughts is fundamentally symbolic and is linked to human language. Symbolic meaning gives words and mental images a reality that is virtually the same as that of physical objects and events in the external world. The relationships we make between words and what they stand for allow us to conjure up the thing a word is related to even when it is entirely absent. When we hear the word *apple*, it produces an image of the fruit so vividly in our imaginations that we can recall the taste and smell. We will probably even salivate a little when we hear the word (if we like apples). This is why our memories of experiences can be so potent, carrying strong feelings of fear or pain or sadness or joy, sometimes much as we felt on the day events occurred.

While this ability to conjure up a reality that is purely one of thought makes astonishing feats of problem-solving, creative imagination, and communication possible, it also means that thoughts we have that may be entirely divorced from reality can be utterly convincing to us. The symbolic reality of language is a big part of why we find the voice of the Dictator so compelling even when it is telling us to believe things and do things that our experience shows are harmful.

What we have lacked in psychology was an account that explained the precise nature of this ability, where it came from, and how to change it. That is the kind of knowledge that can "pull back the curtain" on the mind.

Along with a growing group of colleagues, we have spent over three decades conducting studies to try to answer these questions. We developed a comprehensive approach to language learning and symbolic thought. We've channeled the results of that research into methods for teaching children language, reasoning, and problem solving on one hand, and into methods of breaking the spell that thoughts have over us and our actions on the other hand. These studies clarify why the seemingly logical approach to cleaning up our thoughts that is often promoted in therapy can make about as much sense as trying carefully to rearrange a spiderweb in order to keep it from looking a bit too messy.

The Uniquely Human Blessing and Curse

The way we learn language explains the power of the Dictator. And a core finding of our research is that human language learning does not happen the way that language theorists have posited for three hundred years.

A false idea that has dominated the study of language acquisition is that meaning is derived from a process of association, much the way Ivan Pavlov's dogs learned to salivate at the sound of a bell that reliably signaled just before they were given food. Once that association had been strongly made, the dogs would salivate at the sound of the bell even if no food appeared.

Basic processes of association are indeed the way children learn first words, being specifically trained in the associations between words and their meanings. Parents who are eager for their child to call them "Mama" or "Dada" know this well. We teach them by direct association and by using what psychologists call *contingencies*, learning "when . . . if . . . then" sequences such as *when* I see this face, *if* I say "Mama," *then* happy tickles will follow. To train names with our children, we may say "I'm Mama" or "That's Dada," pointing to ourselves or the other parent. Word after word—*bottle, milk, ball, toy, doggy*—we train our babies when they see an object to expect a characteristic name, or when they hear a name to expect a characteristic object. As they begin to speak, they learn to show the right "when . . . if . . . then" sequences, and can say the right word to refer to an object, or to reach for the right object when they hear its name, or to command the presentation of the right object by saying its name.

But somewhere around age twelve months, children begin to show that language is becoming a two-way street. Any parent who's had a child suddenly say they want something—maybe an apple—when the child hadn't been explicitly taught the word for that thing has experienced the wonder of this natural stage of development. Children come to understand that the relations between words and their meanings go both ways, that if the word *Mama* refers to a particular person, then if someone points to that person and asks who she is, the word *Mama* is the right answer.

No other animal has been shown capable of figuring out that two-way street. If you train a chimp to point to an abstract symbol whenever it sees an orange, and you later hold up that symbol next to a bowl of fruit, the chimp will not know to pick out the orange. The chimp has learned only a one-way association (orange→). If you want the chimp to point to the orange, you will have to teach it the connection in the other direction (→ orange). That seems strange to us because the two-way nature of the relations between words and their meaning is so natural to human adults.

It's once we've developed the ability to make two-way relations that our thinking ability is off and running. By the time children are sixteen or seventeen months old, if they hear an unfamiliar name and both a familiar and an unfamiliar object is in sight, they will assume that the unfamiliar name goes with the unfamiliar object and vice versa (my lab was among the first to show this transition, twenty-five years ago). Parents are often dumbfounded by how quickly children learn new words, not realizing that every word they are saying is now leading the baby to search for events and objects in the environment that are unfamiliar and to derive a two-way relation between those events or objects and these new words.

In the early 1980s I began doing research with a senior colleague, Aaron Brownstein, into how children discovered this two-way street. Association and contingencies, I thought, could never explain it because that kind of learning is one-way learning. Then in a spectacular week it all fell together. Language was not learning to associate, it was learning to relate. Aaron loved it, which was extremely gratifying to me as a young academic.

This seemingly small difference of learning by deriving relations helps explain why human thought becomes so "real." It accounts for why our thought processes become so complex and automatic, and it helps explain why any given new thought, whether triggered by some actual event in the present moment or by a memory, can have ripple effects through elaborate networks of thoughts embedded in our minds.

Aaron and I came up with the term *relational frames* for the many types of abstract comparisons that can be learned because, like a picture frame, they are a construct that all sorts of different objects and concepts can be put into. For example, consider this frame:

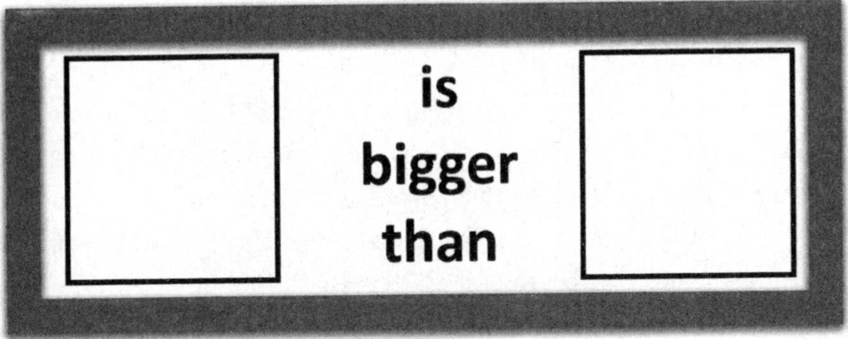

We can say to a child who has learned this relational frame not only "The house is bigger than the car," but "God is bigger than the universe" and the child will understand. The child will also be able to say, "The universe is smaller than God" and "Since I'm smaller than the universe, God is bigger than me." They can combine frames into cognitive networks.

Two-way relations and the networks they produce are the fundamental building block of our symbolic thinking abilities. The kinds of relations we learn quickly become more and more complex, moving beyond direct relations between words and concrete objects to abstract relations, such as that one object is opposite to another, better or worse than another, uglier or prettier, or more valuable. The mind is using language to understand increasingly complex features of the world and how it works.

Without the imaginative ability to understand abstract relations, human cognition would have been hobbled; we realized this was another major threshold of our intellectual development. It takes a number of years for children to master. Three-year-olds tend to prefer a nickel to a dime, because they know that coins are worth something (like candy) and the nickel is physically bigger. Up to that point in their lives, "more" is linked primarily to comparison of physical features, a skill many animals have. But by the time they are five or six, they will prefer the dime "because it's bigger." They now understand that "more" can be abstracted from the physical amount of something and can even be applied to something that is obviously "less" in a physical sense. As this happens, humans enter into a cognitive world your dog or cat will never be able to enter.

As we learn the many relational frames, we move from being able to derive relations by observing events in the world to being able to imagine relations—to conjure them up purely in our minds. At this point our thought processes are becoming extremely complex; we are building ever more elaborate networks of thoughts built out of relations. A good way to appreciate why complexity follows from knowing many different kinds of relations is to think about how enormously complex relations are in an extended family.

Suppose I put a photo of an Asian woman in her early thirties and one of a white woman who appears to be in her late fifties in front of you and I say, "These two people are from the same family. Without asking any questions, can you tell me how they are related?" You'd have to answer "no" because there are so many ways in which they might be. You might guess that the younger Asian woman had married the son of the older white woman. But it might also turn out that the younger woman is a stepsibling of the older woman, because she's the daughter of the white woman's father from a second marriage. The Asian woman might also be the daughter of the older white woman, by blood or by adoption. But she could also be a second cousin, the daughter of one of the white woman's cousins. Perhaps the two of them are married.

You don't need to see the other people in the family who are directly linked to one another in order to spin out these possibilities in your mind. You can work all of those possible relations out because you understand the many types of relations that can occur in families in the abstract (don't we even call all of our relatives "our relations"?). This allows you to *imagine* the many ways the two women could be related. And if you are told the right relation, it could impact information about all of the rest of the family, because relations like that combine in networks.

The bottom line is that relational thought is much more complex than associative thought because it allows us to fabricate relations in the abstract and combine them into vast networks. With associations, we make connections between things or events because they are similar in a physical sense, or because they occurred together in time and space. But with relational thinking, we can connect things that have no physical relation to one another and don't appear together in time and place. Not only can we, but we constantly do, and the connections we make become extremely complex.

This is why any given thought might trigger a thought about something else, such as why having a thought about how sweet your spouse is to you can remind you of how a past relationship ended so painfully in deep betrayal, and suddenly you will start wondering if your spouse is faithful. You've connected your relationship with your spouse to that prior relationship through the "is opposite to" relational frame. Lots of unwanted thoughts are similarly triggered because of such embedded relations, explaining the automaticity of so much of our thinking.

Aaron and I called this new explanation of the way we learn language and higher-order thinking abilities *relational frame theory* (RFT). Extensive research has confirmed that learning relations is crucial to developing our cognitive powers, and also to developing our sense of self. For example, in research with language-impaired children, who have not developed a normal sense of self, we found that if we taught them how to do relational thinking, they would then develop both stronger language skills and more normal self-awareness.

But it was the clinical implications that most stunned me. Trying to unravel these dense networks of relations and reconstruct them, as CBT has tried to help people do, is like trying to rearrange a vast spiderweb. It's futile.

Trying to get rid of thoughts would just *add* to the cognitive networks that surround them. Relating could be abstract: anything could be related to anything.

You can assess for yourself what I mean. Think of any two objects. Anything. Once you have done that, how is the first one better than the second? You will find an answer very shortly. How did the second cause the first?

Think hard. Again an answer! How can you only think rational thoughts if the very nature of thought allows anything to be mentally related to anything else in any way at any time?

I did the math: the relations of just eight things and their names could yield over four thousand possible relations (things to things; names to names; relations to relations; all combinations). That meant it could take an eternity to work out the implications of all of the possible relations any one of us already has in our head! There must be an almost infinite number of inconsistencies in these cognitive networks. And adding a truly new thought could change all others but in highly unpredictable ways.

These implications were sobering. Traditional cognitive ideas were based on an associationistic theory of thought. If that was wrong, traditional cognitive therapy was conceptually wrong, even if some of its methods were helpful. And since we cannot fully restrain how our minds relate things, I realized we would need to focus more on how to alter the behavioral *impact* of our thoughts.

There were other, more expansive implications, especially for our view of human consciousness. I realized that the two-way street of words and objects already implied a kind of perspective taking: from the speaker's point of view an object is called X, but from a listener's point of view if you hear X, you orient toward the object. But that would mean that perspective taking is inside every word we say, and as we speak or tell ourselves stories it could easily begin to establish a "point of view" inside us. I wrote my first RFT paper in 1984 making this claim and called it "Making Sense of Spirituality" when I realized this could lead to a transcendent sense of self—the perspective of an observer within who is witnessing what is being described from a particular point of view (see Chapter Twenty-One).

That was a guess but it turned out to be right. RFT research has since shown that it's not until a particular type of relation is learned that this sense of self, of being a separate being, emerges. This type is referred to as *deictic* relations, which means "to learn by demonstration," but that is an arcane technical term, so here I will call them *perspective-taking relations*.

All of these require a certain vantage point to be understood, such as knowing that you are *here* rather than *there*. A relation like that can be hellacious for kids to learn because the speaker's "here" is the listener's "there" and vice versa. As a result, when you go there, *there* becomes *here* and *here* becomes *there*! (You can almost see little kids in their frustration thinking, "Could you freakin' make up your minds?!") But with enough demonstrations, children do learn perspective-taking relations. The three most critical are *I versus you*, *here versus there*, and *now versus then*. Children usually learn them in that order: person, place, and time.

This magic happens somewhere around age three or four. The perspective-taking relations of person, place, and time merge into an integrated sense of perspective: a sense of observing from "I/here/now" appears. Metaphorically, you show up behind those eyes of yours, and at the same moment, you know that your mother is behind hers. You have developed a sense of awareness of living in the world as a conscious human being, with a point of view. There is a quality of "fromness" to this kind of awareness. You not only see, and see that you see, you also see that you see from "I/here/now." What's more, this sense of self is based on symbolic relations; it emanates from the combination of perspective-taking relations.

Once the skill of taking a perspective in terms of time, place, and person is established, it never really leaves you. Infantile amnesia falls away. This is why you can readily see again through the eyes of yourself at age four or five, but not age one. "Self" as a form of consciousness or perspective becomes the strand you put the beads of experience on. Everywhere you go, there you are. And you can also imagine yourself being somewhere else, say standing on the Great Wall of China. You can even imagine yourself *being* someone else, or what you will be like when you are very old. You can tell yourself stories about other people too, imagining what they are experiencing, even if you are on the other side of the world. In imagination, you can move perspective-taking across time, place, or person.

Perspective-taking also supports storytelling about ourselves that is more content-based and evaluative, and that part is hard to put on a leash. With the rise of our verbal problem-solving ability, the Dictator Within is born, along with the need for a liberated mind. As we begin to create our story of who we are, for example, we also start to compare ourselves to others, and to social ideals of who we should be. Thus, the unfortunate side effect of the same cognitive skills that allow a sense of ourselves as conscious human beings is that we often soon become self-critical, or excessively seek to be attended to, to be important or notable based on the specialness of our self-stories. We have begun to fashion the conceptualized self, and this imagined self often takes on the illusion of being our "real" self. We begin to *become* the content of our stories, and the Dictator comes fully into power.

The problem is not the presence of a self-story; we all need one. But when we disappear into this ongoing storytelling—when we fuse with the story—all sorts of mental health and life satisfaction challenges follow. This is because the Dictator becomes so preoccupied with monitoring the story and defending it, assessing whether we are living up to it or others are believing it.

There is something bittersweet about our entanglement with our minds. Symbolic thinking does not come from a bad impulse. It stems from our deeply rooted inclination as a species to be cooperative, to belong in groups of others and to get along. The three things humans are especially good at, that distinguish us so dramatically from all other species, are our higher-order cognitive abilities, culture, and cooperation.

Human beings are by nature cooperative. If there is a child-sized bench that two toddlers want to move, it is natural for one to try to pick up one end while the other picks up the other. Even our closest animal relatives, chimpanzees (who are quite cooperative . . . just not as much as we are), rarely show such things. Evolutionary biologists argue that we developed the impulse because we lived in small groups, in which cooperation paid off.

It is just the kind of monkey we are: normally developing human babies care about social attachment and social cooperation. Human infants come into life with a certain amount of "theory of mind" skills, meaning the cognitive talents that allow us to know something about what others want based on observation rather than on being told. Even young babies have some understanding of the intentions of others. For example, if an adult and a baby who have been playing with toys together start to do "cleanup time" and the adult points to a toy that is out of her reach but within the reach of the baby, the baby will put the toy in the cleanup box. If a stranger comes in and points similarly, the baby will give her the toy. That shows how we guess what others want and how important pleasing others is to us—just by nature.

The two-way street of symbolic thinking began with a cooperative listener hearing another group member use a term in speech—perhaps asking for an object—and knowing to provide the named object to the speaker. This two-way social relationship allowed an immediate expansion of cooperation and an increase in the well-being of the group. The psychological costs came much later as symbolic thinking became internalized and focused on problem solving. In one sense it was a spectacular success—our problem-solving skills are unparalleled in the natural kingdom—but it led us to view our own lives as problems to be solved. What we gained in environmental control, we paid for in lack of peace of mind. One way this may happen is that we become so intent on being accepted by others that we create a distorted story of how valuable and lovable we are—but then we distrust the affection we receive. We engage in needless comparisons between ourselves and others, which in turn leads to more entanglement in negative self-talk and psychic pain. On and on it goes.

We can see this distorting storytelling process in action if we think about why we lie. Have you ever wondered why you often lie about things you've done or said? We all do, at least occasionally and in small ways. Just for a moment, consider lying slowly, holding the phenomenon in your hands the way a four-year-old holds, say, an unusual item such as a kitchen whisk. And now ask yourself: why do you lie?

Don't answer immediately. Just consider the question, and while you do, review some of the ways you mislead others:

* **You leave out the whole story.**
* **You exaggerate, maybe just a little.**

* **You tweak details to be consistent with the image you want to present.**

* **You deny hard truths.**

* **You ignore what doesn't fit with your current story.**

Why? Why do you do that?

The news offers near-daily examples of big lies: Thousands of Muslims celebrated in the United States after 9/11; I did not have sex with that woman; the investment company is not a Ponzi scheme. Most people are not prolific liars, so as we read these stories most of us can sit back and think, *I'm nothing like that.* That may be so, but that juicy self-righteousness is a kind of mental narcotic that allows us to miss a larger truth: it is hard for us *all* to tell the *full* truth about ourselves. Research suggests that the average person lies in small ways to one out of four of the people they encounter. Teenagers admit to lying several times a day.

Most of us sense that lies come with a cost. Research proves that to be true. For example, we devalue relationships with others if we lie to them, and our brains are less prepared to act effectively while inside an episode of lying. If our lies are tiny or unimportant, the question lands *especially* hard: why do it?

Of course, we tell some lies for material gain or to protect people's feelings. But many lies are told to protect some part of our self-story—the image we present to others that fits with that story. They help bolster the persona we all invent (an interesting word, *persona*. We get *personality* from it, and in Latin it originally meant "a mask; a false face worn by actors").

I remember with some pain the first time my son Charlie told me a lie in order to protect his self-image. A small toy I did not recognize appeared in his room, and I asked where it came from. My sweet four-year-old stumbled over his words as he said nervously that the teacher gave it to him because he was being good. Something was not right and I looked at him quizzically. After a pause, he burst into tears and said that he just took it from the toy box at school. "Why did you do that?" I asked. "B . . . be . . . because I waaanted it," he blubbered.

I felt like crying with him. It was not so much his stealing that saddened me—it was seeing his loss of innocence. In order to protect this tiny ill-gotten gain, he now had to think of others' thoughts about him (from me, for example) and to try to manipulate these perceptions. He was learning not to be fully himself and to present a false self to others. "I'm the kind of guy who teachers give toys to because I'm a good boy, yeah, that's the ticket."

He was starting to create the conceptualized self.

Thoughts Cannot Be Deleted

Much as we might want to stop this storytelling process and to change the story we've elaborated, the activity of our mental networks is largely automatic, much of it subconscious. The thought patterns embedded in our minds become transfixing. We can get hypnotized by them and miss entirely that they are ensnaring us, like the spiderweb I've compared them to. And though we might desperately like to expunge them from our minds, there is no delete button in the human nervous system. There is nothing in all of psychology called unlearning.

Even things you have forgotten stay with you, lurking below your consciousness. That is why you can relearn them more readily later. Psychologists call this the *rapid reacquisition effect*. With Pavlov's dog, for example, you might repeatedly ring the bell without following the sound with food. Eventually the salivation would no longer follow the bell ringing. That effect is called *extinction*. The conditioning went away, right? Well, no, it didn't. As an expert in this area points out, "extinction does not destroy the original learning, but instead generates new learning that is especially context-dependent." In other words, the dog learned that "in that situation before, the bell led to food; in this one it doesn't." Guess what happens if you then present food again at the sound of the bell? Instantly the salivation is back!

You've likely experienced this. Old fears gradually fall away and you feel more confident. Then an unexpected betrayal, or criticism, or tragedy occurs, and instantly it feels like you are a scared little kid again!

A negative thought pattern can even be triggered back into action by a positive thought or experience. When I was struggling with panic I tried to distract my mind from fear by focusing on relaxation. I would say to myself over and over, "Calm and relaxed; calm and relaxed." I think I got the line from tapes I listened to, and I hoped the phrase would remind me of how I felt when I was practicing relaxation. So when I felt anxiety coming I'd say, "Calm and relaxed," in the hope that the anxiety would stay away.

One day I was working down through a pile of correspondence on my desk and I noticed I was feeling pretty relaxed. *Hey,* I said to myself. *That's cool! You're calm and relaxed! Maybe you are making progress!* "Progress from what?" a small voice in my mind asked. I dared not even say the scary words that would be needed to give that answer. About thirty seconds later my heart did a little jump. *Calm and relaxed,* I thought, now a little worried. My heart seemed to skip a couple of beats. *CALM AND RELAXED,* I almost screamed inside myself . . . and within seconds I had a full-blown panic attack.

This is actually a common feature of panic disorder—it is called *relaxation-induced panic.*

I had spent so much time trying to be calm so as to not be anxious that the two states were now glued at the mental hip. Just as I might say *hot* in a rising voice, and hear back from my mind the word *cold,* now I thought *relaxed* and I got back *anxious.*

The unstoppable relation making we do accounts for why if we try to get rid of a thought, we actually create a new relation in our minds between it and our effort to expunge it. Now we'll have the new automatic thought coursing through our minds: *I've got to get rid of that thought.* Great. That's progress—not.

Much research has revealed just how automatic and complex our thought patterns are and how little awareness we often have of what we are really thinking. A classic study done years ago showed people a long series of pictures and then asked participants to name a household detergent. Those who were shown a picture of the ocean mixed in with the many other pictures were more likely to say "Tide" than those who were not. But if asked, they explained their choice by saying things like "My mother used it," not "You just showed me a picture of an ocean mixed in among the many other pictures, and oceans have tides, so I thought of Tide."

RFT labs have figured out ways to find out what is going on in the basement of our minds through an exquisitely sensitive measure of mental habits called the Implicit Relational Assessment Procedure (IRAP). It allows researchers to detect relations that have been embedded in people's minds that they're not conscious of and to show how they influence people's behavior. Say you've got the relation *anxiety is bad* buried in your mind. To detect that, the IRAP would flash the words *anxiety* and *bad* on a computer screen and instruct you to hit a key for *different*, and then after some other word pairs, it would show you *anxiety* and *bad* again and ask you to hit a key for *same*. The computer will detect that you will take about thirty milliseconds longer to respond to *different* than to *same* if you are used to thinking of anxiety as bad. That additional time is due to your mind fighting against the idea that anxiety is not bad.

Research using IRAP tests has shown that our quick relational responses (or subconscious thoughts, if you will) often predict our behavior more strongly than claims we make about what we think—what RFT researchers call our *extended and elaborated relational responses*. For example, people struggling with drug problems tend to drop out of treatment programs if their minds automatically and strongly relate drugs to "fun" as assessed by the IRAP even if they report that drugs only cause pain and they really want to quit.

It's not logical. It's psycho-logical.

One of the benefits of understanding RFT is that it helps us be compassionate with ourselves as we embark on the journey of making the pivots. It's not our fault that our minds work this way. It also helps to accept that what seem to be the obvious logical solutions simply aren't the best psycho-logical solutions, and why the sometimes odd-seeming methods in ACT actually make psycho-logical sense.

To distill down the essence of RFT so that its basic insights can be easily remembered, I came up with this ditty:

> **Learn it in one,**
> **Derive it in two,**
> **Put it in networks,**
> **That change what you do.**

That's the human mind in four lines. The most important line is the last. While we can't delete the unhelpful relations we've made and their elaborate thought networks, we *can* learn to *change what they do.* We can change how they function in our lives, what we allow them to lead us to do.

And that makes all the difference.

Defusion Techniques Break the Spell

Fortunately, as we studied the mental processes that lead to rigidity, we also discovered ways to defuse from identification with the voice of the Dictator, to pull the mental curtain back and expose our thoughts as just thoughts, which we don't have to pay heed to. I'll introduce a number of these methods in Part Two, but let me just show you the way one of them works now.

The exercise of repeating a word out loud to oneself rapidly was introduced about a century ago by Edward Titchener, one of the early fathers of psychology. He used it to show how the meaning of words can rapidly drop away. My research team was apparently the first to evaluate word repetition practice as a clinical method when we started applying it as a method of defusion a hundred years later.

Let's begin with a word that has strong sensory meaning. I'll choose the word *fish*. See if you can remember what cooked fish looks like . . . now what it smells like . . . now what it feels like in your mouth when you chew it . . . now what it tastes like. Take a few moments to create these experiences.

Very likely there is no fish currently in arm's reach . . . but an echo of your actual reactions to fish are here via the magic of relational learning. Those

Chapter Five

THE PROBLEM WITH PROBLEM SOLVING

Take a problem you experience in your life. Any problem. Let's say, for example, you're running late to pick up your kid from school and you know for a fact there is no way you're going to make it on time. Let your mind go to work on the problem, and soon enough you'll come up with a suitable solution—probably several of them: call your spouse or another family member; call a friend; see if the babysitter can go pick her up; call the school and tell them you're running late.

All good ideas.

When we point that same analytical, problem-solving tool at our internal struggles, the outcomes are very different. Imagine being late picking up your kid and dealing with the thoughts it might kick off: *I'm such a loser,* or *I'm not good enough.* Your mind—almost of its own volition—will immediately start looking for a "solution" to this other "problem" as well. It will readily come up with logical-sounding justifications "proving" that you are or are not a loser, you are or are not good enough, and then it will suggest ways to fix the problem, often by trying to deny that it is a problem and involving a good deal of self-recrimination. Our minds often argue *both* sides of an internal argument, and the closer we get to a resolution, the harder our minds will pull in the other direction. Try to adopt *I'm the worst loser of all!!* and you will find your mind objecting: *I'm not that bad.* Try to adopt *It's not my fault* and you will find your mind listing the reasons it is.

One of the most harmful ways in which our minds become trapped in our thought processes is by learning, or inferring, problem-solving rules that we convince ourselves we must follow. The ability to generate and follow rules is among the greatest human achievements. Using them, we can tell others what needs to be done. We can warn our children of dangers, or plan for the future. We can pass down what we've learned to others, or better remember it ourselves. But this powerful tool has a double edge.

One of the earliest and most important insights in the ACT research program was the realization that this enormous cognitive strength could also turn badly against us. Our remarkable allegiance to verbal rules is a major contributor to psychological inflexibility. We follow them so strictly that we never deviate even when they are making our problems worse—sometimes horrifyingly worse.

My own Dictator Within was quite a rule maker, and that was a striking commonality I saw between my therapy clients and myself. My clients had also generated rules they had to follow in order to solve their problems, and their lives had become largely dominated by them. All of us tell ourselves rules to follow as we go about our lives. Many of these rules we tell ourselves are quite helpful. But the problem-solving mind does not know when to stop, and even if it did, it does not know how.

Take a simple string of thoughts from a person struggling with anxiety, such as, *There is something really wrong with me. I have no idea what to do. I can't stand this level of constant anxiety.* We might see these all as simple observations rather than verbal rules. But if we dig deeper, we will see that in saying to ourselves, *There is something really wrong with me,* we're also implying, *If I could only formulate my actions and their history properly and understand what is wrong, I could use that understanding to control the anxiety better.* When we say, *I have no idea what to do,* we're also saying, *If I'm to control this problem, then I need a plan that will work.* Underlying the statement *I can't stand this level of constant anxiety* is the rule that high levels of anxiety are dangerous, harmful, or invalid, or maybe even the rule that if I complain loudly and forcefully enough, someone in the universe will rescue me from this impossible situation.

The strings of thoughts our minds generate as we seek to "coach" ourselves about how to follow rules can be extraordinarily elaborate. This may be starkly seen in the case of people who have obsessive-compulsive disorder (OCD). I once had a client with OCD who would provide exceptionally complex explanations about the many unnecessary ways in which she sought to protect her children, due to her extreme commitment to the rule that she must keep them safe. As an example, the children were prohibited from entering her bedroom—and great energy was devoted to ensuring that this never happened, with constant warnings and questioning when she came home. Why should they not enter? Well, because they might go into the corner of the bedroom.

When I asked her why that was a problem, she said that a year earlier, workers who were painting the room moved a cardboard box into the corner. "So what?" I asked. Well, that box contained soap bars in boxes that came in from the garage. And? And the part of the garage where the soap supplies were kept is the same part where she had seen a caterpillar a couple of years ago. And? And caterpillars like that were also seen on a tree outside in the yard. AND? And that tree is the same tree that was sprayed with insecticide to get rid of the caterpillars three years ago. So? So the corner of the bedroom might have poison in it that would severely hurt the children.

In the name of being a good mom, her mind had become a torment to her. Perhaps worse, she also had become a torment to her children, who will likely tell stories until their dying day of how painful it was to be a child in her home, trying to placate a loving but terrified and constantly overcontrolling mother.

I can never work with OCD patients without a rich mix of wonderment at our cognitive abilities and a deep sense of sadness. My mother was clinically OCD. It was a rare day that I left the house as a small child without a warning not to eat the leaves of the oleander in our yard, a flowering bush common in Southern California (yes, it is poisonous). Parts of the house were off-limits, such as a seemingly terrifying (to her) attic that had once had a poison trap for silverfish bugs in it. At her worst, she would wash her hands so often they would bleed.

I knew what it was like to have a mom like my patient.

Verbal rules dominate our minds so powerfully that creating and maintaining some mental distance from them can be difficult. I was hopeful that understanding the nature of their hold on our minds would lead to insights about how to break their spell.

In launching this line of research I was inspired by a remarkable set of findings in behavioral psychology that I had read about in the late 1970s. Some of the best-known work was conducted in the lab of a well-known behavioral psychologist, Charlie Catania, with whom I studied for a sabbatical year in 1985.

Charlie and his colleagues had conducted a series of experiments that had explored how tenaciously people would cling to rules they had been told to follow in performing a simple task. These experiments were specifically designed to see whether people would cast a rule aside once they saw a better way to perform a task. Remarkably, humans often came across as looking considerably less intelligent in adjusting their actions than monkeys, birds, rats, dogs, and other animals who were essentially put to the same tests.

In these studies, the human subjects were placed before a device that would sometimes, but only sometimes, dispense an item, such as a coin, when they pushed a button. Before they began, they were given a rule like "Push this button to earn money." Let's say that you are running the experiment, and you decide to set up the machine so that on average, people will get a dime after ten button pushes. Sometimes it will be after eight pushes and sometimes eleven or thirteen. The number is varied because you don't want people to figure out exactly how many pushes will produce the dime. That would make the task too simple for testing the effect you're after.

People will readily begin pressing the button rapidly because the faster they go, the more they earn. Now you change the setting so that the money is dispensed not after a certain number of pushes but instead on the first push after so many seconds on average, say after five seconds but sometimes after three or four and sometimes after six or seven. You are trying to discover whether people will detect the change and adjust their rate of pushing the button. After all, now they can do a lot less work to get the dime—just one push will do it instead of constant pushing.

Monkeys, birds, and rats easily detect a change like this, with the machine dispensing food rather than money. They all soon slow down, pushing only once about every five seconds. Humans, however, often just keep pushing like crazy! Hour after hour.

Behavioral researchers gradually narrowed down why humans were so inflexible. When the experiment was run but people were not told the rule "Push this button to earn money" and were instead simply told to interact with the machine as they chose, they were much more likely to show the good sense of a monkey, bird, or rat when the conditions for getting a dime changed. In these cases, people were taught how to get the reward by pure trial-and-error experience. For example, in these studies at first a dime came out when the person's hand was near the button, then with any press of the button, and then gradually with every tenth press on average. When the setting was changed, people fairly readily began adjusting their efforts and landed on the new solution.

The result was definitive—being told the rule made the difference. The field came to dub this intransigence of the human mind when it's given a rule—or has inferred a rule on its own—the *insensitivity effect*, referring to the resulting insensitivity to changes in the situation the rule is meant to address.

In my lab, we performed many similar studies on the impact of verbal rules during the 1980s. Some of the things we found were pretty remarkable. In one experiment, we explored whether people would adjust their behavior, in the same basic setup as in the study just described, if the change in the machine's setting was more obvious. We stopped giving any rewards until people stopped responding for a while (say, ten seconds); the first response after that led to a reward.

Most people still kept charging ahead, pushing and pushing and pushing and pushing, even though they were getting nothing for their labor. As people became exhausted, most participants finally *did* stop for a while, say half a minute. When they then got back to pushing, on their very first push the clock had reset and they got the reward. Did they finally realize that they should change their pushing strategy and that pausing was key to getting the dime? In the main, no, they did not. They started pushing again like mad! Sometimes they would even say out loud about the machine, "It must have been broken and now it is fixed," and then they would say again later, "I guess it's broken again."

To see the insensitivity of rule-following in action in a common daily-life situation, consider a hypothetical case of a husband and wife. Let's imagine that this hypothetical husband, like many men, has overlearned the instrumental rule "If you have a problem, you need to figure out how to get rid of it." Suppose the wife tells her husband about problems she is having at work with a co-worker and her supervisor that are making it hard to complete a project successfully. Her husband immediately offers some possible solutions, and (oddly to him) she becomes annoyed with him.

Perhaps what his wife really wants is a caring ear. What is crucial to her may be the validation from her loving hubby of how bad she feels. His ideas for "solutions" feel condescending, insensitive, and invalidating, so she gets annoyed. But when the husband sees that his approach is not working, what does he do? Regardless of how many times he's been down this path, it may be very hard to shift strategies because underneath the advice is a problem-solving rule. More likely he will double down with his advice, which is unlikely to work any better. Or he might try offering the advice again, only this time a little more loudly. If his wife begins to show that she is upset or even says aloud, "You are being insensitive," the husband may launch into a long explanation of *why* his advice might be useful and explain that after all, he was only trying to be helpful.

Note to husband: shut the heck up!

That is easy to say (and to see from the outside), but it can be reeeeeally hard to do (and to see from the inside) once you've internalized rules like "If at first you don't succeed, try, try again" or "The best way to convince someone of something is with a good explanation." Really hard.

This example had nothing to do with me (ahem).

The Three C's of Inflexibility

As my team and I delved into why we follow rules so rigidly, as did other researchers, three core cognitive processes were found to contribute to the problem. The first of these we can call the *confirmation effect.* We become so enamored of the rules we tell ourselves to follow that we distort our experience to confirm that the rule is correct. For example, a gambler may formulate rules such as "The dice are due" or "I should increase my bet—I'm on a hot streak." In fact, each roll of the dice is independent of the others. Dice are never "due," and it is foolhardy to alter a bet based on streaks—hot, cold, or in-between. But if you play craps it is difficult to avoid the illusion that you control chance. As a Reno resident, I've seen this many times when friends come to visit: the most highly educated folks who know full well about the "gambler's fallacy" still see their mental rules seemingly proven by the dice.

The confirmation effect not only distorts the feedback we receive, it also impedes our ability to learn in a way that is *not* rule based. Some things need to be learned by trial and error—discovering a solution rather than imposing a preordained one.

A wonderful study done over sixty years ago by behavioral psychologist Ralph Hefferline is a fascinating example of this interference with learning. This was before computers and technology made it easy to look at emotional and physical responses. Ralph had to work really hard to build a device that would detect a tiny movement of muscles—so tiny that the person moving would not even know they had moved.

The participants were covered with wires from head to toe, which was a way of masking the real purpose of the experiment—to see if they would learn to move their thumbs a tiny, tiny amount in order to turn off a loud aversive noise. The participants had no idea which movements might be involved in their task (if any), because they were covered with wires and they were just told they were being physiologically monitored while they learned how to turn off the noise.

If participants were left to their own devices, given no rules to follow, most could eventually turn off the noise by trial-and-error learning. They sometimes naturally moved their thumbs a tiny bit but not a noticeable amount, and because that movement was rewarded with the noise being turned off, they started to repeat it more and more frequently. What's really fascinating here is that the movement was so subtle they weren't aware of what they were doing. When asked what they'd done to turn the noise off they would report irrelevant things, such as that they were thinking about a day at the beach.

Another group of people in the experiment were specifically told that they had to learn to move their thumbs a tiny, tiny amount, so tiny that they would not even be able to discern the movement themselves. They were given the same time for the task, but most of them couldn't get the amount of movement right. The movements were consistently too large. In this case knowing an accurate rule actually *interfered* with learning—they were trying to confirm that they were following the rule they have been given, but by the time they did that, they had moved their thumbs too much to turn off the noise.

Anyone who has ever tried to play golf, or hit a baseball, or play rapid and fluent music, or dance naturally knows that your mind can get in the way. All it has to do is come up with a rule and constantly demand that you confirm that you are following it.

This interference with learning is one reason why dismantling control by the Dictator Within is so hard: it cannot just be instructed. Suppose we're given the rule that we must not be so dominated by rules. It would not be that useful because we can become ensnared in trying to confirm to ourselves that we're following that *new* rule, and voilà: we are off into our heads once again.

The second of the three Cs we'll call the *coherence effect*. Because an accurate assessment of the causes of a situation can be extremely complicated, our minds often end up boiling down our assessments to grossly simplified explanations that fit with what a rule or set of rules tells us. For example, the husband who is having a hard time communicating with his wife may conclude that she is a whiner, just likes fighting, or is committed to making him the bad guy. Underneath he may have internalized the rule that "Women are crazy" or "You can never please them." The mind will busy itself trying to make all the rules fit well together, with much of the work being subconscious. What this often leads to is that we create stories about ourselves and our lives that block out the discomfort and ambiguity of the true complexity of situations.

An extreme case of how the coherence effect impedes our psychological health is that of people who experience paranoid thoughts. I've learned never to challenge those thoughts with clients. Suppose a mentally ill person believes that he is being harassed by the government, which is actively but secretly undermining his potential success because the government fears his enormous knowledge and power. People struggling with psychotic experiences (e.g., hallucinations or delusions) often have poor perspective-taking skills. For example, a person with schizophrenia who has created an ID that shows he is a Supreme Court justice may have little awareness that he is making a bit of a fool of himself as he proudly shows the card to strangers at a bus stop. This same poor perspective-taking also means the client does not fully understand the motivations and actions of others. When he finds, say, that he hasn't been hired for a job, he can blame the failure on the government. The mind will work to maintain a consistent and coherent story. If I challenged these thoughts, you can guess where I would be placed in the story (hint: it would not be as a supportive and caring therapist).

The last of the three Cs we call the *compliance effect*, meaning that we follow rules to earn social approval by rule givers. Behavioral psychologists call this kind of rule-following *pliance* (researcher Rob Zettle and I made up the word back in the early 1980s from the word *compliance*, and the field has largely adopted it). The grip of pliance is built into us from early on, as we are taught by our parents to follow all sorts of rules without question. Don't pull the dog's tail; don't play with the toilet lid; don't stick things in the wall socket. Regardless of how interesting that ball in the street is, do not go into the street. Regardless of how tempting a jump on the mattress might appear, do not climb on the bed. This proliferation of rules is exasperating for children at a certain age, even enraging. Their resistance to pliance leads to the infamous parental response to their pushback, *because I said so*. Parents, of course, often have good reason for upholding these rules so strictly. You cannot afford to have your children learn by trial and error that running into the street is a bad idea.

But as an adult, pliance is another issue. Take a commonly taught rule such as "Do what others want or they won't like you." Although trying to gain approval will occasionally produce the desired result, rigidly following this rule can lead people to neglect their own needs, and that can contribute to many psychological problems, such as depression.

All of us are given to these effects to some degree. We cannot avoid absorbing rules deeply into our minds, and, of course, we wouldn't want to avoid rules altogether. Some of them are massively useful to us. The problem is that they become so entrenched that we cannot see a way beyond them even if they are unhelpful.

The good news is that ACT research has discovered a number of simple and highly effective ways to break the excessive grip of rules. To see how dramatic the effect of breaking the spell of unhelpful rules can be, let me tell you one story of an ACT success.

When Alice began ACT therapy, she hadn't worked for nearly a decade. She had been a store manager with a good work record in Stockholm, Sweden. But in 2004, Alice's son died, likely in a suicide. "My world then fell apart," said Alice. "I never wanted to open my eyes again."

In the years after her son died, Alice became something of a shut-in. A physician diagnosed her with fibromyalgia, the poorly understood syndrome that includes widespread pain, difficulty sleeping, stiffness, and other maladies. Many prescriptions for painkillers, sedatives, and relaxants followed; Alice lived for years in a kind of haze.

Then she began therapy with JoAnne Dahl, who has trained in ACT methods and has become an ACT researcher and author of note. JoAnne began therapy by asking what Alice really wanted in life. "I want to feel peace with myself and energy to do what I want to do," Alice replied. That was a great start.

So what was stopping her? JoAnne asked. Part of it was entanglement with a memory from childhood: coming home one day to find her mother bloody after her father had become violent after drinking too much. "I shut down," Alice told JoAnne. "I had to control my feelings in order to survive," she said. "I learned to follow rules, [to be] quiet and on my guard, to suppress my own needs." Just as our studies have shown us, her high level of experiential avoidance came from being entangled with thoughts that told her she needed to be in control of her feelings, *or else*—that she couldn't leave her home or even cry for fear of touching her bottomless sense of pain and loss. JoAnne spent time drawing out these thoughts, but she did nothing to try to challenge or change them. Instead JoAnne had Alice write them down—and then actually stuffed them into Alice's shirt, asking, "What if you could carry these thoughts with you, like words on scraps of paper?"

JoAnne also explored what Alice might want to do if she left the house. To work again, Alice said. JoAnne began to act out the part of the thoughts stuffed into Alice's blouse: "You know you can't do this! Who would want you?" Startled to hear the Dictator Within acted out like that, Alice started to laugh. And then she said she was going to call the public job service.

"What are you doing?" JoAnne yelled, taking another scrap of paper from Alice's blouse and shaking it at her. "Forget about all this. Let's go and take a tranquilizer!" Alice only smiled. She had defused from the voice of the Dictator and could see its rules as absurd. This pivot then helped her on the way to reconnecting with her authentic self and her aspirations.

She no longer clung to her conception of herself as the girl traumatized by her father's violence against her mother, who had to hide any vulnerability and deny any pain. She could see that she wasn't really that stoic, unfeeling person she had convinced herself she was; she was full of feeling. She could also see that no one out in the real world was actually holding her to that standard of stoicism. No one was asking her to comply with that self-concept—it was Alice who was inflicting that notion of who she had to be on herself. This realization allowed her to find the peace with herself she had told JoAnne she longed for.

In other words, she had made the Defusion and Self pivots. She understood that the voice of the Dictator telling her to follow all those rules was not her authentic voice; it was a voice she had imposed on herself. That meant she was free to hear all of its rules not as commands she had to follow but simply as thoughts that had made their way into her mind, which she could acknowledge and use or not, based on whether they served her interests. These realizations in turn helped her begin accepting the pain of her son's death. She was a feeling person and she was going to go ahead and feel.

Alice stopped taking her pills after that session. She began to work again and eventually acquired a job at a dentist's office. Her story shows how readily we can sometimes make pivots.

Once my team and I understood how defusion from our thoughts and our self-story could free our minds to focus on constructive thoughts, we began testing many defusion techniques. One was a brief exercise in which we asked participants to notice their thoughts while not allowing them to control their actions, such as by having them think "I can't pick up this pen" while picking it up. Just that simple exercise proved to profoundly reduce the impact of thoughts over people's behavior, such as whether they would go ahead and have a drink because of the ingrained notion that it would help relieve stress.

We also helped people see that trying to control their thoughts and restructure them could actually increase the power of those thoughts. For example, we'd tell them to try not to think of a chocolate cake, and they would find that the effort would make them think of cake even more, perhaps even buying one. As we walked them through this exercise, people quickly thought of times when they had similarly tried to control their behavior only to experience loss of control (for example, lots of memories of late-night binges on ice cream, chips, or donuts!).

As we were making our discoveries about how harmful to us our thought processes can be, other researchers in psychology were producing similar results. One was the late Neil Jacobson, the founder of a powerful treatment for depression called *behavioral activation*. He discovered that the more people believed in their own mental reasons for behavior, the more depressed and anxious they were likely to be. We began to ask patients to consider that the whole idea of thoughts as reasons for behavior is flawed, and we developed many more exercises to help them accept that idea, some of which will be introduced in Part Two. They facilitate the awareness that while thoughts have a life of their own, their impact on our behavior comes from our relationship to them, from whether we act on them, and that the choice is up to us.

Though sometimes we can make the Defusion and Self pivots quite quickly, as Alice did, that doesn't mean we don't have hard work in front of us. The pains we've been avoiding don't simply vanish, nor do difficult experiences that await us in the future. In making these pivots, we are embarking on developing the ability to keep defusing from our thoughts and the intricate webs they weave. In that journey, we will almost surely find ourselves enthralled to the voice of the Dictator again. The unhelpful stories we've told ourselves about who we are, such as about how damaged by our experiences we've been, are sure to reassert themselves. We'll certainly fall into the trap of lying to ourselves, and others, again to try to shore up our self-esteem and a concept of ourselves we find we're clinging to once again. The point is to catch the slips and notice when we are fusing again with the voice of the Dictator, keeping these lapses to minutes or hours, not months. If we keep our eyes wide open, even lapses are helpful to learning.

Being able to rebalance when situations, thoughts, and emotions knock us sideways is why practice with ACT methods of defusion and connecting to our authentic self is important. The exercises I'll present in Part Two, and the word repetition exercise introduced here, can be easily incorporated into our life routines to keep developing these flexibility skills. Over time, defusing from our thoughts and connecting with our authentic self becomes second nature, and we can call on these skills whenever we face a new challenge that threatens to reactivate negative patterns. They are hugely helpful as we begin to work on accepting our difficult thoughts and emotions.

Chapter Six

TURNING TOWARD THE DINOSAUR

ACT had its fifteen minutes of fame in 2006 when the late John Cloud (a reporter at *Time* magazine who later became my good friend and to whom I've dedicated this book) wrote a story about my work titled "Happiness Is Not Normal." I've never argued that, but I know why he thought it fit. The principle that we need to turn toward our pain can seem to imply that we must abandon hopes of feeling happy. To the logical mind the message of the need for acceptance sounds like "You are doomed to unhappiness. Get over it."

It's amazing ACT ever caught on, I suppose, given how easy it is to infer that sad message.

It is the exact opposite of the true message of acceptance, which is that life can be a rich journey, even with its sorrows. It is just that a truly joyful journey cannot happen until the "feel good" agenda set by the Dictator Within is cast aside.

From my own experience of fighting my anxiety, I knew just how tricky coming to a place of acceptance can be. But why? For one thing, as said earlier, we're massively encouraged by cultural messaging to try to deny or expunge our difficult thoughts and emotions. Some of us heard it in the form of parental commands, such as when parents tell a crying child, "Oh, be quiet, it's not that bad," or "Stop crying or I will give you something to cry about." And of course, self-help books, magazines, and radio and television shows are also full of this advice. Popular books promise that we can and should learn how to feel good, manage our anxiety, or get rid of our depression—but not so much information about how to learn from our own experiences. Our medications are *anti*-depressants, or *anti*-anxiety, or *anti*-psychotics, as if the only sensible goal is to subtract them. Our disorders are called "mood disorders" or "thought disorders" or "anxiety disorders"—once again feeding a cultural view that is often outright hostile to anything painful. We've got to put aside this unhelpful messaging to create some space to try truly new things.

A more pernicious reason why accepting the need for acceptance can be hard is that our fight-or-flight instincts are so strong. They were vital to survival in response to physical threats out in the world, and they often still are. Reacting to our threatening internal experiences—our painful thoughts and feelings—in the same way seems to have naturally developed as those experiences became more vivid, thanks to the development of our language skills. Our symbolic abilities can make *any* situation a threat. In our minds.

On top of this, our biology developed rewards for avoidant behavior. When you evade a difficult or frightening situation, the brain activates the same areas and releases some of the same chemicals that mark the receipt of a positive reward. "Aaaah," your body says. "That's better." While that would be true if you'd just avoided an attack by a wildebeest, what if you'd avoided the anxiety of giving a high-profile presentation at work? That same chemical hit can come from undermining goals for yourself.

So often, when life is not going well, it's because we are doing things that give us smaller, sooner benefits at the expense of larger, later ones. The instant gratification of avoidance tricks us into trading away our future. In healthy development, our short-term gains fit with our long-term aims. So the trick is to use our capacity for symbolic thought to choose the short-term behaviors that will lead to the much richer later rewards that come from persisting even when the short-term steps are hard.

Easier said than done. Once we begin to let ourselves go ahead and feel the pain we've been avoiding, our Dictator will begin urging us to go back to our avoidant ways, often veritably screaming at us.

I could see that a crucial component of developing ACT would be creating some methods to help people first make the pivot, accepting the need for acceptance, and then build their acceptance muscles. By the time my lab and I started to develop ACT acceptance methods in the early 1980s, a good deal of research in psychology was showing that avoidance of difficult thoughts and feelings is harmful to us, both psychologically and physically. Humanistic psychology had championed this notion for decades, and some other psychological traditions had embraced it too, such as rational-emotive therapy, which put forth unconditional self-acceptance as a goal. What was missing were powerful enough methods for helping people stop avoiding and a theory that linked acceptance to other key features of change.

We began crafting ways to apply defusion and self skills to coping with the fear and pain of acceptance. Learning to defuse from the voice of the Dictator helps us keep a healthy distance from the negative messages that pop uninvited into our minds, like "Who are you kidding, you can't deal with this!" It also helps diminish the power of the unhelpful relations that have been embedded in our thought networks, which are often activated by the pain involved in acceptance. For example, the relation between smoking a cigarette and feeling better will be triggered by the discomfort of craving a smoke. Reconnecting with our authentic self helps us practice self-compassion as we open up to unpleasant aspects of our lives, not berating ourselves for making mistakes or for feeling fear about dealing with the pain. We see beyond the image of a broken, weak, or afflicted self to the powerful true self that can choose to feel pain. We learned to help people consciously apply their new skills as they took the plunge into acceptance, such as by placing whatever unhelpful thoughts flared up on the leaves of the stream that carry them away.

We also found that a huge boost of motivation to accept discomfort comes from beginning to see how we've been harming ourselves by avoidance. As we open up to our pain, we begin to hear the lessons it has to offer us.

The Wisdom Within Acceptance

Suppose you have a shiny stainless steel stovetop in your home that has odd-colored marks on it, and you have become obsessed with the idea that you will never be comfortable with that stove in your kitchen until those ugly marks are removed. You scrub and scrub with every tool known to you, but to no avail. The marks remain—if anything they are even more visible! You then try to cover them over with paint, but it quickly peels off. You go back to scrubbing.

Your neighbor walks in one day, and, seeing you scrubbing and scrubbing, she dashes out of the house saying brightly, "I have what you need!" She soon returns with a glass item that looks to you like a scraper. "This will do the trick," she says, and you thank her.

Reenergized, you grab the tool and scrape and scrape and scrape. For a few moments it seems that the marks are finally coming off. But as you keep scraping, you realize that was just wishful thinking. Grrrrr! Another dead end!

If you would instead hold the end of the tool up to your eye, like a magnifying glass, you would see clearly for the first time that the marks on the stovetop are actually written messages about how to cook! Some tell stories of embarrassing failed attempts; some are even painful to read. Others share the delight of mastering cooking skills and tell stories of scrumptious meals you will share with loved ones. You'd immediately see how helpful they'd be.

The lesson here, of course, is that once we stop trying to scrub away the marks left on us through our life history, we receive the gift of vital learning from all of that experience. As I continued to search for methods to help with this, I realized we could adapt some techniques I'd learned about from my work with David Barlow on exposure.

From my experience with David's techniques to help people with phobias, I thought a similar approach might help people learn to cope with other kinds of difficult experiences. Recall that he was having clients experience just the uncomfortable *sensations* they felt because of fears and phobias without exposing them to the actual situations they were afraid of.

He would start with a moderate level of exposure to the sensations and then gradually intensify them. I thought a gradual consideration of difficult life experiences and memories would also be best. But how could I motivate people to keep up the difficult work? What would sustain the effort if we took away the promise that difficult thoughts and emotions would vanish?

When I turned toward the dinosaur as a kid, there was a reward that kept me going. I woke up. In the same way, learning to accept our difficult experiences and turn toward suffering offers rewards; acceptance isn't an end point, it's a means to starting on the path to a more fulfilling life. I had to help people understand that acceptance isn't just about not doing damage to ourselves; it's also about gaining the wisdom to be learned from our experiences. This vital insight was clarified for me through a profound experience I had one day while teaching a workshop on our early ACT methods.

The Messages Inside Our Pain

Within a couple of years of my night on the carpet, there I was teaching a group of therapists about our first set of methods when I suddenly found myself feeling intensely anxious. By this time, I had actually discovered a somewhat positive quality to the experience of anxiety (it continues to this day—I still occasionally get quite anxious). I certainly didn't *like* anxious feelings and thoughts. The closest I can come to explaining why these moments were (and are) at all positive is that I felt a sense of aliveness and curiosity. I felt challenged but also as though I was learning to experience life in a different way that would help me and also help my work with others. The experience was fascinating.

This day at the workshop, however, an unexpected wave of emotion washed through me right after I felt anxious, almost knocking me sideways. Out of nowhere I felt an intense urge to cry. I stopped talking at all for a few moments, practicing my defusion skill, which I had continued working on, and just watching the surprising intensity of the impulse, until I noticed the expectant looks on my trainees' faces. The feeling passed as quickly as it came, and I returned to my teaching.

I didn't think of it again until the next workshop when the exact same thing happened. This time I had a new spark of awareness. I realized that I felt very, very young. A bit puzzled by that, I asked myself (even while still doing the workshop), *How old do you feel?* and the answer leapt back, *Eight or nine.* Then a memory flitted up, sort of like a moth unexpectedly flying out of a drawer you've just opened. I caught just enough of a glimpse of it to know what it was.

What flew up was a memory of an event I had not thought about for many, many years. It seemed to have remained dormant ever since it first happened. I was able to quickly return my focus to my workshop, but that night I deliberately brought back this fluttering moth of a memory and had a good long look at it.

I was under my bed, eight or nine years old, hearing my parents scream at each other. Dad had come home late, and drunk, again. I'd hugged him as he came through the front door, and his cool pressed suit was filled with the lovely smell of juniper berries, as the gin and tonics sweated out through his skin. Sometimes he would settle down and play with me when he'd been drinking (that smell to this day makes me smile), but a play session would not happen this night. My mother had been stewing in a quiet rage as the hours passed and as she calculated how much of the meager family funds from his job as an aluminum salesman were being wasted at Lubach's, his favorite downtown San Diego restaurant and watering hole. Even while I was hugging him to celebrate his arrival, she began to poke at him in an edgy voice. I could sense where this was going, and I quickly retreated to my bedroom.

The words became harsher, and the shouting began. I crawled under my bed. My mother was ripping my dad up one side and down the other about his inadequacies and failures as a husband and father. He responded by repeatedly yelling at her to shut up—shut up *or else.* His threats only sharpened her tongue.

Suddenly there was a horrific crash and then screams from my mother. I would learn only later that the sound was the coffee table being thrown across the living room, but at the time I just trembled at the thought of what it could have meant: *Will there be blood?* I wondered. *Is he hitting her? Are they killing each other?*

These words came clearly and forcefully into my mind: *I'm going to* do something! In the moments that followed, I almost had to physically pull myself back from the intense urge to get up and march my little-boy self into the next room and do whatever was needed to make it all *stop*.

But I didn't get up. I was terrified by the thought of confronting them. A month or two before I'd seen my older brother, Greg, intervene in such a fight and almost get hit in the face. I pushed back *hard* against the urge to do something, scooted back even farther under my bed, and hugged myself and cried.

As I visited with this old unexamined memory, I felt a poignant sense of self-compassion for that little boy, who was a core part of me, and I realized there was something meaningful inside my anxiety that had been totally covered over and lost.

By suppressing how deeply domestic violence had penetrated me, I'd closed myself off to understanding some of the key roots of my anxiety. No wonder the sounds of those old bulls fighting in the psychology department had sent me into a panic! Wanting to see scenes like that stop *and* being afraid I was not up to the job of stopping them had been glued together in my mind since I was very little. Hiding was a wise choice then, but hiding was not what I needed now. I also realized that my fight to vanquish my anxiety had prevented me from feeling a deep connection with my original purpose in becoming a psychologist. I had wanted to *do something* about people's suffering. This was not a decision of the head—it was one of the heart.

I had not been able to save my parents, lovely, loving, and disturbed people that they were. But I might be able to help alleviate the suffering of others.

Yet I suddenly realized that by declaring to myself that my anxiety was invalid, I had, in effect, slapped my internal eight-year-old in the face and told him to *shut up* or *go away*. I had wanted to deny my sense of vulnerability, but that also meant I had to deny not just my own pain but also my own caring—because they were two sides of the same thing.

What had that little boy really done to be treated so harshly? Care about the parents he loved? Care about his own safety? Be afraid in a fearful situation?

This realization also allowed me to see that my failure to be able to see what was inside my anxiety had allowed an unhealthy, avoidant type of ambition to dig into me early in my career. I had become too preoccupied with professional achievement, pushed on by a motive I was unaware of: to avoid the pain and vulnerability of being that little boy who did not feel up to the situation. As I pushed anxiety away with "achievement," I had to push him away—but he was why I was a psychologist to begin with. He sent me there to "do something." Trying to use empty successes to "achieve my way out of pain" was a kind of self-objectification, as if I (and that vulnerable kid within) were a horse to be whipped.

As I did the night on the carpet years earlier, I made another choice. "Never again," I promised my vulnerable younger self. "I will not turn from you and your message to me about my life purpose. I want you here with me."

It was the distance I obtained from my Dictator through defusion and my new ability to accept my anxiety that opened up the room in my mind and heart to recall that little boy with compassion rather than harsh judgment or denial. By learning how to turn toward my anxiety, I was learning how to treat myself—my whole self—in a more loving way and renew a sense of purpose in my work. That little boy had resurfaced, I realized, only when he felt safe to reappear: when I had become ready to accept him.

That is the one-two punch that allows us to escape from the dictates of our evaluative mind. First, we realize that our avoidance is not paying off, and more of the same will have a perfectly predictable outcome. Second, after we "give up" on avoidance, we realize that there are alternatives that are 180 degrees in the other direction, and those alternatives *do* pay off, short term and long term. I realized that helping people onto the path of acceptance meant finding ways to contact both the futility of their avoidant behaviors and some of the rich learning they would receive from acceptance. We didn't want to expose people to pain only to help them accept it; we wanted a type of exposure that helped them begin living in the way they desired.

Dropping the Rope

My early ACT clients were enormously helpful in learning methods that have become staples of ACT. One client supplied one of the best metaphors that help people accept the need for acceptance.

In one of my last sessions with this client, who had anxiety and had responded very well to early forms of ACT, I asked her to explain what had helped her. She responded, "It was realizing what I needed to learn," she replied. "For the longest time I felt as though I was in a tug-of-war with a gigantic anxiety monster who was trying to pull me into a bottomless pit. I fought and pulled, but no matter how hard I tried I could not win, but neither could I give up and be cast into oblivion. It was very hard for me to realize that I did not need to win this war. Life was not asking that of me. It was asking me to drop the rope. Once I did that, I could use my arms and hands for more interesting things."

Since then, many people learning the ACT methods have been asked to picture themselves dropping that rope, or have acted it out in groups using an actual rope. A number of other powerful metaphors have been developed to help with this pivot, and I'll share more in Part Two, when we get into the acceptance exercises.

What we found as we continued to work with people on making the pivot is that once you do, life almost immediately gives you some positive feedback and helpful realizations. I learned to watch for them and trust them as the single biggest indication of progress. People made spontaneous connections with suppressed yearnings and achieved behavior change we'd never deliberately targeted in our work with them. They reached out to old friends long lost. They let go of resentment and cleaned up old messes with loved ones. They started making bold moves—changing jobs, seeking promotions, taking trips, starting hobbies, opening businesses. They started *living*, and the positive reinforcement that followed helped them stay the course of change.

Modifying Exposure

We began rapidly honing our methods for building acceptance strength. After helping people drop the rope, we would begin walking them through the process of exposure through the methods you will learn more about in Part Two, which include labeling emotions; noting urges; feeling feelings on purpose; cataloging memories triggered; and sensing what your body is doing. Vital to the ACT exposure approach is the understanding that it is not a way to get rid of emotions—it's a way to create more flexibility in how we respond to them.

My team and an expanding group of colleagues began testing these methods rigorously in the lab. One study measured how acceptance methods helped anxiety-prone people cope with the discomfort caused by breathing in a high dose of CO_2 as compared to diaphragmatic breathing, a standard relaxation technique used in exposure therapy. The researchers exposed sixty participants to air that was up to 10 percent carbon dioxide (the normal level in the atmosphere is less than a twentieth of that). Within seconds, such a high dose of CO_2 leads to heavy breathing, sweating, and a quickened pulse—exactly the physical conditions that often coincide with anxiety and panic attacks. It's not pleasant.

The participants who had been taught the ACT methods were instructed in a short session before the gas challenge to "watch" these sensations the way they might watch a cloud in the sky, letting go of any attempt to control the sensations, just as we let go of any attempt to make the clouds move slowly or quickly. The control group was taught to relax and focus on their breathing.

All groups showed the same physiological arousal, but while 42 percent of those who did the breathing exercise felt they might lose control of their emotions, as did 28 percent of those in a control group, not a single person in the group who had been taught the ACT methods had that reaction. Those participants were also far more likely to be willing to go through the experience again.

We soon learned that even people with panic disorder responded in much the same way, and that it could impact other aspects of their treatment. A CO_2 challenge for a person with panic disorder is really a form of exposure: deliberately producing the sensations you have avoided. David Barlow's student Jill Levitt showed that acceptance methods did not reduce the sensations from carbon dioxide (shortness of breath, a racing heart), or even the anxiety. What happened was that these symptoms bothered them less, and they were more willing to go through another round. Acceptance made exposure more possible and more effective.

These early studies gradually led to large clinical studies, with long follow-ups (such as a year or more). The findings were confirmed.

Exposure for a Meaningful Purpose

We added another crucial element to our exposure methods—that they were a means to *pursue a more purposeful life*: to live as you truly desire to live. We helped people see that the experiences they'd been avoiding and the memories of painful experiences they sought to escape were painful and scary to them *because they cared*—they cared about living a life enriched by love; about being a nurturing person; about pursuing interests they found intrinsically engaging and meaningful, whether or not society was impressed by them.

This meant, for one thing, that exposure should take place in the service of some valued action. For example, in assisting someone who has agoraphobia with exposure, we would have them go to the mall not only to have them experience the anxiety that would provoke, but to go with the express purpose of buying a gift for a loved one. Or if someone was avoiding thoughts of death, we might suggest they go to the grave of a loved one, not only to defeat their fear but also to honor their love and respect for the person who passed.

With client after client I saw that the exploration of the difficult experiences they were avoiding opened them up to acknowledging that their attempt to avoid the pains of the past had stopped them from living with the richness of purpose they wished to. Think back to Alice, who was so shut down because of her pain over her son's death. JoAnne Dahl not only showed Alice how unproductive the rules about denying her pain were but also helped her reconnect to her desire to make a positive contribution in the world. Her first question to Alice was what she'd like to be doing with her life if she wasn't stymied by her reliance on pain medication, and Alice responded that she wanted to work again. That ultimately led Alice to get out of the house and find a good job.

From Acceptance to Commitment

Once we saw the power of helping people reconnect with their aspirations about the way they wanted to be living, we added more methods to help them make the three additional pivots—presence, values, and action—realizing that they were necessary complements to the Defusion, Self, and Acceptance pivots. ACT can't just be about achieving acceptance; it must also help people reengage fully with life and commit to a new course of action that they set for themselves. To use the language of humanistic psychology, ACT should include ways to help people become self-actualized. The methods of assisting people that humanists had developed had not been tested by the full range of Western science methods. I was determined that ACT would help fill that gap in our knowledge.

Chapter Seven

COMMITTING TO A NEW COURSE

The ability to do what we choose to do in order to live the lives we envision for ourselves is the ultimate aim of ACT—it's called *act* for a reason. At the end of the day, we are what we *do* and *why* we do it. No matter what problems we struggle with—anxiety, depression, negative rumination, self-doubt, chronic pain—they do not have to keep us from acting in a way that brings our lives meaning and purpose.

Consider great figures in history. What do we remember them for? The cars they owned, or the appearance of their spouses? For the rationalizations they came up with for their behavior? Not likely. We remember them for what they did and the values those actions reflected. Some of them certainly struggled internally. Beethoven was well known for his manic fits. Letters survive from Abraham Lincoln's friends that describe him as the most depressed person they had ever known. It was what they did *with* those challenges that mattered.

As my team continued developing ACT methods, we began focusing on ways to help people identify and commit to whatever behavior changes would allow them to live more fulfilling lives. Of course, the notion that to improve our lives we must take committed action is nothing new. The idea is built into our culture to some extent. But as with so many other aspects of human endeavor, the message has been dumbed down to simple slogans. "Just do it!" "Be bold!" "Show your grit!"

Pivoting toward new action is not as those mantras imply. It is not a matter of "just doing it." *How* you do it matters.

Committing to change in an open and flexible way is hard work. Even clearly seeing the new path we want to follow can be difficult. That's partly because attempts at behavior change tend to lead us naturally into avoidance and self-criticism. We're prone to anxiety about whether we've got what it takes to stick to a new path, and the mind screams that this is a problem that must be solved with lower levels of anxiety. With any misstep we make in our new journey, which is inevitable, we further pummel ourselves. The Dictator begins taunting us: "Oh, come on, you're not up for this!"

The first three flexibility skills provide powerful support in staying the course. Defusion disempowers these unhelpful thoughts. Connecting with our authentic self helps us avoid the sway of pliance and becoming preoccupied by what others think of our progress, helping us defuse from thoughts like "They can see that I'm still struggling with my depression; I'm not kidding anyone, I'm a loser." It also helps fend off telling ourselves appealing lies about our progress, such as "I'm fine now, problem solved!" when we've really got a good deal more work to do. Acceptance allows us to stop directing our attention to unnecessary problem solving about the pain we're feeling, instead turning our attention toward the helpful insights these feelings offer.

As we continued to develop ACT, we realized that the three additional skills—presence, values, action—make vital contributions to psychological flexibility, offering great assistance in committing to a new course in life. They provide essential additional motivation and mental agility.

The Puzzle Room of the Past

My kids and I recently spent a fun hour in a "puzzle room." If you live in a decent-sized city you likely have one nearby. You and your teammates are locked in a room filled with various objects. Your mission is to identify the clues that solve the puzzle and get you out of the room. We ran about like madmen, opening drawers, writing down clues, inspecting objects, and trying to decipher meanings. Books and candles and pictures and other objects were grabbed, maniacally examined, and then cast aside if they did not seem relevant. Arduous lists of possible clues were made that later turned out be dead ends. We did not quite solve the puzzle, but we came close.

It was a fun game, but it wouldn't have been much fun if it had gone on for the rest of our lives. I doubt we would have thought it was fun even for a few moments if we had believed the supposed premise of the game: you will never get out unless you figure it out. Win, lose, or draw, we knew that in an hour we would be free.

What if we did not know that?

Many of us live our entire lives struggling to get out of a puzzle room in our minds. We focus entirely too much on the past and how it can help us in the future rather than on enjoying the experience of the moment in its own right. This is natural for our problem-solving minds.

Suppose you were hungry and decided to go make yourself a sandwich but in a blink found yourself in the middle of a beautiful forest. My guess is that you would not stop long to appreciate the trees or flowers—you'd want to know only "How did I get here?" and "How can I get out?" Said in another way, your mind would be totally dominated by the attempt to understand the past ("How did I get here?") so that you might control the future ("How can I get out?"). Said in yet another way, you would likely treat your situation as a problem to be solved.

If you watch your mind as it tries to solve almost any problem, you can detect this strategy: Look at the situation you are in. Figure out what is wrong. Look to the past. Analyze it. Try to understand how you got here. Look to the future. Analyze it. Apply the understanding you have of the past and the present to the process of getting what you want from the future.

Most forms of therapy encourage this process, suggesting that it's the main way to come to terms with past experiences, particularly painful ones. So it is easy to think of therapy as a kind of slow-motion puzzle room, in which our experiences are relevant only as a means to get out of something. You are locked inside anxiety, depression, or pain, and your job is to find the escape hatch and get out.

Clearly it's important to free ourselves from the traps of the past, but in ACT research we discovered that our efforts will be more effective if we learn to keep bringing our minds back to the present and our ability to choose in every moment how we will act.

Developing Flexible Attention

My experience with mindfulness practices helped me understand that the ability to keep redirecting our focus to the present moment allows us to release ourselves from the traps of the past. The impulse we commonly feel to probe into the past and gain understanding from it is not misguided. We do want to spend some time on those considerations. The trick is not getting ensnared; we want to be present with the past, not lost in it. This is where the Presence pivot comes in. It helps us keep our cognitive talents focused on positive possibilities in the present moment.

People are often actually afraid of coming into the present and simply noticing what is here inside and out. The skill of acceptance helps with this, another example of how the flexibility skills support one another. If we accept that fear, we're immediately empowered to begin seeing the possibilities of the present more clearly. When situations spark difficult emotional memories, we can be increasingly alert to the possible relevance of that pain and bring our attention to it in a useful way. We can see the pains of our past as being in the past, but we can acquire whatever wisdom we have to learn from them.

That was how I was able to make the connection between my anxiety and the domestic violence in my early life. I had failed to appreciate the connection because I had been so intent on combating my anxiety with my elaborate "puzzle room" agenda. It focused my mind on getting out, rather than staying put. Once I began learning to accept my anxiety, I was able to pay close attention to the present experience of it and catch that flash of recollection of my parents fighting, rather than impulsively pushing it away. I made fully conscious note of it and was then able to revisit it more deeply later.

Pulling Our Attention Back to the Now

Researchers have found that our thinking often wanders away from the present. We can go for a long time and never actually notice what is here and now, or at least not notice it in a full and useful way.

It is a bit odd that we have to learn to live in the present. After all, there is nowhere else to be. We can have concerns about the future, but these are *present* concerns *about* the future. We can have memories in the present, but these are *present* memories *about* the past. Nothing we can do or imagine is actually in the past or future.

Much has been written about mindfulness and how it can help us cope in life. Unfortunately, some unhelpful simplification has made its way into the popular conception of what mindfulness is. Mindfulness is not simply living in the here and now: teenagers do that when they are playing video games, and they are hardly shining stars of mindful attention at such times. I could fire a pistol behind my son's ear when he is playing Minecraft and he would not flinch. Disappearing into the now is not what we mean by mindfulness—rather it is attention to the now that is flexible, fluid, and voluntary. It allows us to consider the past, and the future also, but to keep bringing our attention back to the present.

Imagine that you are in a dark room with a flashlight you can adjust to have either a narrow beam or a broad one; it can be bright or dim; you can direct it anywhere you wish, or you can remove the cowling and have it light up everything in sight like a lamp on the table.

Attention is like a flashlight. It allows us to focus our awareness. Mindfulness training teaches us how to broaden or narrow our flashlight beam of attention and direct it to where it will be most helpful to us. Said in another way, when the gentle light of present consciousness is trained on our past, we are better able to see the homely and even truly ugly parts of our history with more honesty and self-compassion. That illumination then helps us examine how we have allowed our struggles with the past to divert us from the pursuit of a life in alignment with our values and the purpose we aspire to.

A common training practice is to focus on your breathing, called *following the breath*. It is not long before you notice your attention wandering, and when you do and you bring it back to your next breath, you have just had a moment in attentional control. By doing that over and over, you build the mental agility to focus in a flexible, voluntary way.

Contemplative practice appears in every spiritual, wisdom, and religious tradition, and for good reason. A vast research base shows that contemplative practice has good effects not only on our brains but on every cell in our body. Changes in brain structure and reactivity produced by meditation lead to a greater ability to experience internal sensations, less emotional reactivity, and greater attentional efficiency, among several other important cognitive processes that improved. Meditation also changes the expression of 7 to 8 percent of the genes you have, primarily through epigenetic changes that up- and down-regulate genes involved in the stress response.

I was always a bit afraid of requiring traditional contemplative practice in ACT, though, because as a child of the 1960s, I know that various mindfulness traditions conflict with one another. I wanted to dig down into the essence of contemplative practice to pull out just the elements that would foster psychological flexibility. I could see the value of traditional meditation, and in addition I thought we could adapt some other classic mindfulness processes with our insights from RFT.

Our RFT studies clarified that fusion and avoidance divide our attention into two streams: one that notices what is present, and one that focuses on the problem-solving agenda ("Is it working yet?"). So, instead of classical mindfulness exercises such as following the breath, for ACT we used exercises that would allow people to detect how thoughts "hooked" them and yanked their focus from the present. Here is an example that you can try right now. I would suggest two minutes for this exercise, and you should set an alarm, say on your smartphone.

Imagine that you are sitting in the grandstands at a parade ground, watching people carrying large, blank, white placards. Place your thoughts on those placards as they occur to you. You can transfer them either as images or in words. Your task is to focus on this procession and to catch yourself when you leave the reviewing stand. If you find that you are mentally somewhere else, or the parade stutters and stops, back up a bit and see if you can remember what went through your mind right before you lost the flow. See if you can catch a thought, feeling, memory, or sensation that served as a trigger, then file that away, or perhaps write it down, for later exploration. Then get right back on the reviewing stand and begin again.

Ready? OK, go.

. . . . . .

Welcome back. What did you notice?

For some of you the parade never really got going. You had thoughts like *This is not working for me* or *I'm no good at imagery.* Did you try to put those thoughts on a placard? You might find if you try this exercise again that doing so nicely dispenses with them.

Or you may have gotten the parade going but found that it stopped when thoughts came up that hooked you. That's a mark of fusion. The content of a thought (*This is not working for me*) dominated over your attention to the task. Ironically, an especially common form of sticky thoughts when doing this exercise are ones about the exercise (e.g., *Am I doing this right* or *Is it silly to be doing this?*). That's the force of pliance gripping your mind.

This exercise and others like it have been studied in many clinical trials that have shown it has benefits. In addition to helping people defuse from intrusive negative thoughts, it increases pain tolerance and reduces the impact of urges. Research has also shown that it is not enough to explain how valuable this exercise is and to give people a single exposure to it—people have to practice using it to get the most benefit.

To get some more feel for why building attentional flexibility is so important, try one more quick exercise. Looking around the room—or wherever you are—see if you can see something you do not see *now.*

It is a strange question but just try.

I bet you can't do it. Everything you see, you see now. Correct?

Next let's look around again, but this time evaluate what you are seeing. Compare one thing to another. Figure out which things you want or don't want; which ones are good, bad, or indifferent. If you see something you do not like, consider how it could be changed and how you might go about changing it. Then as you do all *that*, see if you can stay 100 percent in the now.

I bet you can't do that either. If you're at home, you probably started thinking about memories related to the things you were evaluating, perhaps a book you read if you looked at bookshelves, or maybe a time someone visited and sat in a chair in the room. You might even have begun replaying that visit in your mind.

Why can't you look at your thoughts and stay in the present? After all, you can see a picture on the wall now. Right? You can feel your rear end in the chair now. Right? Why can't you, in the same exact way, notice that you are thinking now?

You *can* do exactly that! Noticing thinking is in principle no different from noticing the feeling in your hindquarters. The tricky part is that the moment we focus on *what* a thought is *about*, "the now" slips away at least a little. Interestingly, the original meaning of the word *about* is "near it while outside it." Not in it or on it. It's ab-out, and when you are *out* of the present moment you are not *in* the present moment. So "about" is always "out."

Said another way, once you are in mental evaluation and story mode you are always a little bit off "now." Add in a problem-solving agenda, and you are close to disappearing into a cognitive problem-solving network, with very little "now" left. This is why we can live as human beings for months and years at a time looking almost constantly to the past to figure out what to do about the future. Lost in the puzzle room.

The Past and Future Are Present Fictions

In working on developing attentional flexibility, it's helpful to keep in mind that the future is a matter of pure imagination, while our recollection of the past is largely distorted and wildly incomplete. What we call "memories" are constantly being reconstructed—in the present. When old friends or siblings reminisce about old times, it's not long before they realize that their memories diverge somewhat. One person will remember details this way and another will remember them that way; trips that are separate in the memory of one will be blended together in the memory of another. Inside our own minds, we are usually convinced we are right . . . but of course that cannot be true for everyone. Someone is obviously distorting and revising history.

It turns out that "someone" is all of us. It happens in part because we have an investment in the consistency of the story our memories tell. (Recall the coherence effect from Chapter Five, one of the three Cs of cognitive inflexibility.) So when we look to the past, we are not really looking into the past anyway! We are reconstructing it.

We can't entirely turn off the process of mental fabrication, but we can learn not to become immersed in it, or to buy into our fabrications. We can become more aware of our minds slipping into this mode and choose to look at our recollections of the past and conjectures about the future with a present-focused consciousness. Thoughts are only thoughts. What we do with them is up to us.

Adding in Values Work

So many of us are afraid to risk admitting, to ourselves and others, that we care deeply about our true aspirations. We short-shrift our lives. We don't reach for the stars and instead play small. We often shut ourselves off from expressing the depth of our love, denying ourselves the richness of relationships we might have. Isn't this in large part because it hurts to risk failure or rejection?

As we continued to develop ACT, we wanted to find ways to help people turn toward their deepest caring. Only by doing so would they be able to commit to the new life path they would find truly meaningful. Acceptance makes a start with this process. Recall that acceptance means to receive, as a gift, and perhaps the most valuable gift we get from accepting our emotional pain is that of rediscovering what we deeply care about.

We wanted to find additional ways to help people examine what really matters to them in life, to reconnect with their true values. Many of us get so caught up in pliance, trying so hard to conform to social mandates and to impress others, that we almost entirely lose sight of what's really most important to us. We become overly focused on achievements—or our failure to attain them—and lose sight of the fact that the way to fulfillment is living day to day in a way that is meaningful in itself, not primarily as a means to some other end, such as social acceptance or wealth.

In this regard, research has shown that focusing on our genuine values is helpful. It can reduce anxiety about challenging tasks, reduce physiological stress responses, buffer the impact from negative judgments of others, reduce our defensiveness, and help us be more receptive to information that may be hard to accept, such as about how we have hurt someone we love. And we know a bit about why all of this happens. Considering our values helps us focus on our impact on others, and that in turn helps us transcend our fears about the pain we've been avoiding. Again we see how the flexibility skills reinforce one another. Connecting with our values helps with acceptance.

Values Are Not Goals

ACT defines values as chosen qualities of being and doing. They can be expressed with verbs and adverbs: teaching compassionately, giving gratefully. Values are too often discussed as things that we *have*, but values are not objects. And they are not goals. They are the qualities by which we do things.

Goals are finite; they are achievements, and once achieved, you are done with them. Values are enduring, ongoing guides to living. You cannot achieve a value; you can only manifest it by acting in accordance with it.

Living in accordance with our values is often ironically undermined by our pursuit of goals. Our problem-solving minds direct our attention, and our behavior, too narrowly toward achieving goals. This is harmful in part because the goals we're pursuing are often ones we want to achieve because of the sway of pliance. We think they are a route to social acceptance. Pursuing goals may also be a way of avoiding acceptance of who we are and our authentic aspirations. For example, we may have decided that if we set a goal of getting a law degree, we will have given ourselves cover for not risking the pain of failure in pursuing an artistic calling.

Goals also by their very nature imply that we're not where we should be in life yet. They are most often thought about in conditional terms (e.g., *if-then; when-then*). When I get a degree I'll ____. If I get married I'll ____. When I have children I'll ____. When I make my first million I'll ____. Thinking this way naturally leads us to assess our current state of affairs as inadequate. Meanwhile, if we fail to achieve goals, we too often interpret our failure as proof of our own inadequacy.

Goals can be part of a values journey, and often are. For example, if you value helping people and are getting that law degree so you can help people with legal problems, that's a goal that serves your values. We must not lose sight, though, even with such goals, of the fact that our values give meaning to the goals. I had lost sight in exactly that way by focusing too much on building up my professional reputation rather than my initial desire to help people cope in life.

The Values pivot is about turning away from the pursuit of goals that are socially compliant or avoidant and toward living according to your chosen values. An important aim in ACT became to help people act every day as much as they could in accordance with their values, for the rest of their lives.

To help see how to reconnect with one's values and set this course, we began doing values work. That is, we began to direct people's attention to the qualities of being and doing that they wanted to manifest in their lives by choice. What mattered deeply to them, even if no one was looking or applauding?

Values work helps us take an undefended leap into the wholeness of caring. It is a way to tap into what is deeply inside you during moments such as the following:

* **Hugging a friend.**
* **Smiling at your baby.**

* **Bending your head when you see a great spiritual leader.**
* **Saluting a soldier.**
* **Putting your hand over your heart as a patriotic song plays.**
* **Showing kindness to a person on the street.**

We experience such moments when we act in an undefended way. That's what values are about.

Values Work Requires Flexibility

Exploring our values can lead us right back into avoidance; it can be painful and provoke self-blame and shame. That is why we need our other flexibility skills as we do values work. Knowing how to defuse from the voice of the Dictator allows us to distance from self-judgments about how far from our values we may have strayed. The root word of *value* is also in the judgmental word *evaluate*, and as so much of the public discourse about values demonstrates, values can be held as cudgels, used to beat ourselves and others. Consideration of values can also trigger an inner voice of "have to" instead of nonjudgmental self-examination. Being able to connect with your authentic self helps you stop focusing on "values" based on wanting to please others or to conform to social pressures. For example, someone might claim a value of constantly challenging himself to learn new things, because there's a cultural message that we should, when he really values consistently applying skills he's already mastered to help others. Acceptance skills help us cope with the emotional difficulty of the work, while presence helps us assess how we're actually aligning, or not, with our values in our daily living.

There are many methods for helping reconnect with our values, which we'll explore more fully in Chapter Fourteen. For now, here is one we've often used in ACT that will give you a good taste of how values work motivates committing to life changes, even when they'll be hard. Think of someone you do not know but whose life story you deeply respect or admire. Ponder the person you picked. What about them moved you? Was it their riches, their house, or car? Was it their sex appeal, their clothes, or fine shoes? Was it that they were never sad, or never lonely, or never in doubt? Was it the awards they got, the applause they received, or how long a list of publications they had? These questions help us remind ourselves that these qualities of being and achievements are not the things that really move us.

What does move us? Ask yourself about the qualities of this person: what he or she stood for or represented in how he or she lived.

My guess: these are qualities you want in your life. You would like to see those qualities in your behavior. You would like to manifest them in the world. Your mind may say you do not manifest these qualities, or even that you *cannot* manifest them, but your heart yearns to live according to them nevertheless. That is why you admire these people for their way of being.

We found that the values exercises we developed had a remarkable effect in helping motivate people to do what they really wanted to do. Let me give an example from a study I was part of a few years ago. The exercise in this study is one that you can do yourself right now (it takes only minutes), and as you are about to learn, it can change lives.

We asked 579 college students to be part of a study to improve their academic performance through a short (fifteen-minute) website experience. A total of 132 students volunteered (but we also tracked the grades of the other 447 who did not). The volunteers were randomly assigned to one of three groups: a control group with whom we did no work at all; a group that we taught how to set good, concrete goals; and a group that we had do a values writing exercise in addition to learning how best to set goals.

The exercise could not have been simpler. We asked them to think of values as if they were a chosen direction. If you are headed "west" you can use a road map or a compass to orient you when you get off course. But "west" is not a concrete goal—it's a direction, and no matter how far you go in that direction you can still keep going. Goals are not like that. They are places you land, not directions you take. Chosen qualities of being and doing are like directions: you can always head that way but you never "get there."

After students showed that they understood this distinction (yes, we gave them a test: hey, they were students!), we linked values to action. The website program asked them to think of going to school as if they were tending a garden. Suppose you appreciate the beauty of a garden and you love to see things grow. You soon realize there is no perfect place to plant. By choosing a spot, you can commit to it and work the land even if it isn't perfect, and even if you are not sure of the outcome. Tending the garden is difficult work—it takes constant care and attention. It does not always feel good in the moment, but the doing can be satisfying, because you are, in each moment, working on something that is important to you. We then asked students to consider what their studying for the next week could be like if they approached each moment of studying as such a chosen activity full of life.

Finally, we asked them to stay mindful of the difference between values and goals as they wrote for ten minutes about what was really important to them about education in terms of the qualities of action involved in learning. (You can pick another area of life, such as relationships, work, or spiritual development; whichever you like.) For example, one of those might be freely choosing what to learn, or generously sharing insights with fellow students. We asked them to write about what those qualities were and why they were important, and to reflect on what happens when their actions manifest those qualities, and when they don't. What would life be like if education were a values-based journey, up to you? What would it look like? What would it feel like?

Over the next semester the students in the control group performed about the same as before, just like the students who were not even in the study. The group that got only goal-setting training also performed about the same—goals alone did not improve performance significantly. But the group with the short ACT-based values training plus goal-setting saw their GPAs jump about two-tenths of a grade point over the next semester. The semester after that, we gave the control group the same training and the same thing happened: nearly a two-tenths jump in grade point average.

Not bad for fifteen minutes of writing. It changed these students' behavior in a measurable and positive way over the next fifteen *weeks*.

Once we know the way in which we want to be living, the next step is to make habits of the values-based actions we choose. That begins when we make the Action pivot, away from either avoidant or socially compliant behavior toward persistent action that manifests our values.

Commitment Grows Through Action

The last pivot creates habits of valued living. Making changes in any behavior we've adopted is difficult. Even the smallest actions, such as a nervous habit of biting our nails or tapping our foot, can be hard to change. When we've adopted behavior because we think it helps us avoid emotional pain, whether we're aware of that thinking or not, change is challenging.

We found that the key to making this last pivot, and staying on course with behavior change, is to start small and then to piece together larger habits. Habit development is much more effective when people begin with what might seem tiny, even inconsequential, commitments. You could think of this as prototyping the practice of commitment, which can be done even with behaviors not related to the behavior you're aiming to change. For example, if ultimately you want to change your eating habits, but making changes that a nutritionist has recommended is proving too hard, you might start building up your commitment skill by making a different kind of change that's less challenging.

You could begin by simply practicing keeping your word. Suppose you agree to meet a friend at noon for lunch. That does not mean leaving at noon, or calling your friend five minutes before noon when you are ten minutes away. Being on time means being there when you said you would be there. This is a great commitment to practice with because most people are forgiving if you don't quite come through. If you're a little late, you can give a hundred excuses for being late and a friend will probably forgive you every time. But beware: then you are building a pattern of being unreliable. So you might choose to be vigilant about trying to be punctual, even though the consequences won't be severe.

The basic message of ACT about behavior change is that we can't expect to build competence in a new course of living overnight. If you do not adopt this attitude, the problem-solving mind will become fixated by imagining how you will be when you are different and better, and then judge you for being where and what you are now, pulling out the roots of healthy persistence precisely when they are needed most. If you are trying to quit smoking, and you believe you must stop 100 percent, when you slip, your Dictator will scream at you that you have failed. Many people who try to quit smoking fall into this trap, deciding they just can't do it, instead of realizing that the real problem is that they set their initial mark too high.

One caution: when you do set a small goal, the Dictator will kick in with a thousand reasons why it doesn't really matter. This once again speaks to how the flexibility skills reinforce one another. If you've been practicing defusion, you won't attend to that gibberish.

Commitment is not about never lapsing; it is about taking responsibility even when we do lapse for the larger patterns of living we are creating. I recall vividly a session in our first large randomized trial of ACT for polydrug-abusing opiate addicts. A client of Kelly Wilson's came in with a tale of woe about how he had relapsed and used drugs, which proved he would never succeed. Kelly listened patiently and when the client was done, asked simply, "Which of your values have changed?" After a stunned silence he affirmed, "None of them." "Then it seems to me," said Kelly, "you have a choice about which pattern of behavior you want to strengthen. Will it be commit—slip—commit or will it be commit—slip—quit? I see only those two alternatives." The client sat for a time in silence before recommitting to staying clean and sober.

Commitment involves the acknowledgment that change starts here or not at all. That concrete, humble steps are best. Small is good. Over and over is good. Being responsible for building larger patterns is good. It will lead to remarkable progress. You can indeed pursue your dreams.

Every Step of the Dance

When we add methods for all six pivots with participants in ACT studies, we see improved outcomes. The skills combine to build psychological flexibility into our daily living, very much the way individual dance steps combine to allow a dancer to move gracefully around the floor.

If we keep practicing the exercises—or a core set we find especially helpful—we can draw on them at any moment as challenging situations arise. I often quickly do the word repetition exercise from Chapter Four when I sense negative self-judgments starting to hook me. If you are living with diabetes and you are about to decide to eat a big sugary dessert, you could quickly go through a values exercise to help you reconnect with how important staying healthy is to you.

A recent student of mine, Jennifer Villatte, and my team produced strong proof that the power of ACT is greatly enhanced when all six pivots are made. We conducted a study that tested incomplete versions of ACT therapy with a number of clients dealing with anxiety and depression. In one version we omitted acceptance and defusion work; in the other we omitted values and action work. In both we included work on the self and presence. In essence, we compared two forms of hobbled ACT—one without the A elements and one without the C elements (no, we will not name them CT and AT!).

Both forms led to large improvements in quality of life, but as you might expect, those who had values and commitment training changed their behavior more and saw greater improvements in quality of life. In symptom severity the pattern was reversed. Those with acceptance and defusion training stopped struggling so much when they hit difficult patches and as a result their distress improved more. The lesson? Flexibility processes change only when targeted, and you need all of them.

We have done over seventy studies testing individual components or sets of the ACT components, and the case is clear: all of the flexibility skills are important, and they become even more useful when combined into the whole package that allows us to create a liberated mind, freed from the Dictator Within.

Learning how to make all six pivots may seem daunting, but as I'll show you in the next chapter, you are equipped with the wisdom within yourself that will support you and guide you on the way.

Chapter Eight

WE ALL HAVE THE ABILITY TO PIVOT

All six pivots are within close reach. You knew they mattered, even before you picked up this book. You have this knowledge built into you, both by experience and by genetics.

I can prove this to you in less than a minute.

Think of a profoundly challenging psychological issue you face. I mean an issue that has something to do with how you feel, how you think, what you sense, what you remember, or what you feel pulled to do or not do. This should be a painful challenge that has to do with your inner life. It could be the sadness of a loss; anger from a betrayal; anxiety from a challenging situation; or any of a thousand other such agonies.

Once you have one clearly in mind, peek around to see that no one is looking and then put your body into a posture that shows you at your absolute worst when dealing with this issue. Be a living sculpture, so that if others saw you they might be able to guess what was going on inside. I want your body to reflect you at your most ineffective, or helpless, or overwhelmed. Actually, assume that position, feel what it feels like, and then take a mental snapshot of what your body looks like. Got it? OK, go.

Now do the same with you at your very, very best in dealing with the exact same issue. Imagine you at your most effective, in tune, or empowered with that issue. Express that with your body. Actually do it. Don't hold back (come on, no one is looking, after all), feel what it feels like, and then take another mental snapshot of your body. Go.

If you are like most of us, your first snapshot showed someone closed up. Perhaps your arms were tucked in. You may have looked down, and your eyes may have been slightly closed. Your legs might have been pulled in, or you may have curled up in a kind of fetal position, as if trying to hide, or slumped over as if totally defeated. Your hands may have been clenched in fists, and your jaw and stomach may have tightened. You might even have been in a fighting posture, poised to attack, or alternatively ready to run scared, or flailing about as if actually fighting.

In your second snapshot, you were probably in an open posture. Your head likely came up, your eyes opened wider, and your arms and hands relaxed. You might have stood up and even walked about confidently in large steps, ready to take on the challenge and feeling energetic and centered.

This simple exercise reveals that you already know a good deal about what science shows is and is not good for you as you contend with your problems. Your body assumed first an avoidant posture and then one of flexible acceptance. You know that it does not work to hide, fight, or flee and that it works far better to open up, to have your mental arms and hands free to embrace your problems and learn from them.

I've done this exercise with thousands of people in my training workshops, and my research team has analyzed hundreds of photos we've taken of people around the world doing it. So far the results are the same whether you live in the United States, or Canada, or Iran. People assume dramatically more open postures at their best and more closed postures at their worst.

That's because we have the wisdom of the flexibility pivots within us. But it gets overridden by the rules that seize control of our minds and entrap us in fixation with problem solving.

I can provide more evidence if you will give me just another minute.

This is a bit like that question I asked in the last chapter about a hero you did not know, but this time I want you to think of the most empowering relationship in your life. This should be a relationship with someone who lifted you up, who somehow carried you forward. It could be with a spouse or a sibling; a lover or a friend; a teacher or a coach; a priest, rabbi, or minister; a parent or guardian—it could be anyone. This relationship could even be a spiritual one, as with God or another power you feel close to. And if there truly is no one who has lifted you up (sadly, some people are in this situation), you can answer on the basis of the kind of person with whom you yearn to have such an empowering relationship.

I am going to ask you just six questions about this (which I'll phrase as though the relationship is in the past, but it can also be one that you're still in):

* **Did you feel accepted for who you are by this person?**
* **Did you feel constantly judged and criticized, or was judgment somehow softened or far away?**
* **Was the person generally present with you when you were together or were they distracted, half there, maybe even stealing glimpses at their watch as if hoping to get away?**
* **Did you normally have a sense of being seen by that person, as if they knew you deep down?**
* **Did what you care about matter to that person?**
* **Could you be together in different ways that best fit the situation and what you both wanted, or was it always only one way, determined by the other person?**

Each of these six questions involves one of the six components of psychological flexibility. If your answers are what I suspect they are, then I can say this: you have a model of psychological flexibility available to you in this relationship. You can feel the benefit of living in an open, kind, mentally present, and purposeful way. If you could be the same way to yourself as this person has been to you, and would be willing to be this sort of caring, supportive person to others, you and those you love would reap wonderful benefits.

ACT can be so powerful in part because we are developing qualities of living we already care about and know deep down that we need. By building the flexibility skills, you will be able to consciously bring those qualities into your daily life. To do so optimally, you must work on cultivating all of the skills; remember, they're really six aspects of one whole.

Why Are the Flexibility Skills a Set?

As I realized that all six pivots work together, reinforcing one another, I pondered why they form a set—why these six skills in particular work so well together. The answer came from another area of science—the study of evolution.

Most of us think of evolution only in terms of genetics, but that is a mistake. Culture, thought, behavior, and the expression of genes (the genes you have can be turned on or off) also evolve. In addition, we humans can influence our evolution by the environments we construct and the choices we make; our evolution is not just a matter of chance. We have been given the great gift of being able to adapt our thinking and behavior intentionally, and to change our circumstances deliberately, to better suit healthy, purposeful living. The six flexibility skills form such a powerful set because each allows us to meet one of the six essential criteria for evolution to occur. They provide us with the tools to intentionally evolve our lives.

I can state it more simply. ACT is a form of applied evolution science. I'm not the only one making this point; leading evolutionary scientist David Sloan Wilson agrees, and he and I have been collaborating in exploring new ways to use ACT to facilitate intentional life change (we will revisit that work in a later chapter).

Here, in a nutshell, are the conditions of evolution that the skills help us meet:

1. ***Variation.*** As the saying goes, you'll get what you've got if you do what you've done. Evolution requires alternatives to choose from. That is true with genes, it's true with cultural practices, and it's true with our emotions, thoughts, and actions. We can use this insight to deliberately try new approaches in life. Rigidity is the enemy to change.

2. ***Selection.*** We must have a way to select the variants that are more successful in dealing with life's challenges. While the rest of the animal kingdom can't consciously choose which changes are the best, our capacity for higher-order thinking allows us to do just that. We have the ability to recognize and intentionally pick what works, according to criteria we specify.

3. ***Retention.*** Evolution also requires that we *keep* doing what works. In genetic evolution, that information is stored in our genes and in the mechanisms in our bodies that regulate their activity. In culture, it is stored in our traditions, norms, media, and rituals. In our minds and behavior, we store helpful ways of thinking and acting in habits of responding to the world that get ingrained in our neural networks.

4. ***Fit.*** The selection of what works has to be tailored to the situation. What works best in one circumstance may not be right in another. In other words, we must be sensitive to *context*. When we are, we gain the ability to recognize which approaches to problems work best in which situations and areas of life.

5. ***Balance.*** My mother used to say, "Keep it in balance, dear. Keep it in balance." She was right. Every being is a living system, with many intricately interconnected features or dimensions. You have aspects to you that are biological, cognitive, emotional, attentional, motivational, behavioral, and spiritual. Your overall health depends on you nurturing all of these dimensions and

keeping them in balance. It will do you little good to be more emotionally healthy if you show no care for your physical health, for example.

6. ***Levels of scale.*** All organisms live in ecosystems. In other words, all life forms depend on other organisms. A tree standing out in a field may appear to be living on its own, but it is actually supported by and is supporting a vast community of other creatures, from fungi in the ground to a teeming society of insects in its leaves. In the same way, we are all part of a social community constituting many levels of scale, from the trillions of microorganisms within us that keep our bodies functioning, to the individuals we interact with in our daily lives, continuing up to the communities and whole societies we're part of. Evolution selects for success at all levels, and success at one is insufficient for a thriving life. It will do you a lot less good to be highly evolved at the larger social scale—say, having developed a massive social network—if your close relationships keep falling apart. At the other end of the spectrum, if you killed off all the bacteria in your gut, you would soon die, unable to digest any food.

So that's it; the CliffsNotes version of evolutionary science. All living things adapt based on variation and selective retention of behavior that fits the circumstances, is in balance across key dimensions, and operates at many levels of scale. Again, what's so remarkable for us humans, as opposed to all other living beings, is that we can use our cognitive abilities to intentionally attend to all of these requirements and purposefully evolve ourselves.

The process of evolution can be guided (not just purely random) even in the lowliest of beings. For example, if you have bacteria growing in a petri dish (a good example, because their "generations" can be only minutes long) and you remove an essential food source from the growth medium, the bacteria will show a massive increase in genetic variation. It is as if the bacteria are deliberately trying to find another way forward in this now hostile environment.

Of course, bacteria can't really "deliberate" because they don't have symbolic thought. But people can deliberate! We can consciously adopt the behaviors that lead to healthy evolution. We can go beyond evolution guided by the past to evolution guided by our construction of the kind of future we want.

This is where flexibility skills come in. They support those choices by helping us: let go of the avoidance and fusion that narrow our alternatives (variation); specify through values work what it means for us to be successful (selection); practice and build helpful behaviors into habits of committed action (retention); consciously pick different approaches for different situations by being more mindfully aware of the present moment (fit); stay aware of all the key dimensions of our psychological being (balance); and actively cultivate our social support network and the needs of our bodies (levels of scale).

Combining the Skills

To show you how the skills can be combined and how readily you can begin making progress, let me tell you about results seen in a study evaluating how ACT can help people cope with chronic pain, one of the most difficult conditions to treat.

The study was designed to explore how training in ACT methods could help prevent sick leave and disability in Sweden. It was conducted in 2004, and at the time an astounding 14 percent of the working-age Swedish population was on either long-term sick leave or early retirement due to disability. Public health workers (nurses, care providers for the elderly or people with disabilities, daycare workers, etc.) were the worst off. The average public health worker in Sweden missed 2¼ *months* of work every year, and up to 50 percent of them had already been on disability at one point or another.

The two primary reasons for Swedish "sick listing" were musculoskeletal chronic pain and stress or burnout. The study targeted individual public-sector health workers who were identified as being at higher risk for long-term disability. It was conducted by JoAnne Dahl (the therapist who treated Alice) in collaboration with Annika Wilson, who was a student of hers, and Kelly Wilson, a former student of mine.

All Swedish citizens have free access to medical care including physician, specialist, and physical therapy visits. In the early stages, treatment included explaining how to avoid stress, incorporate relaxation periods throughout the day, and improve exercise, sleep, and diet. Half of the participants were also randomly assigned to receive four individual one-hour sessions of ACT, one each week. The results were stunning.

Over the next six months the high-risk workers who were getting only medical treatment as usual missed fifty-six days of work due to sick leave, or about half of their assigned workdays. Statistics tell us that about half of these workers will leave the workplace permanently, go on full-time disability, and never work again. Those randomly assigned to receive the four hours of ACT training missed on average only a *half a day of work over the entire six months*—a 99 percent reduction in sick leave use. The participants given the usual medical treatment had 15.1 medical visits during that time; the ACT participants had 1.9 visits—an 87 percent reduction. Pain and stress went down in both groups equally, but what is important is that the ACT participants had reductions in pain and stress *while going to work*, whereas the medical-treatment-as-usual participants had so many work absences that they were now headed toward a lifetime of disability, just as the government feared when it identified them as "high risk."

What was in these four sessions that could have had such a dramatic impact? The ACT therapists asked participants to consider what they really wanted in each of ten life areas (work, recreation, community, spirituality, family, physical self-care, friends, education, parenting, and intimate relationships) and barriers that were keeping them from living in accord with those values. Those might be things like a negative body image keeping them from going to the gym or fear of failure stopping them from asking their boss for a new responsibility they'd like to take on at work.

The therapists handed out copies of this figure to fill in:

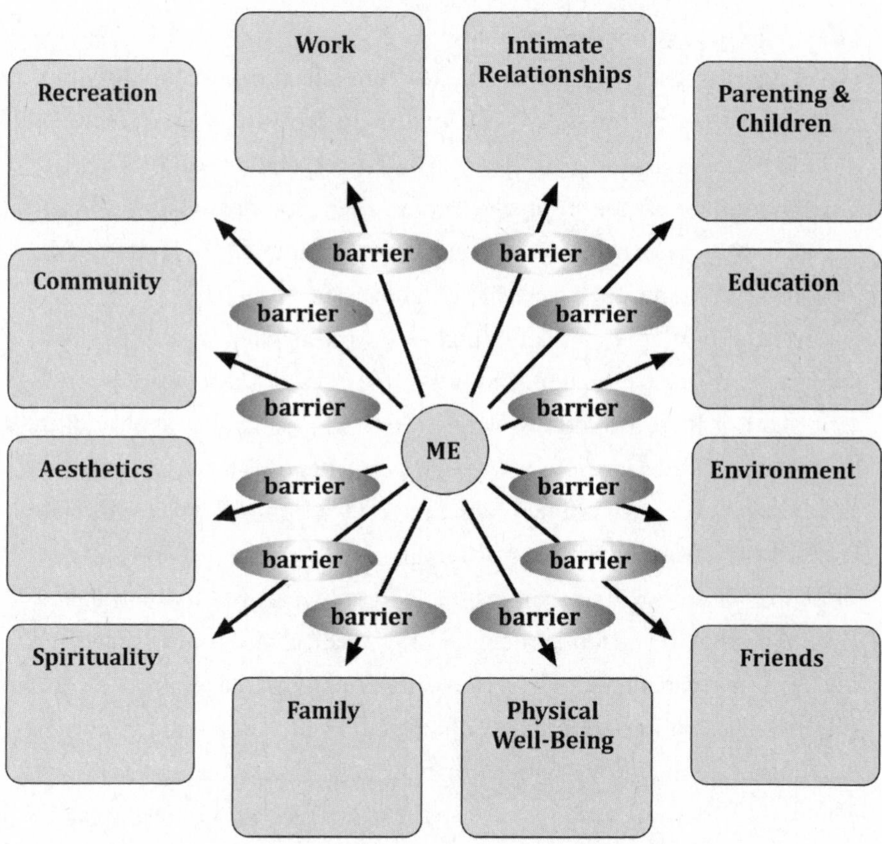

Participants were asked to fill out this Life Compass, writing about what they really wanted in these domains. Attention then turned to considering what internal barriers stood in the way of moving in those directions. An example might be how a fear of pain kept them from exercising. Then they considered the ways they had been dealing with those barriers. One might be procrastinating about going to the gym. Next they took a hard look at their coping strategies and evaluated whether they were actually means of avoidance, and whether the strategies were working. This process helps with accepting the need to "drop the rope" and accept the need for acceptance. It also helps target thoughts and emotions to which to apply the ACT skills.

They applied several defusion and acceptance exercises to the unhelpful thoughts and emotions they'd identified. At the end, they made a commitment to taking one or two actions that would be consistent with their values, such as calling a friend or taking a walk.

In the next session the therapists worked more on acceptance and defusion skills, and added in presence exercises, asking participants to deliberately call up difficult thoughts and feelings and sit with them while noticing them with an attitude of dispassionate curiosity. For example, they were asked to notice where in their body a difficult feeling appeared and to drop their struggle with it. At the end they reported on how they'd done in taking the action they'd committed to and made a new commitment.

The third session involved work on values and self, in which they wrote down what they would most want to see written about them after their death. This helps people look more closely at the self-story they've been weaving and see the contrast between how they've been living and the way they would really like to be living. They also did more acceptance work, playing a game in which they wrote down their mental barriers on cards. The therapists first tossed them at the participants, telling them to bat them away. After noting how much work that battle took, they were told to envision taking the cards and putting them in their back pockets to carry along with them for their life journey. This helps to see that acceptance is actually the easier route. They also did additional defusion and self exercises.

In the fourth session participants reviewed the barriers they needed to address in a defusion exercise, which involved learning to listen to the mind as you might listen to a storyteller rather than a dictator. The session ended with them telling the group their values in each of the domains and how they were going to pursue them.

Given the remarkable results in just those four hours of work, many of the participants clearly made the pivots and continued to apply the learning.

How long do the results of such a simple engagement with ACT practices last? We don't really know. It is common to have follow-ups that go more than a year, and they almost always last that long. But the results from studies with longer follow-ups are promising. A recent example followed over 108 people who had experienced nearly a decade of chronic pain. Three months after brief ACT training, 46.9 percent showed significant improvement in psychosocial disability. Three years later the figure was nearly identical: 43.1%.

Another study followed fifty-seven people dealing with depression who had been taught the ACT skills five years earlier. At the time of their training, their average score on the most widely used depression measure was deep into the clinically depressed range. After just four ACT sessions, 39 percent of the participants were depression free, increasing after six months to 52 percent and after five years to 57 percent. Even five years after only four sessions, two-thirds said they were still using ACT methods and only 6 percent were using antidepressant medications versus five times that number when they started. Their scores on assessments of their psychological flexibility and life satisfaction improved dramatically. When asked what they thought had helped them, responses included "I've been able to influence my own well-being: I don't get stuck in feelings, I see them as separate things" and "A lot has changed in my life, but I've gotten better at handling those changes: no fighting with past matters."

These results may seem startling, but are they really? You just showed with your body that you have the same kind of wisdom these clients woke up to. They stopped avoiding; they backed away from their mind and its stories; they stood up inside their awareness, turned toward what they cared about, and began to walk in that direction with the painful parts of their history coming along for the ride. They learned to pivot.

A Continuing Life Journey

The power of an initial engagement with a set of ACT methods doesn't mean that learning the skills is just a matter of a few hours and *poof!*, you've developed your psychological flexibility. We need to keep practicing exercises to get really good at the skills.

We should also keep applying the skills to more areas of our lives. If you begin by addressing your depression, you might proceed to work on adopting a healthier diet, and then keep going by using the skills to make a career change you've been stalled about. This is how the ACT journey usually unfolds for people; it starts naturally to take you into new and more challenging directions. And guess what? New is always a bit scary, even if it's also exciting. We'll also inevitably face some new difficulties; life all too often doles them out. As we face these ongoing challenges, we'll be lured back into avoidance, fusion, or mindlessness, and we'll have to work hard again to apply the skills. Like any learning process, developing psychological flexibility typically works in fits and starts. For some people substantial change comes very rapidly, but for most it is a matter of two steps forward, one step back, two steps forward.

Ideally, practicing ACT becomes a regular part of our life. Think of this like a physical workout routine. Many people who engage with ACT carve out time in their schedules for ongoing practice of exercises. In Part Two I introduce you to a good set of some of the most effective and popular exercises, and in Part Three, I show you how to create your own ACT toolkit of a selection of those you find especially effective. I then provide guidance about applying them to a wide range of life challenges. Over time, you can continue adding exercises to your toolkit, finding more on your own through the voluminous ACT literature online and in book form. By the end of the book you will know how to find these resources.

One person who has been working on developing the ACT skills wrote a powerful post on a Yahoo discussion list called ACT for the Public that beautifully describes what to expect of the ongoing journey. This is a self-managed list of thousands of people working on the skills, which has lasted more than a decade and includes nearly thirty thousand messages. I think I've read them all. I was particularly struck by this one.

The author calls himself Tim (people can have fake names on the list), and he was offering advice to a new list member who was struggling because "my anxiety is so bad" that she could not cope without heavy doses of benzodiazepines. Tim responded in a wise way, obviously born of practice in pivoting:

> Like most of us, you've arrived here having already programmed yourself up with a lot of harmful nonsense. That's OK. We have all done the same thing. It's a very human thing to do. You didn't do anything wrong.
>
> However, you are still the one that has to take responsibility for setting things straight. This list can be a great help, but you cannot look beyond yourself for solutions too often. You are the most important part of the process.
>
> When I say nonsense, I mean the mind falsely transforming very acceptable things into terrible things. Point is, you've got a lot of work to do to, so summon all the strength you have and get ready to be very patient with the process.
>
> Prepare yourself for ups and downs as you proceed. Your mind will definitely scream to you that you're off course when you're not. Don't believe the hype it gives you. Don't worry about where you're supposed to get to. Assume that you'll be doing this work for life, because you probably will, and you'll be better off for it. You'll likely emerge at some point into a clearing and feel the urge to pronounce yourself healed—that you're now "rid of that stuff." That's a trap, because the next little whiff of "that stuff" has the potential to drag you right down again, and your mind can turn ANYTHING into "that stuff" when the fear alarm is ringing.
>
> Be OK with being a work forever in progress. Allow for a place for pain in your life. That's always been reality. Your mind will come up with crackpot theories about how you can find a new life with no pain or unease at all. That's a lie. What happens if you buy into all that? Well, no version of reality has a chance of ever being good enough, and your mind just keeps saying "Ahhh! Keep running! Keep fighting! We're not there yet!"
>
> I beg to differ. Even now, in the midst of pain, you're so very, very close to the valued and fulfilling life you seek, because what you are

> right now is all that you truly need. Challenge the notion that you have to get to "somewhere else." There are things about our habits that we all need to change, but we can start by just learning to see, to be here, and to care.
>
> That will take time. Though a vital life is a half step away, it's not a step that is easy to take. Fear and sadness and entanglement is hard to turn away from, but it can be done.

I was deeply moved by Tim's message. We human beings have such a hard challenge and yet every wisdom and spiritual tradition says what I believe: we have within us the possibility of a vital life if we can learn to cultivate it.

At the beginning of this chapter you showed with your own body that you have the power within you. You probably already have a better understanding of some of the pain, fear, shame, anger, resentment, or other emotion you've been trying to avoid, and of behavior you want to change.

So let's go learn how to put that mind of yours on a leash.

Part Two

INTRODUCTION: STARTING YOUR ACT JOURNEY

Part Two is your personal workshop in learning the ACT practices. Think of this chapter as the orientation. It also prepares you for the journey by helping you drop the rope in whatever struggles you're caught in. You'll learn a powerful way to identify avoidant thoughts and behaviors, and you will be able to apply the flexibility skills to them as you work through the chapters.

Each chapter is devoted to helping you make one of the pivots and then continue building that skill. I illuminate how each skill helps satisfy a deep healthy yearning we humans all have, but that we unfortunately often try to satisfy in a toxic and inflexible way. Recall, for example, that yearning to belong leads us to lie, resulting in disconnection from others. I try to show how readily we can make each pivot, swinging the energy inside that yearning toward healthy living, often using stories of those who have done so.

Next, I offer a "starter set" of exercises followed by additional exercises to do as you continue building your skills. I recommend that you do the first set and then move on to the next chapter, coming back to do the additional ones once you've worked through all of the Part Two chapters. That way you will quickly experience how all six skills build on and support one another. We've found through many years of teaching ACT that it's best to learn a small but complete set fairly quickly, and then to practice these initial exercises while gradually expanding your skills.

As you read these chapters, you may want to apply the insights and exercises to a particular challenge you're struggling with. That might be quitting smoking, sticking to a diet, dealing with depression, coping with stress, contending with a horrible boss at work, or managing the frustrations of parenting. If you are already engaged in a program of some kind for coping with that challenge or are in therapy or undergoing treatment, learning the skills will assist with those efforts. Studies have also shown that the skills help with following dieting guidelines, staying on a physical fitness routine, and even deepening our sense of spirituality, whether complementary to formal religious practice or outside such a tradition.

If you do decide to apply the skills to one particular challenge as you read these Part Two chapters, you may first want to read the material in Part Three about how ACT helps with that specific challenge. If you are looking into therapy or treatment programs and you want to consider ACT therapists, this link will help you find them: http://bit.ly/FindanACTtherapist. But these days many clinicians know ACT to a degree, and many programs incorporate some elements of ACT. Ask around.

ACT is not just for dealing with specific problems, though. Flexibility skills are a method of evolving as a generally healthier, more fulfilled person. Thus, as you read these chapters, you will have ample opportunities to apply the exercises to whatever daily challenges come up.

Feel free to work through these Part Two chapters at your own pace, keeping in mind that making the full set of initial pivots is best facilitated by fully engaging in the practices. Aim to complete the chapters in about a week or two, ideally reading one chapter and doing the first few exercises in one or two days. You could also, however, go through them faster, say two at a time, or you could spread the reading out over a longer time frame. I strongly urge you, though, to carve out the time to work all the way through these chapters one directly after another without a substantial gap of time in between. I think you will begin to see some positive effects from the practices quickly, which should help keep your motivation strong.

Beware of Using New Tools for Old Tricks

One thing to keep in mind as you work on skill building is that you will sometimes find yourself using the flexibility practices in the service of old harmful habits. Like using the magnifying glass as a scraper. For example, you might find that in doing self work, you begin weaving a fabulous new self-story—*I'm super flexible now!* Don't be too hard on yourself; everyone does it. But do watch out for this. Do not expect your problem-solving mind ever to stop offering its avoidant "solutions." What you can expect is that you'll get better and better at seeing unhelpful thoughts for what they are and respectfully declining to engage with them.

The one absolute mandate I will give you about engaging in the exercises is that it's important to allow yourself to listen carefully to your thoughts and emotions as you go through them, and that you treat yourself with kindness about progress you're making and any difficulty you may be having. The last thing ACT should be about is presenting yourself with more wagging fingers. You are learning a new dance and that's always going to involve some missteps. If you do the exercises in an open-minded spirit—no matter how odd some of them may seem—you should soon see some positive results that will help you keep going. The key is to look through that glass tool and start cooking so you get some good nourishment.

So, are you ready? Let's get started.

How Are You Avoiding?

The first step in learning to pivot is to become aware of your avoidant thoughts and behaviors and to acknowledge how ineffective, and even harmful, they are. To help with that, we developed this exercise.

Consider all of the ways in which you've been dealing with whatever challenges you struggle with and write them down. I gave you my list for trying to defeat my anxiety in Chapter Two, which included the following:

1. Practiced relaxation techniques.

2. Tried to think more rationally.

3. Sat near the door so I could get out easily.

4. Had a beer.

5. Avoided giving talks—letting graduate students do them.

6. Took tranquilizers.

7. Had a friend in sight when I was talking.

8. Pushed myself to do exposure.

Your turn. Write a similar list of the ways you've tried to solve your problems. Actually do it.

The next step is to look hard at whether these methods have delivered results, and if so, whether they were large and lasting or small and fleeting. You will usually find that some—or even all—of them have helped in the short term, but that they haven't contributed to longer-term improvement and might even have made things worse.

Look at my list. When I was at the height of my panic disorder, how did I feel when I, say, turned down an offer to give a talk instead of facing my fear? I felt great! I felt relieved and calmer. Still, the noose tightened. The next time an invitation to speak came, my anxiety was even more fearsome.

Now it's time to look at your list.

Ask yourself one at a time whether each of the methods you've used has actually paid off in the long term. If not, look long and hard at the smaller, more immediate benefits that have made those methods appealing. Often in this exercise you will realize what they were really about. They may have been efforts to control or evade your experience; they may have been driven by the "have to" messages of the Dictator Within; they may have traded away a values-based approach for the addictive short-term pop of chemical reward. Take your time, but cover every single item.

Do not blame yourself as you consider your list. While the purpose of this exercise is to help you "drop the rope" and accept the need for acceptance, it may ironically trigger self-repudiation. Coming to see how ineffectual or counterproductive our efforts to solve problems have been can be painful and lead to self-blame, and even shame. If that's true for you, then make that harsh treatment of yourself a target as you begin to develop the flexibility skills.

Now take a mental step back from your list and ask yourself, if you keep doing what you are doing, is it likely you will keep getting what you are getting? You may hear your Dictator pushing back as you contemplate the answer. Some of your methods may seem incontrovertibly logical. But again, have they worked? Completely? Over the long run?

It's time to answer this question: *Who do you trust, that voice in your mind or your experience?* What could be more incontrovertibly logical than to cast aside "solutions" that don't work *in your actual experience?*

As you proceed through these chapters, you may find it useful to repeat this process of writing down the solutions you're pursuing and closely scrutinizing how they're working short term and long term. I expect you will be heartened that you are adding to your list some highly effective new methods.

One last preparatory step you may want to take is to get an assessment of your degree of psychological flexibility, which you can use as a benchmark for gauging your progress in building the skills over time. This is what we do with the participants in studies; we have them fill out assessments before we put them through the training and then again after the training, sometimes doing follow-ups after several months in which we again ask them to fill out the assessments. A general assessment is provided on my website (http://www.stevenchayes.com), as well as a number of assessments tailored to specific conditions: diabetes, epilepsy, cancer, substance abuse, weight loss, and many more. But you don't have to do an assessment to get the benefits of learning the practices, so if you'd rather not, that's fine.

Finally, you may also want to join one of the many online communities that support people in learning and applying ACT. The oldest is the ACT for the Public discussion list. You can access it at http://bit.ly/ACTforthePublic. It can be very helpful to ask questions there as you read the Part Two and Part Three chapters.

In the entire set of ACT-relevant studies (now numbered in the thousands), I don't know a single example of an improvement in psychological flexibility that was not associated with beneficial outcomes. The bottom line is this: if you acquire flexibility skills, they will help you in many different ways. So if you're ready, let's go!

Chapter Nine

THE FIRST PIVOT

DEFUSION—PUTTING THE MIND ON A LEASH

The defusion methods the ACT community has developed help us use our minds in a more open, aware, and values-based way. We learn to become more cognizant of the automaticity of our thoughts and to watch the ones that aren't helpful from a distance, as if to tell the Dictator Within, "Thanks, but I've got this covered." The critical voice and its commands don't go away, but we see them more as the products of our mental mechanisms, like the pronouncements of the contraption created by the Wizard of Oz. We don't need to argue with our thoughts. It's more like putting the mind on a leash.

Defusion methods are hugely helpful as we begin to probe into the sources of our pain or fear, because that examination provokes many difficult thoughts. We can load heaps of recrimination on ourselves and get caught up in unhelpful rumination. As we learn to defuse from self-judgment, we can replace it with self-kindness. Defusion also helps us turn off our compulsive problem-solving for a while. It opens a door to our power to change, allowing us to acknowledge our unhelpful thoughts while charting a course that goes beyond them.

The Yearning for Coherence

Helpful in learning defusion is understanding the yearning that drives our obsessive self-messaging and problem solving. This is the yearning to create coherence and understanding out of our mental cacophony. It's a perfectly understandable desire that is built into language itself; messy thought processes are discomforting. We feel a sense of vulnerability when our thoughts don't fit nicely together, especially when they are contradictory. We want to know, "Which is it? What do I really believe and what is really true?"

Sometimes we see contradictions in our thoughts that aren't really contradictions at all. Take a thought like "I love my husband but I can't stand living with him." It seems contradictory, and in fact, the word *but* in the sentence declares that. *But* is an ancient contraction of *be out*, and the sentence is implying that because it seems logically incoherent to have such opposing reactions to one's husband, one of the two has to "be out." Yet nothing is really illogical about the statement. The truth might be better stated "I love my husband *and* I have thoughts like I can't stand living with him." We only think there's a contradiction because of a simplistic cultural rule that we should always have positive feelings about those we love. But it makes perfect sense to have mixed reactions to our loved ones. We are complicated beings. Why wouldn't we inspire complicated responses?

Other times our thoughts really are contradictory in a literal sense: we may think both "I'm a good person" and "I'm a bad person," for example, because these thoughts reflect different aspects of our past. Think of the process of trying to give our thoughts logical order as similar to dealing with two quarreling first-graders. If you think you've got to determine who is right and who is wrong, you will have to actively engage with all the back-and-forth between them. But if you step back and watch them with curiosity and gentle amusement, you won't feel the need to choose the winner. You might even be able to help them get past their disagreement, working together even if the core argument is not resolved.

That is the power that cognitive defusion gives us. It frees our minds from rigid thinking in order to find new ways of dealing with our problems and aspirations.

Not only is the desire for coherence natural, but ACT can satisfy it if we stop expecting "untidy" thoughts and feelings to go away. That allows us to let go of "being right" as the primary issue. As the following pivot diagram shows, using the metaphor of a funnel, the agenda of imposing a false order in our thoughts gradually channels a yearning for coherence into living a narrower life. If we're seeking to make our self-story coherent so that it conforms to social expectations, it's time to stop investing in that goal. If we're choosing to follow rigid rules that offer a simplistic coherence of "the answers" in life, we need to let go of that impulse. But there is a constructive kind of coherence that is just a pivot away: that of paying attention to the thoughts that are useful to us for living in accordance with our values,

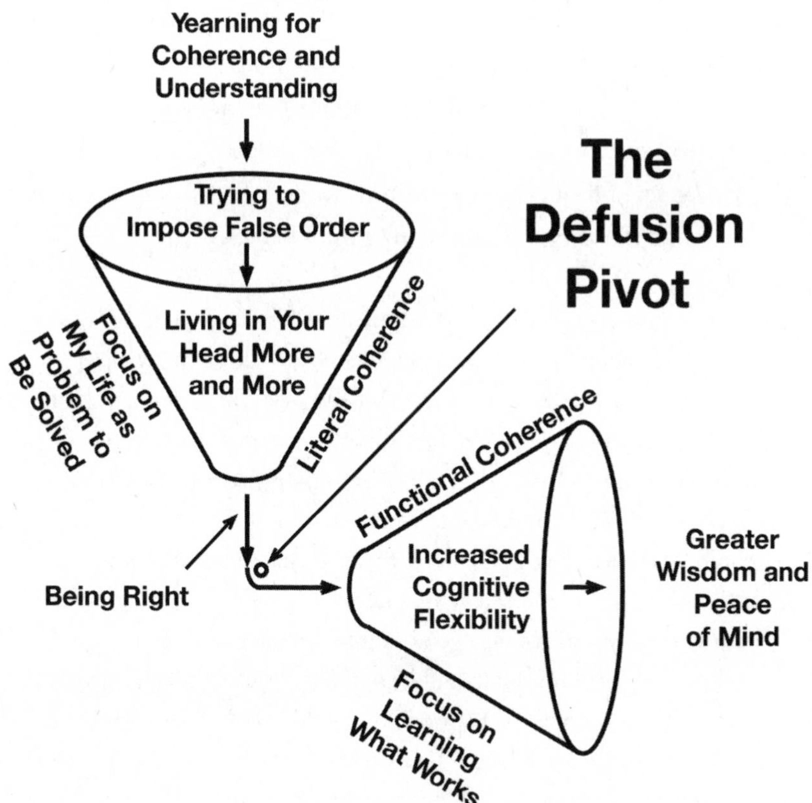

and letting go of a focus on thoughts that are unhelpful. I'll call this *functional coherence*—it channels our yearning for coherence into life expansion, shown in the diagram with the metaphor of a megaphone. Before the Defusion pivot, we grasp at form over function; afterward, we trust function over form. We begin to accept how chaotic our thinking can be and direct our attention and our behavior toward thoughts that are useful.

Ironically as we build a defusion habit, our minds *do* become more peaceful and orderly after a fashion. Because defusion helps us focus on thoughts that are helpful, it also allows the mental chaos to recede into the background. We are broadening and building our useful mental networks.

Catching Automatic Thoughts

The first step in making the pivot is to become aware of just how automatic and complicated our thought processes are. This was a goal of CBT as well, and the ACT community has built on its methods and expanded their range. One is to write down a string of thoughts that emerge when you give your mind free rein for a few minutes.

Here is the set of thoughts I wrote down when I did this exercise as soon as I woke up the morning I began writing this chapter:

> It's time to get up. No, it isn't; it's only 6:00. That's seven hours of sleep. I need eight—that's the goal. I feel fat. Well, birthday cake, duh. I have to eat cake on my son's birthday. Maybe, but not such a big piece. I bet I'm up to 196 lbs. Shoot . . . by the time I run the Halloween candy/Turkey Day gauntlet I'll be back over 200. But maybe not. Maybe more like 193. Maybe exercise more. Anything would be "more." I've gotta focus. I have a chapter to write. I'm falling behind. . . . and I'm getting fat again. Noticing the voices and letting them run might be a good start to the chapter. Better to go back to sleep. But maybe it could work. It was sweet of Jacque to suggest it. She's up early. Maybe it's her cold. Maybe I should get out of bed and see if she is OK. It's only 6:15. I need my eight hours. It's close now to seven and a half hours. Still not eight.

Not only are these thoughts remarkably circuitous, but most of them are about rules and punishment. Many of them are also contradictions of the prior thought. I'm sure you're familiar with that kind of mental to-and-fro. Welcome to the human race.

The old cartoon device of an argument between the devil on one shoulder and an angel on the other is understood even by small children. That's because arguing with ourselves is so natural. We begin to do it not long after our language abilities have developed and our Dictator Within has come on the scene. When we are deeply focused on a mental task our minds can enter into a state of flow, in which thoughts, emotions, and actions are all temporarily in sync. But the more usual state is one of mind wandering, and that is often characterized by a good deal of mental disagreement and disengagement.

The parts of the brain involved in mind wandering are referred to as the *default mode network*, because it is activated automatically when the brain isn't focused on specific tasks. Interestingly, neuroscience scans have recently shown that the executive network of the brain, which is involved in decision making, is also active during mind wandering, physical proof that when you are not watching the mind, it is often engaged in an effort to sort through cacophonous thoughts. The open awareness encouraged by defusion helps calm the default mode network, quieting the mind and helping it focus on thoughts we consciously give our attention. Think of defusion skills as peace-of-mind skills. A kind of mental calm settles in when we experience the functional coherence of a mind focused on what works.

Let me give a personal example. In a talk I gave at Stanford, I was talking about the incredible increase in the use of sleeping medication, but instead of documenting the rise in billions of dollars, I said "trillions." I did not notice the error at the time, but my mind did because in the middle of the night I sat bolt upright and cried out loud, "Trillions?!! You idiot!" Within seconds I was pacing the room berating myself for my stupidity until it occurred to me to do Titchener's word repetition exercise, which I described in Chapter Four. I sat on the corner of the bed and for thirty seconds, I repeated the word *stupid*. Then I was done. Within minutes I was back to sleep. It was not worth any more of my time. I did not need to *convince* my mind of that through argument—that would have only increased the volume.

To get a look at how automatic and circuitous your own thinking process is, right now take a minute to point your thoughts in any direction of your choosing and try to track them as they run their course. You should write down all those that you notice for long enough to capture.

After completing this exercise, repeat it two more times, again letting your thoughts run for one minute. In round two, imagine that your job is to figure out whether each thought is literally true or appropriate. In round three, imagine that your thoughts are like the voices of quarreling first-graders. Adopt a posture of curiosity and amusement as you listen to them, but do nothing else with them than to notice them. Take a minute each and do it.

In round two, you probably experienced the sense of being pulled into your thought networks. Their loudness may have increased; a focus on content may have gone up. You might have noticed yourself getting involved in a kind of argument with your mind.

In round three, you probably noticed more about the flow of your thoughts. Very likely, the specific content of the thoughts seemed less important. You had a sense of being outside the argument.

That difference explains why defusion exercises weaken the link between automatic thoughts and behavior; our ability to step back from our thoughts grows stronger as we practice.

Defusion's Transformative Power

Learning defusion has helped many people make dramatic changes in their lives, even those who have been all but crippled by their negative thought patterns. Two important contributors to developing ACT, for example, found that defusion was instrumental to helping a client overcome the grip that rumination had over her life.

People who ruminate constantly are vulnerable to a variety of anxiety and mood problems such as the seemingly free-floating anxiety that abounds in what is called generalized anxiety disorder (GAD). The two researchers who have done the most in applying ACT to GAD are Sue Orsillo and Liz Roemer at Suffolk University and the University of Massachusetts, Boston, respectively. Sue and Liz target cognitive fusion with mindfulness methods that teach people to back up from their ruminative thoughts and watch them from a distance.

Bea is one of their star clients. You'd never know if you met her that fusion almost ruined her career. She now exudes confidence, but that was not always so. On track for tenure in the political science department of a top university, she was considered a hot commodity because of her intense intellect, her talent in political theory, and her long experience as a social activist—an unusual and vital combination in the world of political science. The sky-high expectations were flattering at first, but she soon felt like a deer frozen in the headlights of her own possibilities.

"The intensities of learning to teach and write at that level were overwhelming," she told me. As she worked to learn the discipline of academic writing, she began incessantly asking herself, "Is this good enough?" and "When will I finish this piece?" She was ruminating, and the more she ruminated, the less she wrote. Soon the negative message "I am going to fail!" became part of the agonizing mental cacophony, and she became totally overwhelmed.

She would focus on inane details for hours on end, such as whether the margins on her page were perfect. Her rumination led to behavioral paralysis that froze her in place for over two years. Desperate to submit *something* she'd written as part of her reappointment package (which would add a few more years before the final tenure decision), she grabbed a half-finished article, attached it to her reappointment file, and hit send.

Her colleagues were horrified. They saw her potential, and they went to bat for her. But this was not acceptable. Something had to change, and change fast.

Something *did* change. For the worse.

Bea turned to beer and Adderall—a type of amphetamine that is sometimes called "the study drug" because it is so widely abused on college campuses for that purpose. When she combined it with alcohol, she hardly knew which end was up.

Bea began making her way out of this free fall into oblivion when Sue and Liz taught her defusion techniques. They showed Bea how to practice watching her thoughts from a distance with a sense of open curiosity. One of the exercises they had her do has become a staple of ACT, which we call "leaves on a stream." You can do it now if you like. It is usually done with eyes closed, as a guided meditation.

> Imagine that you are watching a quietly flowing brook with large leaves on it floating by. Each thought that comes into your mind, place it on a leaf and watch it float downstream. If it reappears, that is fine—just put the second version on a leaf too. The goal is to stay by the stream, watching your thoughts. If you discover you've stopped doing the exercise and your mind has gone elsewhere, which is common, try to catch what led your mind astray. Almost inevitably, what happened was cognitive fusion with a thought. Something popped into your head and instead of placing it on the leaf you started engaging with its content, and it triggered your automatic thought processes. After noting how the "fusion trigger" worked, get right back to watching the brook and begin again.

Bea needed to start with defusion work because she could not make any progress until she freed her mind from her rumination. Once that was achieved, she was able to make rapid progress, learning the other pivots and becoming productive again with her writing after only a month. The happy result was that she was ultimately awarded tenure.

When we learn defusion skills, we can take the energy of our counterproductive yearning and pivot it toward learning to be gently guided by our experience. We become able to prize function over form. As we experience the benefits of focusing on helpful thoughts, we become increasingly motivated to defuse from the Dictator's voice, creating a positive feedback loop.

A columnist at NBC News, Sarah Watts, has personally experienced the power of defusion in her recovery from debilitating anxiety. She described how it helped this way: "Within weeks, after much practice, even the thoughts that once left me paralyzed—my cancer is going to kill me, I'm going to pass another painful kidney stone—had loosened their grip on me. They were neither true nor untrue—they were simply thoughts, and I had the power to do with them what I wished." As her life opened up, she concluded, "This must be how normal people feel!"

Actually, no. This is how people feel after letting go of being attached to mental form over mental function. It is unfortunately *not* normal, but it is within reach.

Getting Prepared to Practice Defusion

It's good to start by getting a basic assessment of the degree to which fusion with negative thoughts may be causing you distress. The first step is to take the following quick assessment, called the Cognitive Fusion Questionnaire.

COGNITIVE FUSION QUESTIONNAIRE

Below you will find a list of statements. Please rate how true each statement is for you by circling a number next to it. Use the scale below to make your choice.

1	2	3	4	5	6	7
never true	very seldom true	seldom true	sometimes true	frequently true	almost always true	always true

1. My thoughts cause me distress or emotional pain

   1 2 3 4 5 6 7

2. I get so caught up in my thoughts that I am unable to do the things that I most want to do

   1 2 3 4 5 6 7

3. I overanalyze situations to the point where it's unhelpful to me

   1 2 3 4 5 6 7

4. I struggle with my thoughts

   1 2 3 4 5 6 7

5. I get upset with myself for having certain thoughts

   1 2 3 4 5 6 7

6. I tend to get very entangled in my thoughts

   1 2 3 4 5 6 7

7. It's such a struggle to let go of upsetting thoughts, even when I know that letting go would be helpful

   1 2 3 4 5 6 7

Now add up the numbers for an overall score. There is no strict correspondence of score to the degree of cognitive fusion, but a rough guideline is that if you score below 20, you are able to think reasonably flexibly. As your score moves into the mid to upper 20s and 30s, fusion is becoming more dominant, and the methods introduced in this chapter will be helpful to you in getting needed distance from your thoughts. Even if your thinking is defused and flexible, however, it is worthwhile to practice defusion methods, for the same reason it is worthwhile to engage in physical exercise even if you are strong. The practice will keep your flexibility of mind in good shape.

Over time, our new awareness of our thought process helps us become more attuned to when we're slipping into fusion. The key signs to keep in mind are as follows:

1. **Your thoughts seem *predictable*. You've had them plenty of times before, so much so that they seem to be part of who you are. Make a note of these thoughts, actually writing them down, and you can practice defusing from them over time.**

2. **You have a sense of *waking up from a reverie*. This means that you have disappeared into your thoughts for a time. You may even discover that a good deal of time has gone by and you're now late doing something you were supposed to get done. When this happens, as in the leaves-on-a-stream exercise, try to back up your thoughts and identify the moment you disappeared. That will help with recognizing triggers.**

3. Your *thoughts become highly comparative and evaluative* and begin wandering. When your mind is just noting what is effective—seeking functional coherence—once you notice it, the review quiets. If you find your mind going around in circles, or your evaluation becomes self-reflective and comparative, you're due for defusion, as, for example, with this string of thoughts: "Can I claim that dinner as a charitable deduction? Yes, I think I can. I'm glad I thought of that. Others would miss it, but not me. I think even my tax advisor would have missed it."

4. You catch your mind in *overbusy mode*, engaged in a wrestling match involving lots of contradictions, self-admonitions, and rules ("You are wrong, you do not need that donut! It will make you fat. Well, even fatter. That's why people avoid you. Oh, come on, it's just a donut . . .").

Cognitive Flexibility Fosters Creativity

Not only does learning the skill of defusion help in coping with painful life challenges, it also helps us consider a wider set of possibilities as we attempt to work on any problem. In other words, it strengthens our cognitive flexibility.

Here is a quick and dirty way to assess how flexible you are cognitively. This is the Alternative Uses Task, which is one of the most common measures of cognitive flexibility. Ready?

Look around the room and pick a common object that you see. A pen, a glass, a paper clip, or envelope—whatever. Grab your smartphone and set a timer for two minutes. Get ready to start the timer when I say "Go." This is the task: say as rapidly as you can everything you can think of that this object could be used for, counting or recording them so you can get an accurate count. OK, ready? Go!

Your score is the number of different uses you came up with. Researchers of cognitive flexibility call this a measure of *fluency*, meaning the relative rate of task accomplishment. If you want to evaluate how you performed, a normal fluency score in this task for two minutes would be around 8 or 9. If you were in an actual study of cognitive flexibility, the researchers would also score how unusual the uses you came up with are. For example, if you were thinking of uses for your glasses, your score would improve if you thought of using them to stir a drink or to magnify the heat of sunlight, or maybe using the lenses as Christmas ornaments, because those ideas are out of the ordinary.

As you tried this exercise, you could probably sense how fusion with thoughts interfered with the task. For example, if you thought of stirring a drink with your glasses, you may have then kept thinking of other things to stir with them, rather than thinking of more different uses. That is called *functional fixedness.*

Ironically, when we let go of the domination of the Dictator Within and its incessant problem-solving mind, we can use our minds to solve problems more creatively. We will return to this topic in Chapter Eighteen, when we look at learning and performance. ACT research has even shown how we can use cognitive flexibility training to increase intelligence successfully.

If we learn to think of our internal voice as that of an advisor rather than a dictator, it can become enormously helpful to us. As in the story of the Wizard of Oz, who said he was not a bad man but just a bad wizard, we can come to see that our mind itself is not bad, or harmful to us, as long as we don't let it rigidly dictate our behavior. It's a tool and when we learn to put it on a leash, it can serve us even better. As I wrote earlier, we have very good minds, just very bad Dictators.

A Starter Set of Methods

Here is a starter set of four commonly used defusion techniques. The first two are general defusion building exercises, and the third and fourth are tailored to defusing from specific problematic thoughts. Consider these four the core of your initial defusion practice. In the first couple of weeks as you learn defusion, repeat each one at least once a day. Additionally, if during the course of the day you notice that you are ensnared by a thought, use a couple of them right then to break free.

It is fine to read about the rest of the methods now if you'd like to, but I suggest you first move on to the remaining chapters in Part Two and then return to actually engage in the additional exercises. Ultimately, you can select a subset you like the best, which you will find you can remember easily and always pull out, on the fly, when you need them.

It's important to work some defusion practices into your life in that ongoing way, using them to help you progressively think more flexibly. The goal is not just to make the specific pivot, it's to learn the dance. You will need to continue developing the skill of defusion for the rest of your life; just as meditators must keep working on their meditation skills, lifetime practice of defusion is needed to keep the pull of the yearning for coherence from tempting us into trying to make all of our thoughts consistent or else. That kind of coherence—let's called it *literal coherence*—is ultimately impossible. But learning to take what is useful and leaving the rest—*functional coherence*—is both helpful and possible.

While it's common, and even helpful, to feel a sense of freedom and distance in a matter of minutes, be careful. Your mind may try to convince you that you have solved the fusion problem and are done with it. Don't you believe it. Fusion is not behind you. The Dictator Within is just giving you a dangerous new thought to defuse from. No matter how good you are at defusion, your mind will keep forming new thoughts that you will naturally fuse with ("I'm the world's expert in defusion!"). It's vital to stay aware of this tendency. I've been practicing defusion for more than thirty years now and I still have to catch myself as I'm getting entangled with my thoughts. Every day. It happens every day. By now sometimes just catching it is enough, but if not, I immediately engage in one of the defusion practices. And sometimes fusion still slips by me for periods of time. That's inevitable. The goal is progress, not perfection.

Fair warning: some of these exercises may seem odd, even silly. No worry; humor is in fact called for here (we *are* funny creatures!). Just work through them with a sense of self-compassion.

1. Disobey on Purpose

Let me start with one that I'm sure will seem perplexing. Just trust me.

Stand up and carry the book around with you while you slowly walk around the room, reading this next sentence aloud several times. (Really do it, *while walking*, OK? Ready? Stand up. Walk. Read. Go!)

Here is the sentence:

"I cannot walk around this room."

Keep walking! Slowly but clearly repeat that sentence as you walk . . . at least five or six times.

"I cannot walk around this room."

Now you can sit down again.

It is such a tiny thing, isn't it? A tiny poke in the eye of the Dictator Within; a little tug on Superman's cape.

This exercise was one of our earliest defusion discoveries, used in the ACT studies done in the early 1980s. Even though it is a silly little exercise, a team in Ireland showed recently in a laboratory experiment that it immediately increased tolerance to experimentally induced pain by nearly 40 percent! I'm not talking about people *saying* they can tolerate pain. People were willing to keep their hand on a very, very hot plate (not hot to the point of injury, mind you, just hot enough to cause real pain) 40 percent longer—after just a few moments of saying one thing while doing the opposite.

Think about that. Even the tiniest little demonstration that the mind's power over you is an *illusion* can very quickly give you significantly more freedom to do hard things. You can easily build this into your life as a regular practice (right now I'm thinking, *I cannot type this sentence! I can't!*).

And we've only just gotten started.

2. Give Your Mind a Name and Listen to It Politely

If your mind has a name, then it is different from "you." When you listen to someone else, you can choose to agree with what they say or not, and if you don't want to cause conflict, it's best not to try to argue the person into agreement with you. That is the posture you want to take with your internal voice. Process work has shown that naming your mind helps with this. I call mine George. Pick any name you like. Even Mr. Mind or Ms. Mind will do. Now say hello to your mind using its new name, as if you're being introduced to it at a dinner party. If you are around others, you can do this entirely in your head—no need to freak people out.

3. Appreciate What Your Mind Is Trying to Do

Now listen to your thoughts for a bit, and when your mind starts to chatter, answer back with something like "Thanks for that thought, George. Really, thank you." If you speak to your mind dismissively, it will continue right on problem-solving. Be sincere. You might want to add, "I really get that you are trying to be of use, so thank you for that. But I've got this covered." If you're alone, you could even say this out loud.

Note that your mind will probably push back with thoughts like *That's silly. That won't help!* Respond again with, "Thanks for that thought, George. Thank you. I really do see how you are trying to be of use." You could also even invite more comments with dispassionate curiosity: "Anything else you have to say?"

4. Sing It

This method is powerful when you're having a really sticky thought. Turn it into a sentence and try singing it—out loud if you are alone, in your head if you have company. Any tune will do. My default is "Happy Birthday." Don't worry about trying to be clever about the wording, like coming up with a rhyming scheme. This is not going to get you on *America's Got Talent*! Just repeat the thought to the tune. See if you can find a thought that is nagging you right now and try it. Try different tunes; sing it fast or slow. The measure of "success" is not that the thought goes away, or loses all punch and becomes unbelievable. It is that you can see it as a thought, and do so just a bit more clearly.

Additional Methods

5. Backward

Take a negative word that is at the heart of a recurrent difficult thought and spell it backward. For example, *I guess I'm just stupid. . . . Say, did you know that* stupid *spelled backward is* diputs? Odd interruptions like that remind you that you are just thinking—and that is the point: to back up and look *at* thoughts, not *from* thoughts. (A fun variant is to apply the old song "The Name Game" to the word: "Stupid, stupid, bo burpid, banana fana fo furpid, fe fi mo murpid. Stupid!")

6. Look at It as an Object

Put the thought out in front of you and ask some questions about it. If it had a size, how big would it be? If it had a shape, what shape would it have? If it had a color, what color would it have? If it had speed, how fast would it go? If it had power, how much power would it have? If it had a surface texture, how would it feel to the touch? If it had an internal consistency, what would that be?

If after answering these questions the power of the thought is unabated, focus on your *reactions* to the thought—especially your judgments, predictions, negative emotions, or evaluations (e.g., "I don't want that! I despise it!"). Hold those in your mind. Then pick a core reaction that seems central. Move the first thought to the side and place the core reaction in front of you. Now answer the same questions: If it had a size, how big would it be? And so forth.

After you've answered them all, peek back at the first thought. Is it the same size, shape, color, speed, power, texture, and consistency? Often you will find that it has changed in ways that give it less of an impact.

7. Different Voices

Say your difficult thought out loud in another voice. You can pick your least favorite politician, or a cartoon character, or the voice of a movie star. Try out different voices. Keep in mind, though, never, ever to ridicule yourself. The voices are to help you look at the thoughts, not to make fun of them, or you.

8. The Hand Exercise

Imagine writing down your thought on the palm of your hand (you don't have to actually write it as long as you know it is there). Then bring your hand close to your face. In that posture, it is hard to see anything else—even your hand and the thought written on it in imagination are hard to see. This is a physical metaphor for fusion: thought dominating over your awareness.

Now move your hand with the thought still on it straight out away from your face. It is a bit easier to see other things in addition to your hand. Now move your hand with the thought on it just a little to the side so you can focus on it if you need to but you can also see ahead clearly. Those actions simulate the stance you want to establish toward your thoughts. Whenever you catch yourself being dominated by a thought, note how close to you it is. Is it like that hand in your face, or off to the side? If it is in your face, see if you can move it off to the side. Note that you do not get rid of the thought this way—in fact, you see it as a thought even more clearly. But in this posture you can do many other things as well, which is the core point of defusion.

9. Carry It with You

Now write the thought on a small piece of paper and hold it up. Look at it the way you might look at a precious and fragile page from an ancient manuscript. These words are an echo of your history. Even if the thought is painful, ask yourself if you would be willing to honor that history by choosing to carry this piece of paper with you. If you can get to "yes," put it carefully in your pocket or purse and let it come along for the ride. During the days you carry it, every so often pat your purse or pocket or wherever you keep it, as if to acknowledge that it is part of your journey, and it is welcome to come along.

10. The Little Kid

This exercise will help you develop self-compassion. It's vital to be aware that defusing from our thoughts should not involve self-ridicule or being hard on ourselves for having such thoughts. You are not ridiculous. You are human, and human language and cognition are like a tiger we're riding that inevitably leads us into some dangerous territory. None of us can entirely prevent unhelpful thoughts from forming in our minds.

Take a difficult thought that goes back a long way in your history, and picture yourself as young as you can while having that thought, or others like it. Take a little time to picture what you looked like at that age—what your hair was like, what you dressed like. Then, in your imagination, have those words come out of that child in the voice of you as a child. Actually, try to do it in his or her little voice. If you are in a private place, try to reproduce the voice out loud—otherwise, try to hear it in your mind. And then focus on what you might do if you were actually in such a situation and your goal was to be there for that child. Picture yourself helping the child, such as by giving him or her a hug. Then ask yourself, "Metaphorically, how can I do that for myself now?" and see if some useful ideas come up.

11. Social Sharing and Defusion

When you've gotten quite good at distancing from judgmental thoughts, you can move to more advanced methods that rely on social sharing. These are more advanced only in the sense that it is important to do the internal work first, rather than to expect sharing alone to do the work for you. Sharing with others can build stronger defusion skills, but forcing yourself beyond your comfort zone can backfire if you are not ready. You are not a horse to be whipped. Letting go of fused judgments is quite emotional work, and it starts with you and the person in the mirror.

Robyn Walser, an ACT expert who works at the Veterans Affairs department in Palo Alto, came up with this first practice while she was working with veterans in group therapy. Many soldiers return from war zones with post-traumatic stress disorder (PTSD), often having experienced a moral trauma, and many have very difficult, judgmental thoughts about themselves and their actions. Robyn was digging into these fused self-judgments in the group, and she kept finding thoughts that the veterans were ready to let go and defuse from but they needed to take that final step.

What she did was very bold. She had them write down the self-judgment in large letters on a label they would then stick on their chests and wear to the group. It would function as a kind of declaration: "I'm not going to let this judgment run my life anymore."

What they wrote down would make you want to cry. *Murderer, Evil, Dangerous, Broken.* If you were still fused with the thought that you were a murderer, merely putting it on your chest would be of little value. It might even overwhelm you, since now what you truly believed would also be known by others. But if you were ready to look at the evaluation as just being a thought, and you'd chosen not to be pushed around by it anymore, then putting it on your chest is a powerful public manifestation of that choice.

I was profoundly impressed by how powerful this practice was the first time I tried it. I was introducing it in a workshop and I decided I wanted to participate too. The impulse came to me to write down the word *mean*, which surprised me because I didn't consciously think of myself that way. I didn't recall ever consciously berating myself for being mean. But there it was.

Suddenly I had a memory of being caught with a magnifying glass when I was six or seven years old, figuring out how fast tarantulas go if you really heat up their rear ends. I lived in an area outside San Diego with lots of tarantulas, and my friends and I were both fascinated and horrified by them. We toyed with the poor things, including on this occasion with magnifying glasses. My mother came up behind us unnoticed, and she was appalled. The look on her face combined disgust, horror, and anger; it could have easily turned a living creature into stone. I'd totally forgotten about the incident, and recalling it provoked a sick feeling of shame. In that moment, I realized that I'd been carrying a fear that I was *mean* around with me ever since!

I wrote *MEAN* in big, bold letters on a sticker and stuck it on my chest. When I went to get coffee at the break, I was startled to notice that I unconsciously turned my body so the camp cook could not see what I'd written—the thought was still that powerful. Yet twenty minutes later, when the workshop was over, I realized it was completely gone. Completely! Decades of hidden shame went poof! In a slightly euphoric mood, I left the badge on my jacket and wore it everywhere for the next couple of days. Some restaurant waiters looked at me so strangely! I just smiled and happily thought, *I'm not going to be running from "mean" for the rest of my life.*

Over the next several years I collected quite a pile of these badges: *unlovable, sick, sad, shameful, untrustworthy, hateful, fraud, empty, cruel, liar, pervert, angry, anxious, dangerous.*

I am not the only one. Rikke Kjelgaard, a Dutch ACT therapist, put together a video of ACT therapists holding pieces of paper with their own negative self-judgments written on them. It is sad and bravely human at the same time, and definitely worth a look: http://bit.ly/OurCommonFate.

I developed a variation of this method for use in large workshops that you could do with a few trusted friends. I ask people to line up facing each other in two long lines, say of twenty or thirty people each, and I request that they each look at the badge of the person in front of them for a few seconds and consider the pain and damage that the person's negative self-judgment has wrought in their life. I then ask everyone to spend about thirty seconds looking directly at the face of the person in front of them, with a sense of compassion for a burden that's been carried and appreciation for the courage it takes to lay that burden down. The two lines then move in opposite directions and new pairs repeat the process until all twenty to thirty pairs have done their work.

By the end of the exercise, most people are ready to weep and to hug everyone in the room. Almost every single person could wear every single badge as their own. A deeply empowering realization thunders in people's minds and hearts: everyone has the same secrets. Yet we become alone in our shame and self-judgment, not understanding that we're all on a similar journey.

There are many other ways you might begin a process of sharing as a defusion method. Have a T-shirt printed or a baseball cap made that includes your fears or self-doubts; write a book and make a list (oh, gee, I just did that!); share some of your insides in public talks (after you've done your work!); have an honest conversation with your children about their judgments and yours; listen carefully when others share their insides with you and share some of yours in return.

If you do this responsibly, you will find a sense of freedom and connection to others, and in minutes or hours you will start laying down unhelpful thoughts that have driven you for years.

Chapter Ten

THE SECOND PIVOT

SELF—THE ART OF PERSPECTIVE-TAKING

Think back to a memory from early elementary school. With a bit of effort you can go behind the eyes of your much younger self, re-experiencing that event.

You have just touched the sense of "you," the observer, who appears when our minds become able to use cognitive perspective-taking. From that point on, a sense of observing from within our mind from the perspective of an "I" is a constant in our lives. I will call this "I" that we become aware of *the transcendent self* because it is always there within us, no matter where we are, who we're with, and what the conditions of our lives are. At the same point when we develop this awareness, we begin to construct a story of our self—crafting the conceptualized self—which can block our awareness of our transcendent self. We become so focused on bolstering and defending this story we weave that we end up trying to hide aspects of who we are and of our experiences, not only from others, but from ourselves as well.

The Yearning for Belonging

Human beings yearn to be seen, cared for, and included as a member of the group. We are the social primates; we evolved in small bands and groups where belonging was literally a matter of life or death. While this yearning is healthy, many of the ways our minds try to satisfy it cause us psychic pain. We lie about ourselves to defend our ego; we play the victim; we berate ourselves for failing to meet inflated standards that might please others; and we become consumed by worries about rejection and perceived slights.

The harm caused can be seen in stark relief when we consider the quest for self-esteem. High self-esteem is a worthy goal. It is generally associated with positive feelings and greater initiative. People who characteristically have high self-regard tend to view themselves as being popular, intelligent, and attractive, and while they will admit to past mistakes, they generally believe they've learned from them and are moving on to a brighter future. That all sounds wonderful, and to a degree it is. The search for self-esteem may not stop there, however; the quest often leads to toxic self-delusion and psychic pain.

Research shows that when people focus on building, protecting, and maintaining self-esteem, they can become *less* able to focus on what they really value. They are more likely to feel pressured, stressed, and anxious and to be less resilient when facing challenges. For example, students who base their self-esteem on academic achievement suffer when they receive a low grade and will be at increased risk for depression—especially if they are already prone to it. Similarly, people who generate rosy stories about themselves begin to think they are better than other people. As that happens, rather than helping us feel that we belong, holding tightly to our self-stories makes us feel alienated and alone.

Genuine self-esteem is soft and open to our own flaws; the kind built on pretense is rigid, defended, and rejecting of self-honesty. The difference is fusion with our conceptualized self-stories.

The costs are everywhere to be seen, from our government to the boardroom, from the TV screen to your workplace. Advertisers happily sell goods that feed our need to protect our self-image. When that image is threatened, we are more likely to become angry, aggressive, and violent. We may also try to prove our worth by taking on tasks that are beyond our talents, suffering more damage to our self-esteem as a result. In these cases, the short-term emotional benefits of pursuing higher levels of self-esteem are far outweighed by the long-term costs in unhappiness and distress.

Connecting with the Transcendent Self

The Self pivot takes the healthy energy of yearning to belong and swings it in the direction of reconnecting with our transcendent I/here/now sense of awareness, allowing that awareness alone to be at the core of what we take ourselves to be. This allows us to relate to others, and to ourselves, in a way not dominated by the distortions of the ego and its self-story. Just as important, it allows us to touch a much deeper sense of belonging that lies inside human consciousness itself.

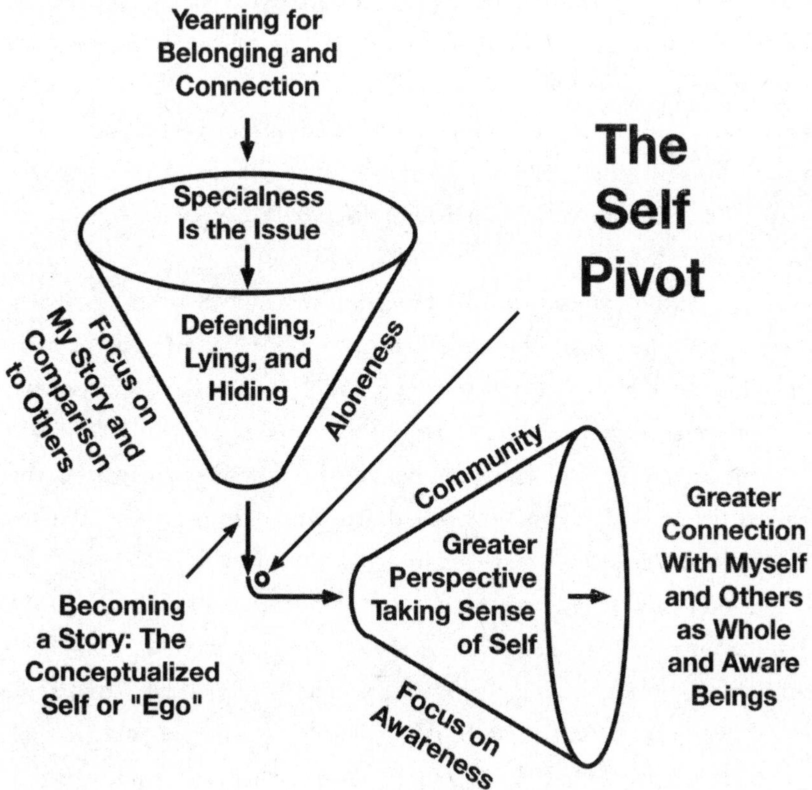

In making the Self pivot, through perspective-taking we connect with our awareness of our transcendent self in the here and now. This frees us from the grip of self-evaluation and the notion that we need to get others to buy into our stories of specialness in order to connect and belong. Instead, we realize we are connected to others in consciousness as our birthright as human beings, no matter how we match up to anyone's evaluations or to our own.

The crucial role of perspective-taking in fostering this awareness of our connection with others is dramatically illustrated in the story of how children with autism have learned to feel that connection through RFT-based perspective-taking exercises.

An ACT colleague who I will call Trudy had a daughter who was diagnosed with autism shortly after her second birthday. She had seen it coming: "There was no connection. I could not make her laugh," she recalls. I suggested that she and her husband take a trip to see one of the world's experts in RFT for children with disabilities, Darin Cairns in Perth, on the west coast of Australia. They were so impressed by the visit that they moved the whole family there—thousands of miles away—to try to save Samantha (lovingly called Sam) from a lifetime of disability. They expected to stay for three years at least.

Darin used a core set of RFT procedures to train Sam to develop her perspective-taking skills of person, place, and time. For example, Sam was told, "I have a cup, and you have a pen," and then was asked, "If I were you and you were me, what would I have? What would you have?"

Within a few months, Trudy was noticing improvement. Years later when I asked her to explain what happened, tears came to her eyes. "We were doing a lot of perspective-taking training. I was constantly grilling her on 'If I were you and you were me.' One day as Sam drove off to the clinic in the van, she turned and looked at me. And for the first time in her life"—Trudy began to stumble a bit on her words at this point—"she raised her hand and waved good-bye. I thought, 'Oh, this is it. This is what parents get.'" She paused and collected herself. "I thought, '*This* is what I've been missing.'"

Her sense of new awareness even let Sam turn the tables on her mother.

One day when Trudy got mad at Sam and scolded her, Sam left the room for a few minutes. When she came back, she put her hands on her hips and firmly declared, "If you were me, you'd know that was not fun!"

Sam was entering the world of *social* consciousness. As she was connecting with the "I/here/now" sense of self, of observing from a particular perspective or point of view, she also learned how to move her perspective across people, place, and time. Said another way, as Sam showed up behind her eyes, she realized for the first time that Trudy was behind Trudy's eyes. Sam could move her perspective over to Trudy's and look through her eyes. *That* was why she waved. She saw Mom seeing her.

After a year and a half the family moved back home. There was no need to stay longer. If you met Sam now, you would never think she had a history of autism. She is a well-adjusted kid.

This may be an exceptional case, but it is not an individual story. A recent study used procedures similar to those used with Sam with a group of children with autism, and all saw improvement in perspective-taking as a result. Entire programs are now being established around the world to work with children in this way, and the early data are very exciting. We will have to wait to see if the science continues to support this approach, but we are now dozens of studies into the journey and it still looks solid.

Making the Pivot

The Self pivot begins by catching the hidden sense of your transcendent self. As with my moment on the carpet, the experience is sometimes catalyzed by enormous pain and a sense of despair. Fortunately, RFT has led us to a set of simple methods that do not require any pain.

ACT has established a formula for connecting with our deeper sense of self that has four parts:

1. Undermine the attachment to the conceptualized self by applying defusion methods, like those described in the previous chapter, to the way we tell stories about ourselves.

2. **See how that opens the mental space to become aware of the perspective-taking that underlies a sense of self that is continuously present. When looking at mental content, notice both that the transcendent self is distinct from content ("I am not my thoughts") and that it contains the content ("I can hold my thoughts in awareness").**

3. **Cultivate habits of perspective-taking through exercises that shift your perspective along the dimensions of time (now is related to then), place (here is related to there), and person (I am related to you).**

4. **Use perspective-taking to build a healthy sense of belonging and interconnection with others in consciousness, in effect expanding the individual transcendent sense of self, *me*, into an interconnected sense of *we*.**

The first two exercises provided next will help you make your initial pivot. The next few in the starter set then help develop increasing awareness of your transcendent self and cultivate your sense of connection with others and of belonging.

On the other side of the Self pivot, your world changes. As you emerge behind your eyes, you begin to see behind the eyes of others. You notice people noticing you; you notice people noticing you noticing them. You sense a kind of awareness that binds us all together. You begin to find that you're making more thoughtful connections with people all the time—in the grocery store, in the elevator, at work, or at home. You will notice an old woman struggling to push her shopping cart through the store, bravely facing her own physical limitations; a waiter taking care to ask a customer what he wants; a child yearning for attention from you but being too afraid to ask.

When we touch our own consciousness in a full and open way, we are much better able to touch the consciousness of others. We see that awareness is far larger and more ancient than the space defined by our own mind and body. In a deep sense it is boundless, timeless; it connects us all to one another. *We* are conscious. That satisfies our yearning for belonging in a healthy, nurturing way, empowering us to be more fully ourselves and yet deeply related to others. You belong, as a birthright.

A Starter Set of Methods

As with building defusion skills, you will find that repeated, ongoing engagement with all of the exercises provided here will keep strengthening your perspective-taking muscle. Don't consider them one-offs; think of them as your set of perspective-taking calisthenics.

1. I Am/I Am Not

A good place to start is with this simple exercise. Following are three unfinished sentences. Take a sheet of paper and write them down. Now complete the top two with one-word answers that represent positive psychological attributes of yours. Don't put in mere descriptive attributes (e.g., *I am male*). Use terms that refer to your most prized personal qualities. Reserve the last for the exact opposite. There, list in a single word a personal attribute that you fear you have or think you have that is negative.

1. I am ____________________.

2. I am ____________________.

3. I am ____________________.

Let's begin by reviewing the top two "positive" answers.

I have a couple of simple questions: Is this true all the time? Everywhere? Toward everyone? Without exception?

You are such a liar!

What about the bottom one. Is it totally true, everywhere? Would someone else say the same thing if they could watch you 24/7?

Now another question: how many of these statements can you turn into a *comparison* with others? Try to do it with each one. If you wrote down *I am smart* or *I am kind*, see if these statements link to the idea that you are smart-ER or kind-ER (or dumb-ER and so on) than at least some other people. This isn't just your story—it's your story in *comparison* to others.

No wonder we begin to feel alone inside our own ego!

The beginning of a solution is to notice your fusion with these statements. Beginning with the first one and continuing through all three, change the period at the end of each sentence to a comma, and then write down these two words: *or not*. For example, *I am smart, or not*.

Now read each sentence again, slowly. Watch what happens. Take your time. If you find your mind filling with negative thoughts as you do this, use your defusion skills on them, saying to yourself, "I'm having the thought that . . ."

You may be able to sense something opening slightly—as if a little bit of air is coming into a room. You may feel that you somehow have more options about how you think about yourself. Don't try to hang on to that feeling—it will come and go—and don't get into an argument with yourself about which version is more accurate. The mental process we are cultivating here is reminding ourselves that we can refuse to buy one version of a story as compared to another. We're opening our minds to possibilities. See if you can notice that this sense of opening happens with both the "positive" statements and the negative one.

Now take the first sentence and cross out all of what you've written after *I am*. Who would you be without that content? Pause to consider the answer. Then do the same with each of the other sentences. What would it be like just to let go of that content?

This process raises the question: Who are you without all of your stories and defenses? Who or what are you trying to protect? If you woke up one day and all sentences like this were just sentences—they all had that open sense of "______ or not!"—would you still be you? If your mind replies, "Heck no!" take just a moment to notice who is noticing that mind of yours. Aren't you noticing that mental reaction? Isn't the you that is noticing a deeper sense of "you"?

As the final act in this little exercise, circle the two words repeated three times—*I am*—and consider them. What if the deeper sense of self we seek is closer to these two words alone? In crafting the story of our lives, we lose sight of this powerful alternative: just being.

There is one more step in this exercise, which helps us become more aware of when we tend to fall under the spell of our self-stories.

Ego-based stories are not just distorted, they also tend to be too general. In actuality, we focus on different aspects of our self-story in different circumstances. For example, when at home with our loved ones, we may focus on our view of ourselves as being caring; while at work, we might focus on our thoughts about being inept. Becoming aware of how our self-story changes according to different situations helps us stay better connected with our transcendent self, and therefore with our ability to choose among possibilities about how we will be.

So now, we're going to transform the "I am ______" statements by rewriting each.

First, instead of *I am*, write *I feel* or *I think*. For example, if you wrote *I am loving*, replace it with *I feel loving*. If you wrote *I am smart*, make it *I think of myself as smart*.

Next, qualify each statement by describing the situation in which you think or feel that way, including how your own behavior is involved, using this phrasing: "When [the situation] and I [your behavior] then [how you think or feel]." For example, "When my wife is disagreeing with me, and I take her perspective seriously, I feel loving," or "When I have a lot to do, and I take time for self-care, I think of myself as smart." You can also write descriptions of the situations in which you do not feel loving or smart. For example, "When I have a lot of work to do and I ignore my twelve-year-old son, I do not feel loving." (By the way, all of these examples are totally random and have absolutely nothing to do with me. Ahem.)

This is a far more useful form of self-description, guiding us about when and how we are not behaving in accordance with our authentic aspirations for ourselves. Keep practicing this exercise as you catch your self-judgments to become increasingly aware of their invitation into an overextended conceptualized self and how many options you have, just to notice and to carry them in other directions from a more transcendent sense of self.

2. Rewriting Your Story

Another way to step back is to write a brief story about yourself and then rewrite it.

Start with a couple of hundred words about something you struggle with psychologically—something that gets in your way and has a bit of a history to it. Be sure to describe some of that history and the internal and external ways that it interferes. Once you've done that, get a pen and draw a circle around all words that are reactions: thoughts, feelings, memories, sensations, urges, or actual behavior. Don't circle explanations for *why* you reacted: just the reaction itself.

Now do another run through of the story and underline every external situation or fact. I'm asking you to note reactions (circled) and external facts (underlined) because the mind sometimes mixes the two, which makes the next step harder.

After those two tasks are done, here is your challenge: rewrite what you have just written so that the theme, meaning, outcome, or direction is totally different, but every item that is circled or underlined is included in your new story. Mind you, I am *not* asking you to write a better story, or a happier one, or a truer one. It only needs to make sense, to fit well with the underlined and highlighted material.

Here is an example of the first story written by a client of mine. The external facts are underlined and reactions are "highlighted" here in boldface.

> I was **sad** as a child. I felt **alone** and **neglected**—my mother seemed more interested in her own misery than her children. I did poorly in school because I was more **focused on my fears** than on learning. The other **children didn't really like me** and the teachers were as inattentive as my mother. I was frequently the object of bullying and I **thought I was stupid**. It wasn't until middle school when I **realized I was smart** when I entered a team academic competition and we won the whole county. They then tested me and sat me down to say I should be in the gifted class. All of a sudden, the teachers saw me differently—but the kids not so much. I got the sense that even my parents now saw me differently—like "who is this kid?" Other children seemed to think I was strange, though. In high school the boys discovered me, and I learned I could get a lot of attention from them, which made me **feel great** on the outside—but I still **felt inadequate** on the inside. Somehow school success happened, but **I think it was in spite of myself**. I'm **surprised** I could get out of my way enough to even let that happen. Externally I guess some would say I'm a success, but with this history I live more with my own **self-doubts**.

Her rewrite was a revelation to her. What shocked her was that though not a single fact or reaction was changed, her conclusion changed considerably. You will recognize an ACT flavor in this rewrite, which makes sense since we had been working together within an ACT model.

> I was **sad** as a child. When I felt **alone** and **neglected, I focused on my fears** which may have contributed to my initially doing poorly in school. I think I had initially internalized an idea that I saw my mother pursue—when you are miserable, focus on that, not on what you have in front of you. That cost her a lot in terms of her ability to focus on her children and take in the love that was around her. I learned a lesson from watching that. When I felt that the other children really **didn't really like me**, or the teachers were inattentive like my mother, or when I **thought I was stupid** and even when I was bullied, I focused on what I could actually do something about. For

> example, in middle school I entered a team academic competition and we won the whole county. The decision to enter that competition had a profound effect, because after that success, the teachers saw me differently, and I was tested. Soon they sat me down to say I should be in the gifted class. Even my parents then saw me differently—like "who is this kid?" That got things rolling in a very different direction, and it all came from these little choices I was making to try to learn from my mother's mistakes. If some kids didn't appreciate me or thought I was strange, I found ways to get to do the positive things that brought me healthy attention. I think my confidence and achievement attracted others—for example, in high school the boys discovered me. I learned, whether I was **feeling great** or **feeling inadequate**, to focus on what I could do, one step at a time. I've had a **surprising amount** of school success as a result—I just got out of my own way and did what needed to be done. My mind tells me it was **in spite of myself**, but I guess we all have **self-doubts**. Bottom line, I'm a success.

Be careful with what your storytelling mind will do with this. Again, the point is not to write a positive story. This client ended up having a positive realization, and it's just fine if that is an outcome, but that is not the aim of the exercise—the point is to instill awareness that we are always story-*ing*. We are creating a narrative that is but one of many possible narratives. To heighten your awareness, you might even want to rewrite the story another time.

When we attribute our interpretations of our experiences to the situation rather than to our own way of seeing the situation, we shove our own meaning-making out of view. It's a form of self-delusion. This exercise is one way of applying defusion skills to our self-story so that we can take responsibility for the consequences that follow from the way we've interpreted events and how we've reacted to them. This rewriting process helps us see that we have a great deal of freedom and creativity in how we weave the story of our life situations, even very difficult ones.

One last step in this exercise really helps to drive that realization home.

Ask yourself: What if there is no one, true story, but only a variety of different stories that can be used in different settings and circumstances to promote different ways of being in the world? Which storyline will lead you forward to where you want to go? Which storyline seems most useful to you and under which circumstances? Who would you rather determines which storyline gets your attention? The Dictator Within, or your transcendent self?

3. One Truthful Conversation at a Time

Another good way to begin to let go of your self-story is to practice being yourself more fully and openly with another person. You can do this exercise during any conversation with a friend or co-worker you trust, and you can easily keep practicing it on a daily basis and with additional people.

Bring your full mindful awareness to your next conversation with the person you've selected. When a discussion regarding you comes up, such as how you are doing at work, notice any subtle ways that you are pulled to lie in response. Look carefully for exaggerations, overstatements, half-truths, statements of certainty when no certainty exists, or pretending you know more than you do. As you notice any pull to lie, direct compassion toward yourself for falling into this trap of human nature. Look at yourself the way you might if you were very young and just beginning to learn to lie. See if you can let go of the attachment to lying. If you feel safe with this person, see if you can speak more honestly. If that does not seem safe in this particular conversation, mentally note what you might have to do to be more honest in the next conversation with this person, or with someone else you trust. As these opportunities arise, try to expand the space you have to speak a more complete truth.

Also try to see if you can identify why you're feeling that tug. The point is not that we must strive to always be absolutely honest. That is simply not realistic. The point is to open the door to places that are hard—insecurity, inadequacy, fear of rejection, and so on—and to learn what is fearsome about them. If you can be mindful of any places where this is hard, you can use your acceptance and defusion skills to keep carving out more space for you to be you, with those feelings, more genuinely connected to others, one truthful conversation at a time.

As you feel more certain that you can speak the truth when it is safe to do so, deliberately seek out a conversation with a person who is a little less safe, especially if in the past you have succumbed to exaggerations or half-truths with this person. In order not to push too far past your comfort zone, discuss a topic that you feel confident will allow everything you say to be the truth as you know it. Keep your eyes open to what thoughts and feelings come up that make discussing the subject with this person harder.

4. Catching Self-Awareness on the Fly

Begin to regularly ask yourself the following question as you go about your daily life: "And who is noticing that?" You can set reminders on your phone or computer to do this. Or you could set a rule for times to ask it, such as whenever you touch your phone, or keys, or wallet. When the cues appear, take a moment to notice your experience and touch awareness for a split second as you ask, "And who is noticing that?" Be careful not to let the question lead to an extended mental treatise about who you are—that is your judgmental mind trying to tell a self-story. Shut that process down if it kicks in by using your defusion skills, such as by listening to the mental treatise in the voice of Donald Duck, or imagining that you are a pompous professor holding forth.

The goal is to touch the "I/here/nowness" or your transcendent self, even if just for a millisecond. Over time you will find that asking yourself this question becomes second nature and your connection to your authentic self keeps strengthening.

Keep practicing this set of exercises as you now move on to Chapter Eleven. You will quickly find that you are treating yourself with more compassion and feeling more genuinely connected with more and more people in your life. Then it's important to keep developing your perspective-taking skill by coming back to do the following exercises.

Additional Methods

5. Distinction Between Awareness and the Content of Awareness

You can do this next mini-exercise with your eyes open or closed, and you can practice it anywhere it is safe to engage in reflective thinking. Take a breath or two, notice who is noticing that sensation, and then note your experience. Whatever your mind settles on—an external object, an internal sensation, a thought, a feeling, a memory, or so on—get clear on it. Then restate the experience in three forms: first, "I am aware of [state the content]," and then, after a pause, add "I am not [state the content]," and then after another pause, add "I contain awareness of [state the content]." For example, "I am aware of the television. I am not the television. I contain awareness of the television" Or "I am remembering a memory of being five. I am not a memory. My awareness contains a memory of being five." Five or ten minutes is plenty of time for this exercise, and after the first engagement with it, you should practice it regularly for several days. Then, for ongoing practice, you can simplify the task. Just notice the experience and then state "I'm not that; my awareness contains that." Don't get drawn into an argument—instead see if you can touch a deeper awareness that your attachment to *any* content is distinct from awareness itself.

6. The Meeting Coming Up

Begin to practice perspective-taking regularly at work, socially extending this sense of "you" to include the awareness of the awareness contained in others. Suppose you have an important meeting coming up in a few minutes with a colleague. It could be challenging and you need to be at your best. You are prepared but feel a bit anxious. As you wait in your office, a wonderful way to spend those two or three minutes is just to consider this list of points and questions, which you could copy and post by your desk:

* As you sit here waiting, who is noticing you waiting?

* As you notice that, don't grab at it—just for a second touch that you are here, now, aware.

* As you think of this meeting coming up, search for a memory—in childhood if you can go that young—that is somehow related. Don't get there by cognitive analysis. Just let any memory pop up and then notice it for a few moments. Notice who else was there and what you were doing/feeling/thinking.

* In the original memory, who was noticing these things? See if you can catch your original sense of awareness as an experience, not a preconceived idea.

* You've been you your whole life. Whatever else may happen in this meeting, you will notice what happens there too. See if you can promise yourself to stand with yourself, becoming more aware of the rise and fall of experiences in the meeting.

* Picture the person coming to meet you. Imagine where they might be in this moment. Take the time to go behind that person's eyes and picture what they are seeing right now as they come to the meeting.

* What might that person be feeling? Take a moment to feel that.

* What might that person be thinking? Take a moment to think that.

* What might that person be worried about? Take a moment to notice that worry.

* What does this person deeply care about? See if you can sense that.

* **And what might this person care about specifically in the meeting coming up? See if you can experience these things.**

* **Now come back to yourself here and now. What do you most care about in this meeting?**

* **Then, as you come back into the moment, consider this: Is there a way for *both* of you to accomplish your deeper purposes of meeting?**

This exercise is essentially about developing empathy, as you will surely have understood. It is an extended form of the perspective-taking practice that Trudy taught her daughter, Sam, building your ability to connect with others not only more authentically, but with more compassion. This is a powerful means of developing your sense of connection with others.

7. Applying Perspective-Taking to Acceptance

This exercise allows you to use your perspective-taking ability specifically to help with acceptance of a difficult experience (I will expand on this skill in the next chapter). Go through this first by applying it to an experience that you struggled with. Then, by practicing it repeatedly, you will find that you can engage in a version of it even in the midst of a new difficult experience. It will become a powerful drill that you call to mind when hard things are happening in real time. To follow the instructions, record them on your phone as an audio file, leaving gaps between each bullet, and play it back.

* **Close your eyes and get in contact with whatever you struggled with. Take some time to feel what you feel, think what you think, and remember what you remember. Don't try to fix it—try to contact your pain.**

* As you do that, notice that a part of you is noticing that suffering.

* Take that noticing part of your awareness and imagine leaving your body and looking back at yourself. Notice what you look like from the outside but realize that inside you are hurting.

* Ask yourself (but do not answer . . . just hold the question in, in awareness): "What do I think of that person I see called 'me'? Is this a lovable person? Is this a whole person?"

* Take that point of consciousness to the other side of the room, leaving yourself sitting there. Now look back at yourself from afar. See yourself sitting there, suffering. You might notice also that there are others not too far away (in your house or neighborhood) and for sure some of them are suffering right now as well.

* Ask yourself again (but do not answer . . . just hold the question in, in awareness): "What do I think of that person I see called 'me'? Is this a lovable person? Is this a whole person?"

* As you picture yourself from across the room, imagine that you are reading a book that asked you to look at yourself from across the room while feeling something that was causing suffering. But it is ten years from now and you have grown far wiser. If you could pass back two or three sentences from that wiser future about how to be with yourself with this issue, what would you pass back to yourself?

* Sit with that for a few moments and mentally write yourself a short note of advice. Then come back to your body and open your eyes.

One of the interesting things about this exercise is that the notes people write usually conform to the wisdom the flexibility skills teach us: just be you; go for it; it's OK—this will pass; you are lovable; you can let it go. I believe this indicates that our natural consciousness is psychologically flexible, which means you have a constant ally in learning how to develop your own psychological flexibility: you have you. The whole, complete, genuine, authentic you.

Chapter Eleven

THE THIRD PIVOT

ACCEPTANCE—LEARNING FROM PAIN

In Chapter Nine we learned that the first step in turning toward acceptance is admitting to yourself that the things you've been doing to cope with difficulties haven't been working because their aim is avoidance. Now that you've begun practicing defusion and reconnecting with your transcendent self, it's time for the next steps in acceptance—turning toward your pain and beginning to open up to experiencing it and learning from it.

The defusion and self skills are powerful aids in the difficult work of learning acceptance. As we begin to allow ourselves to feel our pain, our fight-or-flight instinct will kick into high gear. Our minds will begin virtually screaming at us to go ahead and take that drink or push down that anxiety. All of the unhelpful rules we've been following will assert themselves ("It's better not to feel the pain, just numb yourself") and our negative self-talk will flare up ("You're not strong enough for this" or "This is too hard" or "Who are you kidding, you're just a failure!"). Our ego-defending self-deceptions will call out to us, pushing back on making behavior change and telling us we're a victim—"Why should you have to stop smoking, it's not your fault cigarettes are addictive."

Knowing how to acknowledge and then let go of those unhelpful messages empowers you to begin tapping into the wisdom of your pain. You can begin probing into the underlying motivations of the behavior you want to change. Just as I was able to catch that glimpse of my young self hiding under the bed as my parents fought, by building your acceptance skills you can begin to listen to your painful memories and cope with current distress in a less defensive, impulsive way. You'll start to hear helpful messages in place of the avoidant ones. You'll also be able to appreciate the central piece of wisdom our pain offers us—that our pain is due to a healthy yearning.

The Yearning to Feel

The great irony of emotional avoidance is that it denies one of our strongest human desires. We yearn for experiences that make us feel. It also denies us one of our greatest strengths. Feeling is a key to our survival—not only in helping us learn about dangers but in guiding us to the sources of joy and fulfillment.

Even newborn human infants will work for the opportunity to see, taste, hear, and feel. Every parent has watched and cringed as their small ones reach out and explore their environment. They rub, lick, stroke, poke, and fiddle. They bang, clank, roll, and throw, sometimes even in ways that are dangerous.

That yearning to feel does not stop with the five senses. Babies love to be surprised with a peek-a-boo or "threatened" with an imminent tickle and a smiling "I'm gonna getcha!"

As we grow up, we watch sad movies, horror movies, and comedies. We read love stories and daydream of the sweet moments we've experienced. You cannot name a single emotion, whether "good" or "bad," that people do not seek out (in a safe way) through song, literature, or art.

Of course, we like for feelings to stay within a range of intensity and predictability. We yearn to feel, but not excruciating pain. We like surprises, but would not want to be in a tall building on the verge of collapse. While babies laugh at peek-a-boo, they cry at a severe startle.

Avoidance is provoked when our emotions move beyond that comfort zone. Our problem-solving mind thinks it knows how to eradicate that discomfort by redirecting our inborn motivation to feel toward the effort to figure out how to feel *good* and avoid feeling *bad*. In effect, the "answer" the mind presents to the problem is to kill off the yearning to feel unless the feeling is good. Acceptance instead helps us spread our arms wide and take the bad (so-called) with the good (so-called) and open up our capacity to feel, sense, and remember. We learn to FEEL good, instead of trying only to feel GOOD. We say to the Dictator Within, "You can't make me turn from my own experience." We develop emotional flexibility.

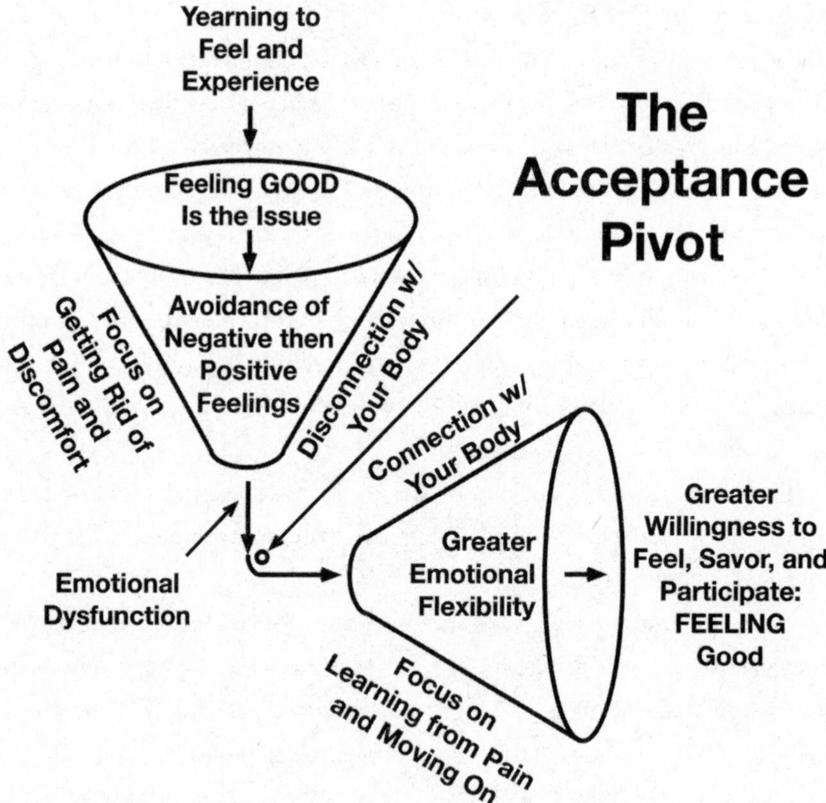

This pivot is not easy. No one should ever claim that it is, or expect it to be. But powerful methods have been developed for helping make it. And here is the wonderful future that this pivot can bring: as we develop the skill of acceptance, we can keep doing a better job of feeling and experiencing. I had a panic-disordered client once who said it this way: "I used to see my emotional life in black, gray, and white. Now I see in color."

We can even begin accepting the pain of our most damaging experiences. As I began writing this chapter, I decided to talk to one of our earliest ACT clients, whom I'll call Sandy, about how learning to accept the scorching pain of an abusive childhood has helped her heal and flourish.

The single hardest burden for a human being to carry is a lack of nurturance in childhood. Physical or sexual abuse, neglect, constant criticism: in the face of such treatment, our bodies and minds brace for a tough life ahead, even down to the level of how our genes are expressed. Genetics research has revealed that our life experiences influence which of our genes will become more or less active. For example, a specific group of genes is involved in responding to stress. A lack of nurturance intensifies their activity, making us less able to handle stress and decreasing our resistance to disease. We can also experience emotional instability or emotional blunting that can be lifelong.

ACT research has shown that these effects lead people to become psychologically inflexible—every one of the inflexibility responses has been associated with experiencing early abuse. Sandy knows all about that. But when I sat down with her to see where life had taken her, she was energetic and confident, and she showed great facility in talking about her difficult life experiences.

Sandy's father was bipolar, meaning his mood swung from periods of deep depression to outright mania. He abandoned the family when Sandy was three years old after nearly choking her mother to death in a rage. Shamed by his actions, he moved to a distant town the next day. Less than a year later he swooped in and kidnapped Sandy and her brother and sister. "He did ask me," she remembers. "He said, 'Do you want to live with me?' and of course I said yes. I wanted to see my father. But had he asked, 'Do you want to live with your mother?' I would have said yes to that too." She would not see her mother, let alone live with her again, for several years.

Her father eventually remarried, but his instability made for a chaotic home life and long periods of neglect. An older family friend raped her at age ten. Though she was terrified, she put up a fight, but he overpowered her. Even though he did not threaten her, "Somehow I knew the drill," she says. "I knew to keep my mouth shut." He raped her several more times. Years later as an adult she found out that her stepmother knew the man had molested other children. "I'm hearing this and I'm mad," she told me. "They knew! They left me with him!"

Sandy responded to the abuse, neglect, and instability around her by playing to her intellectual strengths while trying to suppress any sense of emotional need. Enrolled in a school program for gifted and talented students, she became the tomboy geek. "I was bright. And I knew it." Unfortunately, that was a kind of cover. "Deep down I think I felt I deserved to be abused. I wasn't worth much."

How can a young woman who was repeatedly raped when she was ten simply vanquish that emotional pain? How does she take her hand off *that* hot stove? She can't eradicate the pain; echoes of that experience will go with her to her grave. As we've seen, our memories are so deeply ingrained in our mind's complex thought networks that they can be triggered again and again, at any moment, even after we think we've dealt with them. They can be triggered by things we don't consciously realize have become related to one another in our minds. They are even triggered in our sleep.

Consider one of the ways this might occur for Sandy, which helps us see why our thought processes become so avoidant. Hearing the word *love*, or thinking about a loving moment, might trigger for her thoughts of rape, because the two might be joined in her mind by the relation of things being opposite. That relational frame can be easily brought to mind, which I've done sometimes in workshops in a very subtle way to make this point. I start talking in a low tone of voice and then slowly raise my voice. Just that change is enough to prime participants' minds to think of opposites, and when I then say the word *cold* and ask them to tell me what it made them think of, many respond that they thought of the word *hot*.

Our problem-solving minds think avoiding painful memories and current experiences is eminently logical, but this shows again why it is an impossible task. Cold reminds us of hot; love can remind us of rape. Sandy's experience with avoidance also demonstrates how denying our pain shuts us off from the wisdom it has to offer us. One of the horrible outcomes for sexually abused children is that they are likely to be revictimized if they suppress the pain of their abuse. That was what happened to Sandy.

When she was sixteen she was having a fantastic conversation at a social gathering at her church with a man in his midtwenties. Her intellect was on full display, and he was all ears. She felt warmed by his attention and flattered by his appreciation of her mind. As the party began to break up he asked if she wanted to come home to continue the conversation. Of course she did! "I was so stupid," she says. "I thought that meant he wanted to continue the conversation. I could not read the situation. It was like I had emotional blinders on."

Within a few minutes of arriving there, she knew something was wrong. He smiled oddly as he talked and he stood too close to her. Soon he was unbuttoning her blouse and pushing her toward the back bedroom. She put up resistance, but he was stronger. "As I did when I was ten, I knew the drill," she says. She protested feebly, whimpering slightly as he raped her on the bed.

After he fell asleep she assembled her clothes and left, walking home and crying softly. Again, she was reluctant to tell anyone. He was respected in the small town she lived in. "I thought it was my fault," she says. "I thought they would ask what I did to deserve it."

When she did tell a few friends, they were aghast at his behavior, but in a way they also *did* blame her. "What!" they asked in horror. "Go home for a conversation?! Didn't you know what he was going to do?!"

No, she did not; at least she could not consciously access that information, because she had unknowingly checked her emotions at the door long ago. That is true for many survivors of sexual abuse or interpersonal violence. They tend to be both experientially avoidant and alexithymic, which you may recall from Chapter One is a condition in which people do not know how to identify and describe their feelings. It's one of the most pernicious ways in which people deny emotions. If you do not know how to name your emotions, you can't talk about them, and from there it's a short step to convincing yourself that they don't exist. Children are especially prone to this defense mechanism, but it can easily extend into adulthood.

What is especially sad is that those who become alexithymic as children because of sexual abuse (which is a totally normal and understandable response to a horrible situation) are then more likely to be revictimized as adults, as Sandy was. Disconnection from emotions leaves people with less capacity to feel. That is dangerous. Like a person who could leave a hand on a hot stove and not know it, Sandy was more likely to go home with someone unsafe because she had hidden her feelings from herself. Her alexithymia meant that she had a harder time being responsive to cues that he might attack her as a result of her understandable attempt to push down the pain of her past abuse. She also experienced anxiety, depression, substance use, social isolation, and loneliness—all linked to avoidance.

In a way it seems almost unfair to ask survivors to learn new ways to hold their pain (and it *would* be imbalanced if the ACT community were not also finding ways to stop perpetration of violence and abuse—steps we will cover in a later chapter), but in the interests of love and life we have to do that, because the costs are so high. The cost is not just things like anxiety, depression, substance use, social isolation, and loneliness either. Experiential avoidance produces other long-term results that are just as upsetting. If we become more and more determined not to feel bad feelings, we have to begin to avoid positive ones as well!

My friend Todd Kashdan, a psychologist at George Mason University, was one of the first to show this clearly. He had socially anxious people report throughout the day on their smartphones about what they were doing and how they were feeling. The results showed clearly that anxious people are not anxious all of the time; they have periods of joy and happiness, such as when they're given compliments, invited to social gatherings, get good grades, and so on. But Todd found that those who were most experientially avoidant could not sustain these emotional highs as long as most people do. When good things happened, they did feel good about them, but their positive feelings rapidly plummeted! If you are not willing to feel pain, you cannot risk much joy. After all, the bigger you are, the harder you fall. Better just to be numb.

We found a number of ways to help people progressively become less avoidant. I wanted to talk to Sandy precisely because I knew she was able to turn her life around using some of the classic ACT acceptance methods. In the twenty-five years since Sandy had been in ACT therapy, she had married and raised three children. She has a good job as a respiration therapist and in her own words is "healthy and happy."

She told me that those twenty-five years have been filled with all of the usual ups and downs of raising children, and also filled with the work of learning to accept her past and her feelings. "I've learned there is more to me than my intellect," she says. "I've learned how to feel." After her husband died, she developed a long-term relationship and continued to apply her improving skills: "I've learned to tell him more of what is happening to me and more of what I want. I can talk about sex, I can talk about intimacy. I've been on an exciting journey of learning that it is OK to be me."

Almost every day she continues to work on her psychological flexibility, and she says of her journey, "I know it will never be done. It doesn't have to be. I'm not damaged goods. I'm not broken. I'm learning and growing, and that is enough."

The Gift of Acceptance

Recall that the word *accept* comes from a Latin root that denotes "to receive; as if to receive a gift." We still have that meaning in English, as when we say something like "I hope you will accept this as a token of my appreciation."

The gift we receive when we choose to accept our experience, pain and all, is the wisdom of being able to feel and remember fully in the present, without disappearing into a negative thought network about the past. The other flexibility skills are vital in assisting with this. Defusion, for example, helps us let go of the judgment that we should not feel pain. The result is that we can appreciate the gifts our pain is offering.

What gifts could possibly have arrived with my panic disorder? Once I began to work vigorously on developing my psychological flexibility, I received many of them. The first was that rediscovery of the eight-year-old hiding under the bed who reminded me of my life purpose. Soon, other difficult childhood experiences came to the fore. I recalled being sexually abused by a group of teenage boys at age four. Remembering my fear helped me be kinder with myself. I remembered how sad it had been to watch my mother sink into depression and struggle with OCD, and how anxious and awkward my father seemed when he was sober. Opening up to these memories helped me better understand clients who were experiencing the same struggles. Acceptance also helped me renew a loving relationship with my mother. I realized I'd blamed my mom for my dad's problems, and I sat down with her and asked her for forgiveness for the years I pushed her away (which she lovingly gave). I've received countless more gifts. They are not all sweet smelling—some of them are tearful and fearful—but they are all precious.

Exposure the ACT Way

After the impressive early results we saw in developing ACT-based exposure exercises, we continued to develop and test methods, and we now have many highly effective exposure techniques. Recall that exposure involves people deliberately putting themselves in emotionally difficult situations. In the traditional CBT approach to exposure, a person with agoraphobia might be instructed to go to a mall; someone with a fear of heights might be helped to climb a tall ladder. Since the idea had been that exposure worked by damping fear enough to engage in behavior without avoidance, people were constantly asked during exposure to rate how distressed they felt. The message was clear: exposure is a means to the end of not feeling anxious.

Research (much of it inspired by ACT and other Third Wave CBT methods) has shown that's not why exposure works. Instead, exposure assists with developing a new *relationship* to the source of pain or fear by being able to observe, describe, and accept our emotional reactions. That change in turn allows more response flexibility so that new learning can take place in the presence of fear or pain, and new ways of responding to them can be learned. The mainstream CBT community has now come around to this understanding of exposure, and CBT exposure methods have moved strongly in an ACT direction by including acceptance, mindful noticing, and new learning, rather than focusing on anxiety reduction per se.

Keep in mind that fundamental to the process of exposure is the understanding that progress will be gradual. The fruits of developing the skill of acceptance take time to ripen, and incremental steps are best. When you make the pivot, you are headed in a new direction, but walking in that direction is indeed a walk. And no matter how well you've developed your acceptance ability, experiences may come along that will continue to trigger your problem-solving mind's fight-or-flight instinct. That's why ACT adds the practice of defusion to exposure: to quiet the Dictator's commands to avoid. I'll introduce a number of exercises that do this, such as labeling emotions while revisiting a painful experience; making note of urges and distancing from them; and cataloging memories triggered.

Over time your acceptance muscles become stronger. New experiences become less threatening. Learning from both bad times and good ones becomes more possible. The emotional flexibility you develop is vital in committing to the new course of values-based living you chart for yourself.

All of the ACT acceptance methods are premised on three underlying principles:

> 1. ***Avoidance causes pain.*** The single biggest step in embracing acceptance is appreciating how dangerous avoidance really is. ACT uses a number of ways to make that message compelling, one of which is the quicksand metaphor. If someone steps into quicksand, the logical thing to do seems to be to pull a leg out and try to step forward. But the last thing you want to do is lift up a foot. That halves the surface area bearing your weight. So guess which direction you'll go—deeper down. Instead, you should lie flat on top of the mud and then gradually pull yourself to solid ground. That metaphor helps people see that it is actually safer to

increase contact with what is feared, rather than struggling to "get away."

2. ***Acceptance is in the service of valued living.*** An important modification that ACT made to exposure is to instruct that it take place in the service of valued action. Don't go to the mall just to expose yourself to the anxiety of being in a mall; go with the purpose of buying a gift for a loved one. If you're avoiding thoughts of death, don't go to the grave of a loved one to defeat your fear, but to honor your love and respect for the person who passed. In fact, knowing more about what your values are is one of the gifts that is fostered by acceptance, and acceptance skills will be critical when we begin to explore values in Chapter Thirteen.

There are many ways to make exposure more meaningful and even enjoyable. For example, if going to the mall is an exposure practice for you, in addition to doing it to buy gifts (after all, continually buying presents can get expensive!), you could focus on people watching, which is a way to build *now skills*, attending to the present moment rather than slipping into avoidant thoughts and emotions. When I am in a mall with a person who has agoraphobia, I'll wait until the person seems present and then ask, "Look at that guy over there. What do you think he does for a living?" or "Who in here has the worst hairdo?" The point is not to simply distract them from their anxiety. It is to show them that they can be OK enough with their anxiety to refocus their minds. That is why I always wait until they seem present, so that I'm reinforcing the value of that acceptance they're demonstrating. If you do this with the awareness that it's for the purpose of acceptance rather than avoidance, it can have good effect.

You can also slot in lots of other valuable activities, such as helping someone with a disability get through a doorway or engaging in conversation with a store clerk to brighten that person's day. Even having some tasty food counts as being valuable.

> 3. ***Acceptance is not about control.*** People often approach acceptance as though they're using a wrench that will adjust how much they open the valve of their emotions. They want to be able to control the process. This is understandable but misguided. Acceptance involves an abandonment of conscious control—you just open the valve in safe circumstances. You have to let the emotion be what it will be.

Sometimes people try to stay partially emotionally closed as they practice exposure. That will seriously undermine getting the benefits, and when you need to accept the most difficult experiences, the skills will not be there.

The most common limits people set are to try to impose a threshold on the strength of the fear or pain they'll open up to and to rule out ever facing certain issues. An example of the first is "I'm willing to practice acceptance as long as I'm not too anxious." That never turns out well. Why? As soon as anxiety ticks up a little, your mind will begin to worry that it might go higher and cross the threshold you set. That fuels more anxiety, and voilà, you are "too anxious."

This does not mean you can't set other kinds of limits. You can, for example, limit deliberate exposure by time ("I will go into the mall for five minutes") and by the type of situations and emotions you tackle. You can take your time and take incremental steps. There is no speedometer glued to your forehead. Overwhelming yourself by trying to tackle your most difficult feelings right away is counterproductive. Start with feelings, memories, and current experiences that are less intense. Others can wait until you've developed greater flexibility.

We use the metaphor of taking a leap not from a cliff but from a chair, or maybe the roof. You can control the circumstances of acceptance and therefore, to a degree, naturally limit how much emotion you'll expose yourself to. But that is because less is provoked, *not* because you're denying the feelings or trying to tamp them down. A leap is a leap—even if it is from a low stool. When we choose to accept, we've got to go "all in" or the benefits will not flow.

Starting out with less intense sources of fear and pain does not mean that you should rule out ever needing to face certain issues. Suppose you decide you will never face your sexual abuse history, and then you find the love of your life and discover you cannot open up a place of real intimacy because that place reminds you of the abuse? Suppose you decide you will never face the death of your father, and then your mother gets a terminal illness and you can't be there for her? We are all forced to "receive the gift offered" inside some kind of incredible tragedy. If you've worked on accepting your most difficult experiences, you'll be much better prepared for these shocks.

Applying acceptance methods to the most difficult experiences is best done after all of the flexibility processes are in place, however. Your growing psychological flexibility will guide you about when to tackle the next challenges. For this reason, in this chapter I'm providing only a core starter set of practices for you to do now. A number of more advanced additional practices will be introduced in Chapters Twelve, Thirteen, and Fourteen, which combine acceptance with presence, values, and action skill building.

One last point to make is that taking acceptance to the max is often best done with professional help, and you can find a list of several thousand therapists who do ACT at http://www.bit.ly/FindanACTtherapist.

A Starter Set of Methods

1. Say "Yes"

A core skill in acceptance is to be willing to have events be what they are. You can start practicing just by looking around. As your eyes land on anything, see what it feels like to look at it from the point of view of "no" meaning "no, that's no good; that has to change; I want that the hell out of here; that is unacceptable." Simply look at a specific thing you see, and mentally adopt a "no" approach to it, then move to another item as you scan the room and do the same, over and over. Do this for a couple of minutes.

Now repeat the scan but this time do it from the perspective of "yes" meaning "yes, that's OK; that is just like that; it does not have to change; I can allow that to be just as it is." Simply look at a specific thing you see, mentally adopt a "yes" approach to it, then move to another item as you scan the room and do the same, over and over. Do this for a couple of minutes.

Take a pause and see if you can sense how different the world seems inside "yes" versus "no." Back in Chapter Eight, I asked you to put yourself in a physical posture expressing you at your best and then you at your worst when faced with difficult experiences. If you were like most people, at your best your body assumed a more open posture (e.g., head up, arms out). The "yes" and "no" ways of looking at the world tap into a similar mind-set: the open and accepting one and the avoidant and controlling one.

A way to ratchet up this "yes/no" exercise is to add to it the physical postures exercise. This time, when you are doing the "yes" cycle, put your body in an open position—standing or sitting tall, palms up, arms out, head up, eyes open, legs apart—and when you are in the "no" cycle put your body in a closed position—arms in, head down, eyes lowered, legs closed, fists and jaw clenched, stomach muscles tightened. Notice very carefully how your experience differs.

You can move on to do this exercise with specific thoughts, emotions, urges, and memories. Over time, you will begin to notice as you go through your daily routines that sometimes you settle mentally and maybe also physically into a "no" posture without meaning to. Noticing the mental and physical cues can help you catch yourself and consciously adopt a "yes" posture instead.

2. A Caring Exercise

Pick a feeling or experience that you have a hard time accepting, one that's leading to unhelpful resistance. Start small. Then envision one of the following for at least one minute.

* **Hold your experience as you would hold a delicate flower in your hand.**
* **Embrace your experience as you would embrace a crying child.**

* **Sit with your experience the way you would sit with a person who has a serious illness.**
* **Look at your experience the way you would look at an incredible painting.**
* **Walk around the room with your experience the way you would walk while carrying a sobbing infant.**
* **Honor your experience the way you would honor a friend, by listening carefully even if it was hard.**
* **Inhale your experience the way you would take a deep breath.**
* **Abandon the fight with your experience the way a soldier might put down his weapons to walk home.**
* **Take in and carry your experience as you would drink a glass of pure cold water.**
* **Carry your experience the way you carry a picture in your wallet.**

These metaphorical ways of treating your feelings, memories, and current experiences are often powerful in building acceptance. That's true even if as you consider them your mind says, "I don't know how to do that." Give them a try over time with different memories, experiences, emotions, urges, or thoughts.

3. A Wider View

Feeling something painful or difficult tends to cause us to focus our attention narrowly, allowing pain or fear to loom large in our minds. If we bring a wider perspective to the experience, we can more effectively open up to the gift buried inside it.

Take some time to conjure up a difficult experience, bringing it fully to mind, and then consider these questions.

* Is there a specific bodily sensation that is associated with this experience, and can you say "yes" just to that sensation? Give yourself a minute to consider that and to see if you can. Don't rush.

* Have you seen anyone in your family struggle with something like this experience, and if so can you bring that memory to mind with the purpose of looking at their experience with compassion? Again, don't rush. Extract what you can from the question and then move on.

* Is there a specific thought associated with this experience, and can you say "yes" just to that thought? Think that thought as a thought and drop any sense of struggle with it. Just notice it.

* If you were to look back on your life from a wiser future, would you say there is something in this experience for you to learn from? Pause with this question. Don't get all mind-y. Don't try to figure it out or second-guess yourself. Just gently look to see, from a distant and wiser you, what might be inside this experience that would help you on your path?

* What does this experience and your struggles with it suggest you deeply care about? In your pain you find your values: what does this painful area say about your values and vulnerabilities? What does it suggest about what you want?

* If this experience were in a book you were writing, how might the character experiencing it become wiser or more alive as a result? In other words, if you were on a hero's journey, and this were a challenge, how could the hero use it to foster vitality and wisdom?

* Are there other memories associated with this experience? Can you say "yes" just to one more? Give yourself a minute to consider that and to see if you can. Don't rush.

* If you blame someone for this experience, can you think of times that you have done something like what they did? Perhaps in a lesser way? Sometimes we hold others responsible for our difficulties. Sometimes we even do so as a way to avoid seeing how our behavior is similar to theirs.

* If someone else you care about were struggling with an experience like this, how would you feel? What might you suggest that they do? Picture a friend with the same issue and allow yourself to connect with both of these questions. How do you feel about them, knowing they have this issue? What would you say to them about what they might do?

* What would you have to do to let go of a struggle with this experience? You picked something you say "no" to—what would you have to give up in order to let go of an attachment to that "no"? This is a subtle question: don't rush your answer. Open up all of your channels of sensing and being aware. Try to feel the answer more than overthink it. Is there something there you are holding on to?

* If you could feel this experience without defense, what would you be able to do in your life? Allow yourself to reach out and dream. Imagine you could take the experience along with you for an adventure. If you could, what journey would that be?

4. Practice Opposites

This is a more advanced skill that is a playful variation on the last method. Begin practicing this exercise whenever you find your mind telling you not to do something or think about something. This is a way of using fearful emotions and thoughts as guides to good exposure experiences.

If I'm working with someone on exposure to being at the mall, for this exercise I'll ask, "Where does your mind say we cannot go?" If the person answers, "Up the escalator," then it's up the escalator we go. It's always a choice—there's never a need to force it. You could choose an alternative, such as taking the stairs if that's less difficult, leaving the escalator on an action plan list of behaviors to commit to later on. But don't underestimate this exercise, especially if it has a playful mood. I've seen clients grab back territory they've abandoned for many years. It's a bit like deciding to ride a zip line or bungee jump for the first time—often once you begin, within seconds your fear is overtaken by a joyful sense of life expansion. Who knows? Maybe a parachute jump is next!

Chapter Twelve

THE FOURTH PIVOT

PRESENCE—LIVING IN THE NOW

I'm not usually chatty on planes, but on a recent flight the man next to me was, and I went along to be polite. Soon I was fascinated. He was a commercial pilot who lived in New Orleans and loved to sail boats competitively. He claimed spectacular success as a racer, particularly in his hometown. "You must understand the local currents and winds," I offered. "Of course," he answered a bit dismissively, adding, "but all locals do." After looking from side to side in a conspiratorial way, he leaned close and in a semiwhisper said he would divulge the secret of his success. Enjoying the drama, he paused and said, "I smell the coffee."

I looked at him a bit slack-jawed but no, he had not lost his mind. He explained his sailing advantage with a story that I checked out soon after I landed.

New Orleans is the second-largest coffee port in the country, and there are a few industrial-sized roasters spread along the Louisiana coast near the river. Each roaster is known for particular beans and qualities, and for that reason, each has a distinctive aroma. When miles offshore all he had to do was to notice the characteristic smells and voilà, he knew the wind direction! Using his well-trained nose and knowledge of the city, he could sense small wind changes far more rapidly and accurately than competitors who had to watch wind socks or hold up a wet finger. He tacked into these changes before others knew what was even happening. Sometimes his crew members would yell at him over what looked to be a totally irrational choice of direction, only to quickly settle down as the wind change became clear.

We are all surrounded by vast and potentially important information, both inside and outside of us, that generally sits there unnoticed and unused, especially when our attention is constrained and rigid. How many of us would think to smell their way through a sailing race? Perhaps very few, but a dog or cat needing to use this information would have no problem accessing it—not only because they are better smellers but because they live more in the present, which keeps them primed to learn by experience.

The inability to live in the present enormously reduces the information available to us. It's as if we're playing tennis while wearing sunglasses with a lens that's been rubbed with sandpaper. We're distracted by preoccupations that mar a clear view of the current moment.

I can show you in less than a minute how our attention becomes limited. Look around the room for thirty seconds and find everything that is colored black. Catalog every black item and then bring your eyes **BACK HERE** to these capitalized words.

Now, close your eyes and recall absolutely every item you saw that was a rectangle. No cheating!

■ ■ ■ ■

Are you back? Did you have trouble remembering rectangular items?

If I had asked you to count all the black things you'd seen, you could have done pretty well. But though you probably saw plenty of rectangular shapes—take a look around now for them—your attention was dominated by the rule to find black things, so your mind saw only *part* of what your *eyes* saw. There is a lesson here: our judgmental, problem-solving minds constantly pull our attention away from full awareness of the present moment.

Another way to demonstrate this is to look around the room and try to figure out what is wrong with everything you see. Look for flaws, item by item. Do it now, again for about thirty seconds.

■ ■ ■ ■

I bet the journey into a "now" that you were evaluating made you feel like you were more in your mind than in the room. You might have thought about how visitors who came recently must have noticed all the flaws, and you might have wondered what they thought of you because of those flaws. Maybe you berated yourself for not being more vigilant about fixing up your home, or for not having better design taste. And while you were busy with those thoughts, I bet you hardly noticed how your toes felt, or whether you were breathing freely, or whether the room was cool.

If the aroma of coffee was wafting through the room, you probably didn't notice that either. What if, like our sailor, there was something to be learned from your present experience? Too bad . . . you missed it.

The first three flexibility skills are all vital to empowering us to live much more in tune with the present and the learning it affords. All of these skills support us in making the pivot toward presence, away from preoccupation with the past and future to the possibilities of today. We can also build a number of practices for cultivating attention to the present into our life routines. This helps us stay on the path of living, day-to-day and moment-to-moment, in accord with our values.

The Yearning for Orientation

As you begin working on developing presence skills, it's important to understand that the pull into the past and future comes not only from the impulse to avoid suffering but also from a positive yearning—the deep desire to know where we are in our life journey.

Yearning for orientation makes sense. No one wants to be lost. If you suddenly found yourself in a strange place, you'd look around hard, trying to figure out how to get back. The problem is that instead of orienting us to where we actually are and the opportunities we have, our problem-solving mind tries to orient us by ruminating about what's happened in our past and worrying about what will happen in our future. We get fixated on questions like "Why am I here? and "How can I get somewhere else?" and "What's going to happen? How can I control it?" We are mired in the cognitive weeds of our minds.

We may be so involved in this supposed problem solving that we fail to appreciate that today someone was kind to us, or that we could make the time to call a loved one or to take a walk in the woods and revel in their beauty. Our desire for a mind-y form of orientation actually leads to *disorientation*: keeping us from appreciating the full range of our life choices that are here, right in front of us.

The Presence pivot redirects our yearning for orientation toward mindful focus on the here and now. The mindful part is vital; it helps us keep our attention on the potential to live every day with more meaning and purpose.

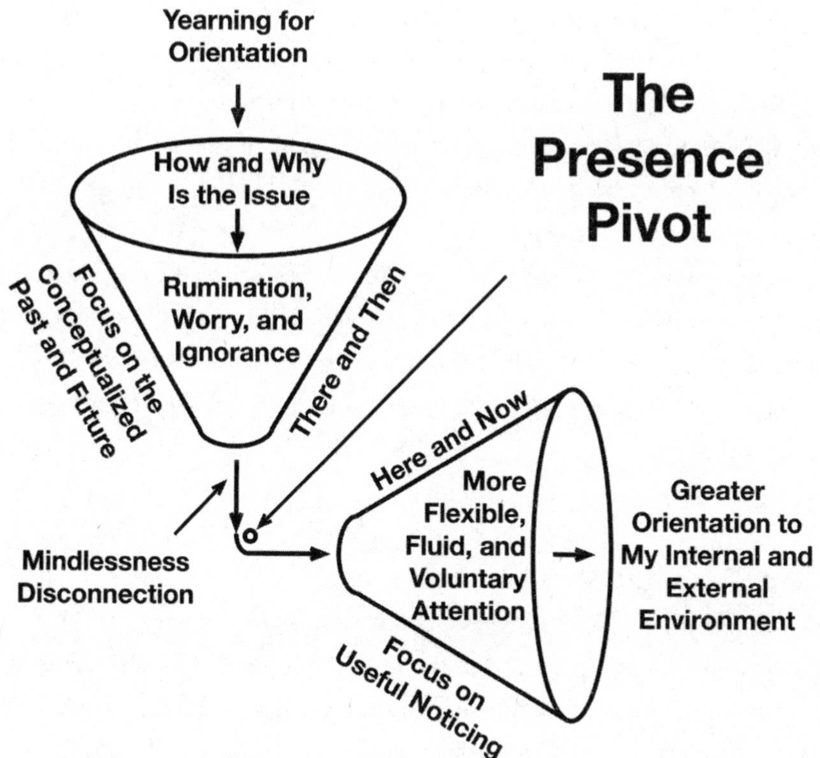

To understand what mindfulness means, it's helpful to turn to Jon Kabat-Zinn (a fellow traveler and professor of medicine emeritus at the University of Massachusetts Medical School). He is widely recognized as a path breaker in bringing an understanding of mindfulness to Western society, drawing from the rich tradition of Vipassana mindfulness training in Asia. Jon defines mindfulness as "paying attention in a particular way: on purpose, in the present moment, and non-judgmentally." ACT adds that this is fostered by the perspective-taking nature of the transcendent self. Jon agrees that mindfulness includes perspective-taking but avoids "self" altogether.

It's important to highlight Jon's emphasis on *purpose*. I think he is saying that our awareness should be directed toward being here and now so as to live the life we intend. Mindfulness is in no way an escape from the pressures and worries, hopes and fears of our lives. Traditional mindfulness methods are used to empower "right action"—being present in a way that helps us live in accordance with our chosen values.

Our talkative sailor's racing technique is a fine example of how purpose can guide presence. If he noticed the aroma of the wind because it was a way to distract from the race, his nose would not help him be a more effective captain. Instead, he used the aroma to be more attuned to his surroundings and decide which route forward was best. That is, in essence, what presence helps us to achieve.

With this understanding of mindfulness, we can see better how the other flexibility skills we've covered help enable it. Practicing defusion, connecting with our transcendent self, and opening to acceptance all assist with being nonjudgmental and keeping our minds from slipping into rumination or worry.

Being Mindful About Mindfulness

The last few decades have witnessed an explosion of interest in mindfulness, and ACT has been a part of the rise of that broad cultural interest. In fact, about 40 percent of the studies on ACT have included explicit attempts to encourage contemplative practice, and virtually all include some methods that are well-established components of mindfulness training. The ACT community has also added insights of its own about the value of mindfulness, and some cautions about not practicing mindfulness as a form of avoidance or unhealthy attention to self.

Consider the practice of meditation, which is a central element of most forms of mindfulness training. Meditation is now a widespread enough practice that you may know some people who demonstrate the potential problems with it. People can become selfish meditators ("You take care of the kids! I have to go meditate!") or avoidant meditators ("I'm feeling anxious! I need to go meditate!"). Some even become obsessive about their contemplative practice, turning into virtual meditation junkies. Research shows that meditation is most fruitful when practiced with the aim of building flexibility skills, not as an escape from the pressures of life and a way to try to suppress feelings. Meditation's benefits come specifically from using the practice to build attentional flexibility *on purpose*—to become more fully engaged in life, not to "get away from it all."

One recent study, for example, looked at how meditators and nonmeditators dealt with the challenge of performing the Stroop Task, which is a commonly used (and very frustrating!) measure of people's "executive control," the ability to organize information in our minds and effectively act on it. The Stroop Task requires extremely careful focus on the present moment. People look at words for colors, such as *red* or *blue,* that pop up on a computer screen. They have to say as fast as they can what the color of each word is. The trick is that the words are not in the color that they stand for. So the word *red* might appear in blue and vice versa. Until you've looked at the word *blue* printed in red and had to quickly say *red,* well, you've simply not lived. It is hard as heck not to blurt out *blue*!

In the study, the meditators scored better. And when the researchers looked into why, they found that the meditators with particularly superior performance had higher levels of emotional acceptance. Why would that be? Well, if you are trying not to be upset about a wrong answer, guess what you are focusing on? The emotional impact of the last word, not the work of identifying the one that just popped up.

In short, as we work to become more mindful, we need to watch out that our minds don't turn this helpful process into yet another method of avoidance. As a kind of warning, one study recently showed that a focus on observing what is present can lead to *more* rumination, which can lead to more depression. It matters what mindfulness is for.

I talked recently to a college teacher who learned this lesson the hard way. I'll call him Fred. He'd done well on his own developing his psychological flexibility skills with ACT self-help books, but he e-mailed me some time ago asking for assistance in finding an ACT therapist. About a year later, he sent me a thank-you note saying how well it had gone, and I called him to learn more.

Fred's story was so much like mine it was downright spooky. He even had a variation of the dinosaur dream as a kid! In his version he was trying to defeat a monster by finding the right spell in a big book, and finally learned to put the book down and hug the monster instead.

Fred had spent several desperate years inadvertently using mindfulness practices as a method of avoidance or problem solving. He was trying to overcome intense anxiety attacks that had started while he was giving a lecture to one of his classes. Within months he'd built that experience into a terror of speaking in public (more that we had in common). He'd also developed an obsessive fear of poor sexual performance after having one obsessive thought show up with his girlfriend—"I hope that same thing happening in class does not happen here!"

For Fred, mindfulness work was "the search for the silver bullet." He told me, "I did Vipassana meditation; I studied Buddhism; I read Thich Nhat Hanh; I went to his retreat center. But always in the back of my mind was whether this was going to solve my problem. At my lowest point, I remember being on the verge of a panic attack while trying to tell a story to my best friend. My world had shrunk down to an inch or two beyond my own skin."

When he read about ACT shortly after that low point, he remembers, "I was washed over with the relief of knowing that I could drop the search for the magic bullet." He said he realized he had to shift how he used his mindfulness skills. "One of the biggest changes was that I would just sit and watch all the fear inside me, moment to moment, and not ask it to change one bit. I just wanted to see what was going on, and when fear came up linked to something I care about, I refused to buy into 'no.' Instead, I said 'yes.'"

Within three months of adding acceptance to his mindfulness practice, he had applied for a competitive teaching fellowship that required a weekend full of intense interviews in front of panels of big players in the educational world. He told me that doing so "would have been unthinkable three months earlier." He won the fellowship, and he has continued to make good progress in his ACT journey. Last year he developed a successful invention and went on a demanding business tour to sell it. "My life has a richness that simply wasn't there when I was struggling to find the cure for my anxiety," he said to me. "To be honest, it is a richness that I thought I would never know again."

His mind is still telling him he needs to worry: about talking in public, about whether he will embarrass himself sexually. "The mind is still the mind," he says. "There are days when it feels like my mind is just throwing the kitchen sink at me. But it's easier to take it less seriously now. It's easier to focus on what I care about most deeply, welcome all the fear, and let my heart make a choice about how I want to live."

Using Your Mind as a Flashlight

Learning to attend to the here and now can be compared to boosting the range of your vision, but in a specific way. The roots of the word *attend* mean to stretch out toward something. In developing mindfulness we want to increase the range of our awareness and ability to focus it in a chosen direction.

Do you recall that I earlier compared expanding our awareness of the present to using a flashlight to see better? Well, I like that analogy in part because I'm a flashlight nut. I love them, and I have many cool ones. My wife gave me one last Christmas that has a beam that can be adjusted to be very narrow or very broad and everything in between. I've got another that can be converted into a camping lamp that casts light in all directions. Still another is actually three flashlights clustered together—each of which can be cast in a different direction.

Training our attention is like learning how to use such high-tech flashlights. We can practice adjusting our focus in all sorts of ways. Meditation is just the best known of these methods. These practices don't have to be complicated or time-consuming. Many types of meditation have been popularized, including mindfulness-based stress reduction (MBSR), developed by Jon Kabat-Zinn, Transcendental Meditation, and bodily focused traditions such as yoga and zen. Those would be fruitful for you to learn, but when starting out to use meditation for psychological benefit it's best to keep it simple and brief. The research on meditation, for example, shows that only about 7 percent of its benefits are determined by the sheer *amount* of practice.

The *quality* of the practice is more important than the time devoted. A little meditation done right can go a long way. Some of the benefits come immediately. A recent study found that having people meditate just once for fifteen minutes led them to make better financial decisions. One of the researchers explained the finding this way:

> A brief period of mindfulness meditation can encourage people to make more rational decisions by considering the information available in the present moment. Meditation reduced how much people focused on the past and future, and this psychological shift led to less negative emotion. The reduced negative emotion then facilitated their ability to let go of "sunk costs" [throwing good money after bad when a poor financial decision is made].

A Starter Set of Methods

I am going to focus here on simple methods that have proven effective. If you do not yet have a more complicated form of practice, I recommend starting with these, each of which can be performed in just a few minutes, which helps with doing them regularly. Consistent practice is key to lasting results.

Ideally, you should make a few of these part of your flexibility skills toolkit, practicing them often enough that you can do them by heart. That will allow you to call on them at any moment when you find your attention being unhelpfully pulled into the past or future. You can make them part of your daily life routine, whether that's in the morning right after waking up, while in the shower or having breakfast, or perhaps in the middle or at the end of the day. You will immediately begin to see the positive effects on your ability to focus on the things you want to be attending to, and that is often highly motivating in continuing with daily commitments. Consider sticking to a daily flexibility practice as your first commitment to living your more values-based life.

For the initial set I'll begin with a simple meditation technique and then introduce a few attentional flexibility exercises. Once you've read the rest of the Part Two chapters, you can come back here to do the rest and then decide which you want to keep practicing.

1. Simple Meditation

A wonderfully simple method of meditating was laid out by a friend of mine from graduate school, Raymond Reed Hardy, in his book *Zen Master*. What he suggests is not new—it is just the simplest possible beginning. Here are the instructions. Sit down, back straight, eyes slightly open, cast your eyes downward at a forty-five-degree angle, and maintain a soft focus (don't sharpen your visual attention to any particular point). If you are uncomfortable sitting cross-legged, sit in a chair with your feet flat on the floor. Allow your mind to come to rest on your breath. Each time you find your mind has drifted away, release it from that train of thought and then allow it to settle again on the breath.

That's it. Do it for a few minutes a day.

How can such a simple practice work? It builds your attentional muscles. Each time you notice that your mind has wandered, you are strengthening your ability to notice and to regain focus.

2. Single and Multiple Targets of Attention

Get your smartphone or another type of timer and set the alarm for two minutes. You can do this sitting or standing. I will give you the instructions and then you can start the timer and close your eyes and focus.

For the first two minutes direct your attention to the sole of your left foot. Focus on what it feels like. What are the sensations you can feel there? See if you can sense that blood is pulsing through it. See if you can notice how warm or cold it is. See if you can be aware of the amount of space that is taken by your foot. Notice if your attention wanders and gently bring it back to the sole of your left foot. Continue to focus on what your left sole feels like. Don't stop until the two-minute bell rings.

OK, start the timer, close your eyes, and begin.

▪ ▪ ▪ ▪

If you are like most people your mind did wander, but sooner or later you noticed it wandering and brought it back. You probably also noticed things about the sole of your left foot that you don't usually think about: sensations, qualities, features. You may have noticed its size or its shape or a tingling or warmth.

Now set the timer for two more minutes and do the same with the sole of your right foot. See if you can deepen the awareness of sensations and observations this time, such as noticing even more aspects or features. Again, if your mind wanders, gently bring your attention back.

OK, start the timer and begin.

▪ ▪ ▪ ▪

What did you notice this time? Did the time seem to pass more slowly? Did your mind start telling you there was nothing new to learn?

Now set the timer for two more minutes and see if you can be continuously aware of the soles of *both* your left and right foot simultaneously. Try not to alternate, but instead broaden the beam of your attention to allow you to see both at once. If your mind pulls you away, gently redirect it back.

■ ■ ■ ■

What did you learn? What did you notice? Did your observations and awareness come and go? Did you find yourself sometimes focusing only on the left and then the right, while at other times you could do both? That's great! Directing your attention first to one foot and then the other not only builds attention in the present, it builds *flexible* attention. Remember that the goal is directed attention that is both flexible and voluntarily.

This is a version of one of the most effective and yet simplest mindfulness exercises, developed by mindfulness researcher Nirbhay Singh. Studies have shown that it helps reduce aggressive behavior in children or in adults struggling with chronic mental illness. It can help people stop smoking. It can help children with a biological inability to feel full to keep from overeating. This exercise helps focus awareness by grounding it, very much as a boat is stabilized by an anchor. Your feet become anchors. Grounding awareness undercuts the automatic thoughts and behavior processes that pull people quickly from anger to aggression, from having an urge to actually smoking or eating. It opens up a tiny window of choice while damping down emotional and cognitive reactivity. I prefer it at times over the more common practice of following the breath. For one thing, you can use it anytime and anywhere—even while talking (try *that* with a "follow the breath" approach!) For another, many forms of anxiety involve difficulties with breathing, and focusing on breathing can be an invitation into panic.

3. Broaden and Narrow Attention

As an extension from the soles-of-the-feet exercise, you can train your mind to broaden and narrow its focus by doing attentional work with any rich sensory experience. Listening to music is a great example, and successful attention training programs such as metacognitive therapy have commonly used it.

If you want to try it now, put on some music you like, which must feature multiple instruments. You're going to shift your focus from one instrument, or a group of them, such as the strings, to others. It's best to have a plan for where you'll put your attention before you start, so that the music doesn't take charge and dictate your focus. You can use a one-minute timer on your phone to remind yourself to shift focus. As you listen, first note the combination of instruments and then focus all of your attention on just one of them, say, the bass, or one group of them. After a minute, focus on another, maybe shifting to the drums, and so on. Finally, shift your attention back to the entire band or orchestra. Then cycle through these different focuses again once or twice.

4. Open Your Focus

Many attention practices teach you to narrow your attention, instructing you to focus on and repeat specific words (a *mantra*), or to look only at a small spot on the wall. But as I've been saying, it's just as important to broaden your attention. One practice I rather like is called Open Focus. In this approach you consider entire sets of events at once (you have to soften the focus on any particular event to do this). The set can be composed of people, objects, sequences of thoughts, notes in music—really anything. Once you have a set you are interested in, focus on the physical or temporal space between the events: the physical space between objects, for example, or the empty gaps between thoughts or the notes.

To clarify how to do this: look at the room you are in, focusing sequentially on specific objects. Then soften the focus on any particular object, and focus on the relationship (the "space") between most or all of the objects in the room. With a few minutes' practice of alternating between these two sets you'll sense you're using different attentional strategies. You can feel a softening and expansion of your attention as you adopt an open focus, and then a sharpening and narrowing as you focus on each particular object.

A good way to practice this in daily life is during work meetings. In the next meeting you are in, see if you can flip back and forth between focusing on a specific speaker or listener and then on all the attendees at once.

Additional Methods

5. Getting Present with the Past

One of the most difficult challenges in focusing on the present is that our minds are so often "hooked" by the past—memories, emotions, and thoughts are all embedded in our mental networks and easily triggered. A helpful way of reminding ourselves of these hooks is the acronym I'M BEAT. If you notice you are being pulled from the present moment, see if you didn't just get hooked by Interpretations, Memories, Bodily sensations, Emotions, Action urges, and Thoughts of other kinds (such as predictions and evaluations). Once you make yourself aware of them, you are back in the present! Said another way, the way to get unhooked is to bring full awareness to the hook itself. Almost always you will find the hook inside the I'M BEAT list (which is not a bad acronym since without awareness, these reactions *will* beat you down).

Here's a great exercise for learning to counter the pull of the hook.

Deliberately bring a memory to mind and then say to yourself, "Now I'm remembering that . . . ," continuing the statement by briefly describing the memory in one short sentence. For example, you might say, "Now I'm remembering that my boss told me I would never amount to anything."

As you do this, be on the lookout for any emotions triggered; any bodily reactions, such as a tightening of your gut; thoughts that may arise; or an urge to do something. Also be alert to other memories that might pop up. When you're done with the statement of the memory, attend to these emotions, thoughts, and other sensations one by one, saying, for example, "Now I'm having the emotion of sadness." If you had the thought, "That should never have happened," you should state it as "I'm having the thought that that should never have happened." If you lost track of the responses you wanted to describe, go back to the memory and restate it to capture them again if you can. For other memories that pop up, go through the same exercise.

This simple phrasing "I'm having the thought that . . ." is a powerful means of bringing defusion into mindfulness, creating a little distance from our thoughts and emotions and impulses that allows us to be in the present moment with them. The thought or feeling may be *about* the past, or the future too, but by these tags you are alerting your mind that this reaction is occurring in the now. Cultivating that awareness develops a powerful habit of mind that can help us stay on course even when the most difficult memories, thoughts, and emotions present themselves.

6. Inside/Outside

This last exercise helps build our ability to be aware of our internal experience while also attending to whatever tasks we're engaged in, not getting rigidly fixated on either.

While you're engaged in some task, say gardening or a household chore, keep paying attention to what you're doing but also shift some focus to what's going on inside your body. This is very much like focusing on both your feet. Allow any physical sensation to step forward but without grabbing all of your attention. Where do you feel this sensation? Notice the edges. What is the quality of the sensation? Hot/cold? Tense/calm? Throbbing/constant? Tight/loose? Rough/smooth? Remember to stay with the activity as you do this.

Now bring your attention more fully again to the task, but also continuing to be aware of the sensation. How is the sensation related to the task? How are your feelings about the task, and your degree of focus on it, related to the sensation?

Your insides are reacting to the task, and your feelings about the task are impacted by that. Maybe you're feeling deeply satisfied by seeing how well your flowers are growing and you notice that you have a physical internal sensation of pleasure even while you are also feeling some pain in your knees and arms. Or maybe you're feeling bored with the task and you notice that you're also feeling a slight sensation of hunger. It's important that you allow your awareness of these interconnections to emerge from just shifting your attention around from inside to out and that you don't start problem-solving and giving yourself a rule—"I've got to find a connection!" This exercise is one of attentional focus, not of diagnosis. It helps us keep our attention limber so that we're more fully present in the moment, with both our bodies and our minds. Over time, this helps us experience the present moment more fully, staying alert about whatever information may be presenting itself to us that can be useful, like that scent of roasting coffee my sailor friend picked up on.

Chapter Thirteen

THE FIFTH PIVOT

VALUES—CARING BY CHOICE

One of the greatest sources of psychological distress is losing touch with the values that are truly meaningful to us. I had a client who, when asked about her deepest values, paused for a long time before pushing out the words, "That's the scariest thing I've ever been asked." After another long delay she added, "I've not thought about that in a long, long time," and began to cry.

That is the most common emotional reaction to connecting deeply with values. I've seen it scores of times in therapy. I suspect it's also why we cry at the sight of a newborn baby, and why tears flow at weddings. It's why sometimes our eyes tear up at a spectacular sunset. We're feeling connected to aspects of life we treasure.

The Yearning for Meaning

There is no yearning more important to human beings than to freely pick and pursue our life direction. A clear sense of self-directed meaning provides us with an essentially inexhaustible supply of motivation. But we can easily lose sight of what is actually meaningful to us, pursuing socially compliant goals and superficial gratifications instead. Every tick of the clock can mock us with the emptiness of such a life.

We misdirect our yearning for meaning for a number of reasons. One is that we don't trust ourselves to make good choices, and we escape from the freedom life gives us. We fear we might pick a life course we don't have the necessary qualities to pursue. Maybe we value dedicating ourselves to raising children but doubt we'll be a good parent. Or perhaps we aspire to get a graduate degree to explore new knowledge, but we question that we have the intellectual prowess. We also worry that our values may be out of step with cultural norms, leading us to be looked down on, left out, or even ridiculed. Maybe we would prefer to leave our high-pressure, well-paying job and spend more time with our family, but we stick with it because we're convinced people will think less of us if we quit. We cling to our conceptions of ourselves and fear being free to pursue a life direction—perhaps because our sense of self is fused with being that successful lawyer or business manager, while deep down we know we want to be a therapist. Most commonly of all, we turn away from our true values because of past pain we want to avoid. We might convince ourselves that we don't value loving relationships because someone we loved hurt us. Thus, all forms of psychological rigidity show up inside our mishandling of the yearning for meaning and self-direction.

In the main, our culture doesn't help people choose their own sense of meaning. Instead, we're encouraged to define what gives us a sense of worth by chasing superficial wants. We mistake a quick hit of gratification for a sense of meaning, and we accumulate things and achievements, pursuing a long list of socially mandated "shoulds." The dominant social message is that our worth is evaluated by our possessions and by culturally approved forms of achievement or compliance with social expectations, whether that's work success, getting married and having children, or even "being happy." We may find those things authentically meaningful, but if we are pursuing them in order to avoid the pain of social censure and of our own self-criticism for failing to make the grade, they will be an empty sack.

Consider the effects of materialism, the belief that possessions and their acquisition will lead to life satisfaction. Studies have been done in which people fill out surveys asking if they agree with statements such as "Some of the most important achievements in life include acquiring material possessions;" "I'd be happier if I could afford to buy more things"; and "I like to own things that impress people." Agreement correlates significantly with anxiety, depression, negative self-assessment, and low life satisfaction.

Fame, power, sensory gratification, and the adulation of others all are unfulfilling "wants" and "shoulds." Once we are grasping for them, enough is never enough. Billionaires asked what it will take to have enough money have been known to answer "more." Buddhists call this state of focusing on achievements and material wealth "attachment," and they identify it as a core cause of suffering. We lose sight of what actually motivates us in a lasting way, and the more we grasp, the more miserable and out of balance we become.

The Values pivot allows us to redirect our yearning for meaning toward the pursuit of the activities that align with what we truly find meaningful.

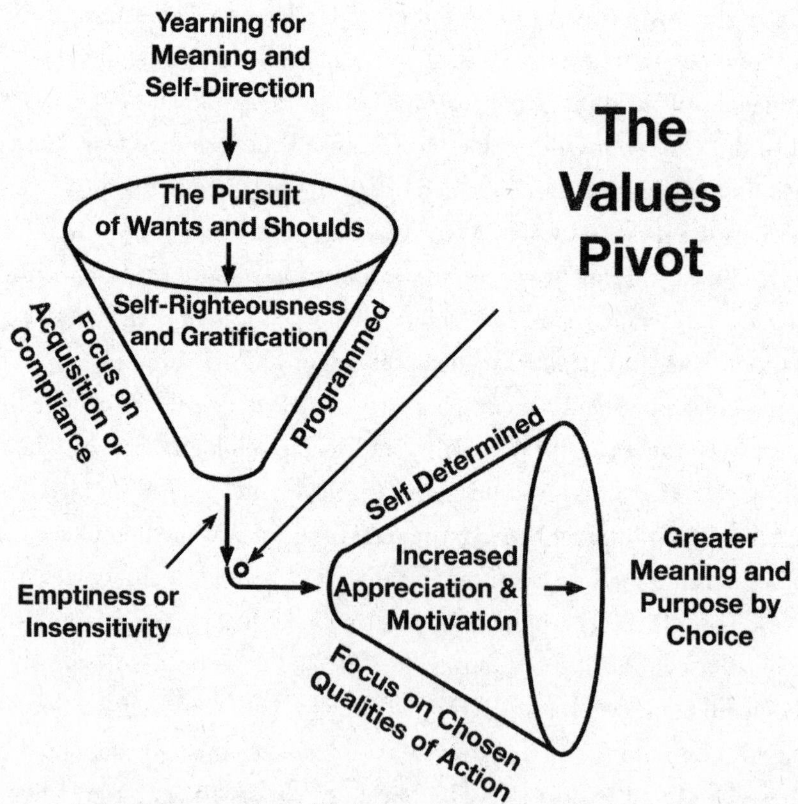

The four flexibility skills you've now been developing are of great assistance in making this pivot. Here's how.

Acceptance Allows Us to Listen

If we're blocked from connecting to our values because we're trying to avoid pain, we ironically only contribute to our pain. By listening to our pain instead, and moving toward that yearning to feel, we can identify the discrepancies between the way in which we're living and the way we want to live. Pain is like a flashlight if we know where to point the beam.

I once had a depressed and anxious client, whom I'll call Sam, who told me fairly early on in therapy that the effort to help him was pointless because life was empty and there was no real reason to live. As I tried to explore with him things he cared about, he was slippery and at times even provocative. For example, he said in a matter-of-fact way that he really did not care about family, or children, or even having intimate relationships. "I just don't think that life is for me," he claimed, and shrugged as he shifted in the chair, as if to say with his floppy body: *Who cares? Who cares if I have love in my life? Who cares if I ever have rugrats? Prove to me it matters.*

As his eyes caught mine, though, I did not see indifference. I saw pain.

I did not confront him then and there. Instead I sent him out with a simple homework assignment: to notice places he was hurting and to consider the possibility that these places were ones he cared about. He said he'd do it but did not expect much from the exercise.

When he came back the next week he said, "I'm such a liar, even to myself." He reported sitting in a fast-food restaurant having a hamburger when a family came in and sat down at the next table to eat. As he watched the mother, father, and two small children unwrap their burgers, he was surprised to notice a feeling of sadness. Instead of shaking it off as he would usually, he remembered what I asked of him and looked more closely at what he was feeling. Metaphorically, he opened a long-closed door to his inner self.

A wave of intense sadness washed over him and he turned away from the family, trying not to show his tears. Next he felt a shock of yearning. He *longed* to be in a loving relationship and to be a father.

As he told me this in session, the tears began again and he had to choke out his words. He then told me about his long history of childhood neglect and traumatic betrayals by his parents and stepfather. He had for many years dealt with that pain by trying to shut down his caring and focusing instead on his work and success.

But his "success" was not sustaining him emotionally. He was like a person lost at sea who has decided to drink ocean water because he was thirsty: the immediate effect might be quenching, but the net result is greater thirst.

To help clients see how their pain relates to their values, I tell them that as they open up to pain they should flip it over and ask, "What would I have to not care about for this not to hurt?" I've never met a person with social phobia who did not deeply desire to be with people in an open way. I've personally never met a person with depression who did not deeply desire to be vigorously engaged in life again. In your pain you find your values, and in your avoidance, you find your values disconnection. Without emotional flexibility and openness, it's impossible to live according to chosen values.

By the way, I saw Sam a few months ago for the first time in nearly twenty years. He went on to have a family and to found a business that allowed him to work with scores of children over the years. His two sons, now adults, run his business with him. He is proud of them and happy about their time together. All of that never would have happened had he not used his pain as a flashlight to help him find his values and the direction he really wanted his life to take.

Defusion and Self Skills Allow Us to Stop Judging

The problem-solving mind loves to sort through reasons that we should or should not do things, which is great when doing your taxes or choosing which stock to pick. But it's a *lousy* way to pick values. That's because coming up with justifications assumes we need some reason to make a choice—other than that it is simply intrinsically meaningful to us. If I tell myself I should value being a good father because that's what society expects, then I'm robbing myself of a connection to the fact that I actually choose to be a good father, because it's so richly meaningful to me. Once we focus on justifying our values, we're falling under the sway of pliance, and that often pulls us away from what we really care about. By defusing from judgment, we can satisfy that yearning for coherence that sits inside that we really want; by connecting with our transcendent sense of self, we can foster the yearning for belonging that resides inside our values.

When I want to show my clients how tricky it is to have all sorts of reasons for their values, I stick out three fingers of one hand and put it behind my back. Let's say that a client has told me that he is happy with himself because that day he chose to eat a salad for lunch rather than the cheeseburger he craved. I would ask him why, and the dialogue would proceed something like this:

> ***Steve:*** Why did you choose the salad?
>
> ***Client:*** It has fewer calories. [Justification 1]
>
> ***Steve:*** Why is having fewer calories important?
>
> ***Client:*** It keeps me from being unhealthy and overweight. [Justification 2]
>
> ***Steve:*** Why is avoiding being unhealthy and overweight important?
>
> ***Client:*** Because I will live longer! [Justification 3]
>
> ***Steve:*** Why is living longer important?
>
> ***Client:*** . . . I don't know. It just is! Everyone wants to live longer!

I bring my hand out from behind my back, with my three fingers still stuck out, and I explain to the client that usually this questioning goes no more than three rounds. By the fourth question, if not sooner, almost everyone has answered with, essentially, "I don't know." This helps them to see that they've been buying into the need for all sorts of culturally scripted reasons and not really appreciating that the answer is not really all of the *whys* anyway. It is far closer to the truth just to say "because I *choose* to."

I recall once working on weight control with a client with diabetes who, after a values conversation, said she was going to work on her health so she'd have a better chance to see her daughter grow up. It rang true; I sensed that this was her authentic motivation. Just to test that, though, I asked her why seeing her daughter grow up mattered. She wasn't fooled. "It doesn't," she said a bit flippantly, and then after a short pause she peered down at me over her glasses and with a clipped intensity added, "except . . . to . . . me!"

Saying that we freely choose our values doesn't mean that our choices aren't shaped by family and cultural influences, such as parental guidance and being taught religious beliefs. We absorb these teachings, but as we do, we exercise our ability to choose, even if we don't acknowledge that to ourselves. All choices are informed by our history. But justifying our choices with the rationale that they're what we were taught is a way of avoiding personal responsibility. This is a precept of all the world's major religions. They emphasize that human beings have the capacity to choose to live in accord with religious teachings or not. The affirmative leap to do so is often called a "leap of faith."

Defusion and self skills help us stop the justification process from kicking in and connect with others in a deeper way. We learn to catch ourselves as our minds begin spinning out compliant reasons for our behavior. They also help stop self-recrimination as we begin doing values work. The Dictator can become quite harsh as we begin acknowledging to ourselves that we haven't been living in accord with our values. It will start berating us—"See I told you, you're no good. You're a hypocrite, a charlatan." We may also get caught up in excessively evaluating whether we've chosen the right values, ruminating over whether they're really our "true values." With the ability to disregard these unhelpful messages, values work is freeing rather than punishing.

Presence Helps Stay Focused on the Ongoing Journey

Recall that earlier I discussed that values are not goals but rather are qualities of living—such as living lovingly, playfully, kindly, compassionately, protectively, persistently, and faithfully.

Goals can be helpful to staying on course in your values-based journey, once the distinction between goals and values is clear. The key point is that values-based living makes goals meaningful, rather than goals being valuable in themselves. If you value alleviating the suffering caused by addiction, you might set a goal of becoming a certified addiction counselor. The certificate will enable the expression of your value; it's a stepping-stone on the journey. I have taught in universities for more than forty years and I've seen many a graduate student forget why they initially pursued a degree. The goal of getting it overshadows the value of getting it; once they graduate, they ask with a bit of shock, "Now what?" Keeping attuned to the here and now helps avoid this pitfall.

Goals are in the future until they are achieved, and then they're quickly in the past. Values are always in the now. And that is crucial to their motivational power. Living day to day according to our values is enormously rewarding.

When people are focusing primarily on future achievement, or what they want or "must get," they miss the richness of life in the present; the yearning for orientation is thwarted. This important wisdom is actually contained in the word *want*. By definition, wants are something you do not have (the word came from the Old Norse *vant*, which meant "missing"). Once we achieve our wants—we get that car, or spouse, or job that we've taken to *be* a value—life calls our bluff. We soon feel how empty those aspirations were because they were not connected to living according to what was truly meaningful. Our thirst for chosen meaning and purpose will be unquenched.

As we work to make the Values pivot and then stay on our new course, attention to the present helps focus on our current behavior—on the journey rather than reaching the destination.

A wonderful benefit of values is that at the very moment we identify them, we are already beginning to *live* them. There is no wait period, no certificate you've got to earn. You will never "get there," you can only "be going there." That also means we don't finish with them; they are an inexhaustible source of meaning. Suppose you value being a loving person. No matter how many times you do loving things, there are more loving things to do.

The effects of making the Values pivot can be dramatically transformative. And sometimes it does not even require extensive work once the other flexibility pivots are in place. A case in point is a client of JoAnne Dahl, the ACT therapist whom you met in Chapter Five. Niklas was a respected, elderly author who lived on a distant small island. He had become powerfully agoraphobic; as he ran from his fear, fear demanded more and more of his freedom. His life was a horrible irony. He wrote soaringly beautiful stories about the natural world around him, and yet he was terrified to step out of his house into the landscape he so loved. He had been housebound for many years.

Things came to a head when he needed to go the hospital to get treatment for a worsening case of diabetes. He reached out to JoAnne for help. It was hard to get to his home—she had to make something happen in a single day.

Instead of trying to restructure his fearsome thoughts or damp his difficult feelings, JoAnne focused first on her genuine curiosity about his anxiety. Within minutes of meeting him she asked if he was anxious; of course he was, and she said that was wonderful. She wanted to understand it, and that meant she had to see it as he did. "Close your eyes and let it come," she asked, adding, "Let it do anything it wants to; we are just going to sit tight like two kids watching the stars at night and just explore it." He agreed. It came but as she asked with great enthusiasm exactly what it was like, and where he felt it, it slowly began to disappear. "Oh, no," JoAnne cried, playing dumb. "Get it back! Hold on to it this time . . . hold its tail tight so that we can explore it." It came but disappeared even faster this time. "What else can we do?" JoAnne pleaded. Over a riotous few hours they locked the door to the room, lay on the floor, went outside, walked far from the house, did somersaults down a hill, got in a car (for the first time in thirty years), went over bridges, and finally went to the ferry (the boat he needed to ride to get to the hospital), and both stood at the front on the railing like in the movie *Titanic*. For each step forward, anxiety would come but as together they tried purposefully to feel it fully and see it clearly, it was felt and then faded.

Meanwhile, he was becoming almost overwhelmed by the beauty of his island that he loved so but had to write about from memory. As he ventured farther from his house, he literally cried tears of joy at the beauty of nature. As he held his anxiety the way you might hold a precious baby, he saw that he could once again freely choose what mattered. Values work was more like a somersault down a hill than wielding a mental lash.

Closing the deal, JoAnne asked Niklas what he might do if the diabetes proved to be controllable. What were his growing diabetes symptoms costing him that he cared about? "A walk on the beach during the first signs of spring," he said. JoAnne had Niklas tell her what nature walks were once like, and why they mattered. In the future, if his condition worsened, what would that cost him? "Sharing beauty through my writing," Niklas answered.

JoAnne had playfully and cleverly drawn Niklas into the possibility that feeling fully liberated him to do what he really cared about. I personally think she'd also shown with her own playful caring for him that values matter. She'd modeled what needed to be done as she herself stood on that railing with him. From there it became obvious that the potential cost of this disease was far too high for him to leave it untreated. He saw in clear relief that appreciating and sharing beauty was his very lifeblood and he had the ability to pivot toward what mattered without anxiety first having to go away.

Niklas faced his fears and went to the hospital for treatment. Going turned out not to be a difficult "grit your teeth" affair. The words he used to describe the trip was that he chose to "hug himself and go."

JoAnne is a brilliant clinician and no, most decades-long anxiety struggles are not abandoned in a long session in a single day. But there is a deep wisdom inside Niklas's story. What is standing between us and caring deeply? Why can't our values-based journey be more like "hug yourself and go"?

Taking the Valued Living Questionnaire

Another person whose life was transformed by reconnecting with his true values is Kelly Wilson, who entered my lab as a graduate student in the late 1980s and has been an important contributor to the development of ACT methods. Kelly altered the direction of ACT's development to include more emphasis on values. Before pursuing a psychology degree, he had experienced a harrowing struggle with addiction, including lying on a bed in a detox ward in four-point restraints wondering how he might kill himself. It was only a couple of years after that, as he fought his way from addiction to succeeding in school, when he realized that he wanted to devote his life to helping others overcome psychological challenges. He read some of my early work on ACT and sought me out to help continue to develop it. After getting his degree, he created the Valued Living Questionnaire (VLQ).

The VLQ asks a series of questions about what your values are and how much you have been living in accordance with them, evaluating that measure in a set of life domains, on a scale of 1 to 10. Taking the VLQ is a good first step in doing ACT values work, and you should fill it out now.

It is best to plan not to let anyone see this so you can answer as honestly as possible, setting aside as best you can social pressures and the wagging mental fingers of *should* and *have to*. This is between you and you. So perhaps rather than filling in your answers in this book, download the VLQ, which you can do at my website (http://www.stevenchayes.com). If you find you are beating yourself up in the process of filling it in, step back and remind yourself that values are what you choose to work toward, not what the mind says you have to do or care about, or else.

VALUED LIVING QUESTIONNAIRE

The following are domains of life that contain values for some people. We are concerned with your quality of life in each of these areas. One aspect of quality of life involves the importance one puts on different areas of living. Rate the importance of each area (by circling a number) on a scale of 1 to 10. A score of 1 means that area is not at all important. A score of 10 means that area is very important. Not everyone will have notable values in all of these areas, or care about all areas the same. Rate each area according to your own personal sense of importance.

1. Family (other than marriage or parenting)

   1 2 3 4 5 6 7 8 9 10

2. Marriage/couples/intimate relations

   1 2 3 4 5 6 7 8 9 10

3. Parenting

   1 2 3 4 5 6 7 8 9 10

4. Friends/social life

   1 2 3 4 5 6 7 8 9 10

5. Work

   1 2 3 4 5 6 7 8 9 10

6. Education/training

   1 2 3 4 5 6 7 8 9 10

7. Recreation/fun

   1 2 3 4 5 6 7 8 9 10

8. Spirituality

1 2 3 4 5 6 7 8 9 10

9. Citizenship/community life

1 2 3 4 5 6 7 8 9 10

10. Physical self-care (diet, exercise, sleep)

1 2 3 4 5 6 7 8 9 10

11. Environmental issues

1 2 3 4 5 6 7 8 9 10

12. Art, creative expression, aesthetics

1 2 3 4 5 6 7 8 9 10

In this section, we would like you to give a rating of how consistent your actions have been with your values in each of these domains. We are not asking about your ideal in each area. We are also not asking what others think of you. Everyone does better in some areas than others. People also do better at some times than at others. We want to know how you think you have been doing during the past week. Rate each area (by circling a number) on a scale of 1 to 10. A score of 1 means that your actions have been completely inconsistent with your values in this area. A score of 10 means that your actions have been completely consistent with your values.

1. Family (other than marriage or parenting)

1 2 3 4 5 6 7 8 9 10

2. Marriage/couples/intimate relations

1 2 3 4 5 6 7 8 9 10

3. Parenting

1 2 3 4 5 6 7 8 9 10

4. Friends/social life

1 2 3 4 5 6 7 8 9 10

5. Work

1 2 3 4 5 6 7 8 9 10

6. Education/training

1 2 3 4 5 6 7 8 9 10

7. Recreation/fun

1 2 3 4 5 6 7 8 9 10

8. Spirituality

1 2 3 4 5 6 7 8 9 10

9. Citizenship/community life

1 2 3 4 5 6 7 8 9 10

10. Physical self-care (diet, exercise, sleep)

1 2 3 4 5 6 7 8 9 10

11. Environmental issues

1 2 3 4 5 6 7 8 9 10

12. Art, creative expression, aesthetics

1 2 3 4 5 6 7 8 9 10

There are a number of ways to assess the results. The first is to look at all domains that have relatively high importance scores (a score of 9 or 10) and also have relatively low consistency scores (6 or less). These are clear problem areas, and I suggest doing your initial values work with any one of them. Then you can move on to other areas.

It's also good to calculate your overall score. Multiply the two numbers from the first and second parts for each domain. So if for family, in the first part you scored it as 10 and in the second part you circled 4, for that domain you'd get 40. Add all of those numbers and then divide them by 12 to get your composite score. To get a rough sense of how your score compares to those of the broad public, the average composite result is 61. Do not begin beating yourself up if your score is lower than that. Practice some defusion from that negativity. This is a discovery process, not a critique, and after all, you've embarked on this journey—give yourself some credit for that. You're here to embrace change.

If you scored quite a few of the domains as low in importance to you, you should consider whether you were being fully honest with yourself about them. It is perfectly reasonable to have some domains that are unimportant. You may not care about citizenship, or the environment, and if you do not have children, you may not care about the parenting practices of others, and so on. That being said, research suggests that if many of these domains are unimportant, that's a contributor to psychological distress. Use this assessment as an opportunity to admit your true values to yourself.

Now, with a good idea of the values domain you'd like to start working on, you're ready to get going.

A Starter Set of Methods

I recommend that in this reading session you do at least the first exercise. Then you can either read the others but return to work on them later on, or if you want to, jump to the next chapter on committed action and come back to them. You will find as you move into committed action that all of the flexibility processes now become relevant, but values especially so, because they provide motivational energy to go ahead with behavior change. For example, the second and third exercises in this chapter are great ways to start identifying actions that you want to commit to change.

Don't be surprised if this work stirs things up. There is a palpable sense of vulnerability that comes from doing values work. Don't be surprised if you find yourself getting unexpectedly emotional over the next few days, or cranky, or anxious. If you do catch yourself getting caught up in rumination of past difficulties and self-recrimination, go right to a little defusion, self, and presence practice. If you feel yourself pushing back against emotions, or procrastinating, practice some acceptance exercises. Remember, we hurt where we care, and values work is all about caring.

1. Values Writing

I want to ask you to write about your values, answering a small set of questions I will ask. This values writing will help you explore further, in an open and unregulated way, the story you've been telling yourself about your values and how you can reconnect with your authentic values.

Research has shown that values writing has more impact on behavior and health than just asking people to pick their values from a list or state them in a few words. Values writing can reduce defensiveness, making us more receptive to information that suggests changes we need to make in our lives. It reduces physiological stress responses and buffers the impact of negative judgments of us from others. And we know a bit about why all of this happens. Values writing is most powerful when it leads us to care more about transcending our own ego and self-story and helps us link our caring to the good of others. Values work helps build socially positive emotions, like gratitude and appreciation, and the feeling that you are making a meaningful difference in others' lives.

If that sounds preachy, please remove any sense of "should" from it. You don't need a wagging finger from me any more than you need one from anyone else, including you. I'm advocating values work because science shows that it improves our lives. It's just the way we are wired.

To start, take out a piece of paper and write for ten minutes about a value you care about deeply in any domain from the list I just gave you. Really do it—ten minutes is not very long! As you do so, address the following questions:

What do I care about in this area? What do I want to *do* in this area that reflects that caring? When in my life has this value been important? What have I seen in my life when others pursue this value, or not? What might I do to manifest this value more in my life? When have I violated this value and has that been costly?

Try to focus your writing on the qualities of your life as *you* want to live it—qualities of your own that you hold as being of intrinsic importance. This is between you and you; it's not about seeking approval or following a bunch of rules. You are not trying to avoid guilt or tell a self-justifying story.

If it feels like you are beginning to write a holiday list to Santa—a list about what you want *from* life or others—redirect your writing in the direction of describing the qualities of actions you would like to manifest in your life. If you get bogged down, just rewrite things you've already written until new things show up. Since this is between you and you, you cannot get it wrong.

Don't continue reading until you've written for at least ten minutes. Trust me on this. Just do it.

▪ ▪ ▪ ▪ ▪

Now we can look back at what you've written. But before turning to that, consider that I asked about times in your life when this value was important, because that helps reaffirm your commitment to it. For me, one of these times was crying under my bed as my parents fought, which helped me see how I longed to help others in a new way. To this day, I sign off on most of my e-mails (especially ones in which I'm trying to help others who are looking for ACT resources and the like) with the phrase *peace, love, and life*.

I asked what you can do to act more in accord with this value, to help you identify specific actions to commit to. Finally, I asked the painful question about times you've fallen short and how that affected your life, because we have much to learn from the pain we inevitably experience.

OK, now read what you wrote and see if you can distill out of it a few examples of things you want to *do* in this area. Actual behavior. Next look for mentions of the qualities you want to manifest in your actions. You might want to do things genuinely, lovingly, carefully, creatively, curiously, compassionately, respectfully, openly, joyously, industriously, healthfully, adventurously, thoughtfully, justly, supportively, learnedly, peacefully, humorously, simply, honestly, spiritually, fairly, charitably, traditionally, dependably, and so on and so on. We are not used to writing about the qualities of action, so don't expect these exact words to show up—I'm trying to give you a set to help you see what I mean by qualities. It's hardly a complete list . . . just use it as a rough guide.

With this first set of actions you'd like to take, you might want to move now to the next chapter, to gain guidance about how to commit to them. Or you might want to do the other two starter exercises here first. If you decide to move on now, be sure to come back to do at least these next two exercises. They have proven very powerful for people in developing a deeper awareness of their values and continuing to chart a course of more meaningful living.

2. Drawing Out Sweetness

Pick a values area you want to work on—say family, education, or work—and allow yourself to recall an event, a day, a moment in that domain that was especially sweet. See if you can find an actual moment when you felt especially connected, vital, or alive; when you felt in flow, or supported, or empowered. Who else was there? What were you doing? What were you feeling or thinking? Notice how consciously in the now you were. Relive that moment as fully as you can.

Now, as you reflect on that special moment, consider what it suggests about the qualities of being or doing that you want to put into the world. But don't formulate an answer in words, not yet. Allow the question to hang in your mind; now pull out a piece of paper. Draw any picture that comes to mind that somehow speaks to you about that value. Allow your picture to form without forcing words on it. This is not an art class, so let go of any self-criticism or self-praise about the quality of the drawing. The point is to break out of a verbal evaluative mode of mind and to envision that sweet moment and what it suggests about how you want to live. Now, sit back and reflect on what you drew.

What does the picture tell you about what you care about in this domain? What would you have to do to manifest that value in your actions? See if you can connect in a gut way with what you are yearning to stand for in your life moments, starting even in this moment, now. Awareness is the first step. See if you can put what you are feeling and sensing into a few words. If you have a sense that they resonate, write them down under the picture.

I call this process of awareness, recognition, and remembrance *driving a nail into the wall*. That last part, connecting with what you yearn to manifest, is metaphorically like the support of a nail that helps you keep this picture in place in your awareness. By linking that picture to a verbal statement of what matters to you, you affix the awareness more securely in your mind. I like to display these pictures on my phone or desk, or actually hang them on my wall, to even more firmly anchor them in my mind.

3. Flipping Pain into Purpose

Recall that one of the gifts of acceptance is the guidance we receive from feeling our pain. This exercise helps you see the values that are hiding in plain sight inside your pain, so that you can identify ways to live more in alignment with them.

I had a client once who had been verbally abused and neglected as a child. She was constantly told she was dumb, and she believed it. Her mother would also leave for weeks at a time, even when she was very young. She'd been passed around among relatives like a sack of potatoes. As an adult she worked as a low-paid secretary; her relationships were a mess.

ACT work helped her see that the pain of feeling worthless, lonely, and helpless revealed how strong she'd actually been and how much she cared about living a life that fulfilled her values. Even with her sense of helplessness, she had in essence raised herself. She put herself through community college. And she had sought therapy, diving into ACT headfirst. After only about six sessions she joined a women's group, and a few weeks later she applied to college. She began advocating for candidates who embraced women's issues and became a community leader. In college, she was an honors student and went on to get a full scholarship for graduate training at an Ivy League school.

She found her motivation to change her life trajectory right inside her pain. Inside worthlessness was a value of being kind and accepting of others and standing up for those who were downtrodden. Inside helplessness was a value of being competent and knowledgeable. Inside loneliness was a value of connecting with others and caring for their suffering.

Now it's your turn. Take a values domain that's of high importance to you but where there's a large discrepancy between its importance to you and how much you're living in accordance with that value. See if you can identify painful thoughts, feelings, memories, urges, or sensations that function as barriers to living as you'd like in this area. Write them down. Then take each barrier and flip it to uncover the purpose that the pain it causes you has to reveal, and write that down. Ask yourself, what would you have to not care about for that not to hurt?

The client I wrote about might have selected the domain of citizenship and identified her sense of worthlessness as a barrier to advocating for women's rights. This exercise would help her see that she would have to not care about fairness and opportunity for women. She would also realize that she'd have to not care about her mother's disparagements of her. The first was unacceptable to this woman, while the second proved more possible than she had imagined.

Next, for each of the barriers, write the following statement: *If in [situation] I [feel, think, remember, sense X], let it be a reminder that I care about [value]*. For example, my client might have written this down: *If in a social situation I start to feel worthless, let it be a reminder that I care deeply about making a difference in the world, and that I want to do that by supporting women's rights.* Don't expect it to remove the pain—expect it to help you live more as a whole person.

Additional Methods

4. Writing Your Story

This is a slight modification of the values writing task. Before I ask you to write, though, I want you to think. Imagine that the next year is going to be a key year in defining who you are in your life. If you were to become more fully you during this year, while at the same time still supporting those you care about, what would your process of "becoming more fully you" look like over this next year? Where do you wish to grow? What kind of person are you yearning to be? If you were writing the chapter of the next year of your life, what would the theme be?

Now that you have the set, do ten minutes of writing about the next year and what you hope to become.

5. I've Got a Secret

The purpose of this exercise is to strengthen your awareness of how meaningful it is to act in accord with your authentic values in contrast to acting in the service of getting social approval or an ego boost.

Pick an action that manifests a deeply held value, and see if you can plan a way to do it in total secrecy. For example, do a favor for a friend without disclosing you're the one who has done it, make a large contribution to a charity you love without telling anyone you know that you did so, or show compassion for a stranger in need but anonymously.

At some point that same day, do ten minutes of values writing about what that experience was like for you and what it suggests about how you might build more values-based actions into your day-to-day life. Make sure not to talk to others about what you've learned from this exercise. This is about you doing things you care about doing only because you care.

If this exercise is hard, that is important to reflect on. You may find yourself letting your plan leak out to a friend, or telling her about your good deed later. Dig into why. If that dig-in is emotionally upsetting to you, I suspect that the need for social approval may be overshadowing your capacity to find your own sense of meaning. In that case, do a very small version of this exercise almost every day until it is easy and you can maintain your secrecy about your actions 100 percent. Then you can gradually increase the importance of the actions you take.

Many more ACT exercises have been developed for connecting with values, and I highly recommend you seek them out (follow the search strategy I listed in the Author's Note, before Chapter One). Building your connection with your values is a journey that can last the rest of your life, and every step will make your life more meaningful.

Chapter Fourteen

THE SIXTH PIVOT

ACTION—COMMITTING TO CHANGE

We have reached the last step in the dance of living the life we want to live. Without this last pivot, we're at risk of backsliding on all of the progress we've made in the previous steps. But once we commit to building values-based habits of action, we secure our progress with all of the flexibility skills. Taking action that helps us get where we want to go requires us to employ the other skills, reinforcing their importance. As in a real dance, in which all of the movements you've practiced flow together into a smooth and seamless pattern, committed action brings the six pivots together into a healthy, ongoing process of acting as you choose.

Recall that psychological flexibility is really one overarching ability, not six. It can't be learned all at once, any more than how to dance the tango could be learned all at once. Ultimately, as you continue working on the skills, they combine into the one skill of living with psychological flexibility. Choosing more meaningful ways of living is the payoff that comes from integrating the skills—I even emphasized that idea in the subtitle of this book. It is habitually pivoting toward what matters that makes the other flexibility skills foundational. It is hard to truly commit to a new way of living without having developed some other flexibility skills, and all of that work begins to come to fruition once we begin making changes in our patterns of daily living.

As we embark on committing to behavior change, of whatever kind, the key is to do so with psychological flexibility. What does that mean exactly? It means moving forward with self-compassion, not berating ourselves for inevitable missteps, and buying in when our judgmental minds label them, or ourselves, as failures. It means embarking on your new course with a clarity that you're not doing this to impress others, bolster your ego, or conform to a new version of a conceptualized self. Rather, you're committing to change because doing so is helping you connect with your deepest values from your most authentic sense of self. It means accepting the pain and risk that is inevitably involved with change, whether that's the physical pain of withdrawal symptoms or cravings, or the emotional pain sure to come from opening up to experiences we've been avoiding, such as rejection by someone we ask on a date, or criticism from a difficult parent with whom we reconnect. Finally, it means keeping our attention on the richness of making an effort and learning new habits rather than fixating on a static state of success and how far we are from it.

The last realization needed to engage in building new life habits in this psychologically flexible way is that we're not going to be immediately competent in our new chosen actions. We will without doubt stumble as we pursue our new course. We'll backslide in our behavior and we'll probably grasp again at avoidance. That is *OK*—that is how change happens. Stumbles are no reason to berate ourselves or to flee back into self-delusion or give up in despair.

The Action pivot moves us away from an unhealthy desire for perfection and toward a flexible appreciation of the intrinsic satisfaction of developing competence.

The Yearning to Be Competent

We yearn to be able to act effectively in the world; to live, and love, and play, and create skillfully. This is the yearning for competence—to be *able*.

We do not have to learn to want it; the desire is inborn. If you watch young children explore and play you see that they are willing to spend many hours learning to do very simple things like open a box or bounce a ball. No one has to tell them this needs to be done or provide much in the way of external rewards to get them going. They want to know how to do things. The reward is built into the action itself, and as children grow they will spend endless hours learning a new jump-rope trick or how to build a taller tower with wood blocks. Evolution built this yearning into us, and good thing too, given how much we have to learn.

Learning a new skill can be fun, satisfying, fascinating, even a relief. But we have probably all felt how difficult it can be to learn something we don't find intrinsically interesting and satisfying. We don't feel engaged; we may even push the task away. Used carefully, extrinsic rewards—rewards that come from the outside—can help greatly in these instances. Your parents' excitement at seeing you tie your shoes was probably key to your learning how; their encouragement may have kept you going to piano lessons. But it's important that such rewards not *overwhelm* intrinsic motivation—which comes from within—especially once you are the one determining how to motivate yourself.

We can be the ones overwhelming our own intrinsic motives. We can easily become entranced by the desire to impress, to be admired, or to please others quite apart from whether the accomplishments we're undertaking are actually meaningful to us. The satisfaction from those rewards will diminish over time. If, for example, we're pursuing applause from others, rather than focusing on serving others, the day will come when applause feels empty. When the going is tough and we're not doing well, we'll be quickly frustrated, getting angry with ourselves, and impulsively thrashing about trying to find a reason to keep going. We may become obsessive about trying to prove our competence or avoidant of the shame of not being perfect. Procrastination is one way we avoid these situations; we mistake it for a way to keep feelings of failure or anxiety about the prospect of failure at bay, but it only ultimately intensifies them. Of course, often we also just abandon the effort altogether.

Simplistic cultural mantras like *Just do it* don't do the process of committed action justice. They imply that the process isn't really so hard. But it is, and we're simply not going to be immediately competent in building values-based habits. One of the difficult aspects of learning new skills or habits of any kind is delayed gratification. We're not going to see big payoffs right away, and we will experience plenty of frustration, even pain, during the competence journey.

One of the most famous studies ever done in psychology looked at whether four-year-olds could sit with a marshmallow in close reach for several minutes without eating it, in order to earn two marshmallows later—in other words, whether they could delay gratification. The children who could were more likely to be successful in college, more than a decade later. It's a critical skill, and unique to humans. When nonhumans act in accord with a distant future, like hiding seeds to eat next season, it is primarily as a result of genetic programming. They do not have the symbolic-thinking ability to conceptualize the future. The fact that we do is a wonderful asset. It allows us to devote ourselves to years of school, to take on multiyear projects, and to save for retirement. But it is also fraught with danger.

Envisioning a future in which we've mastered the new behavior we're committing to leads us into the *competency conundrum*: our problem-solving mind wants to get us to that future *now*, and that fixation on future success and external achievement undercuts the will to stick with the process that builds competence.

Let me give you an example.

I've taught dozens of people to play the guitar, and I've learned to predict who will learn to play well: those who enjoy the (pretty bad, maybe even atrocious) music they produce as a beginner. If someone tells me in the first session how they picture themselves being applauded for their great skill or how they want to be famous and play in a rock band, I know there is heavy sledding ahead. They're a long way from any such outcome, and grasping at it will make learning the basics like fingering or playing simple scales that much harder for a biologically built-in reason: immediate consequences dominate over delayed consequences. Even at the level of underlying brain chemistry, if the immediate consequences are not reinforcing, behavioral habits are devilishly hard to establish.

Many years ago, I bought a ukulele (the only instrument I could afford as a twelve-year-old). I learned a single song, "Ain't She Sweet," and played it for at least a month without respite. I loved it! Although I gradually got better, during that month people literally ran the other way when they saw me coming (or, rather, *heard* me coming). My family banished me to playing in a closed room, well away from them. No matter. I was thrilled at what I could do, and, yes, that I was getting a little bit better.

A major problem with building competency is that the Dictator Within judges us so harshly for falling short of what it thinks our progress should be. It also convinces us that success is an end state, rather than an ongoing process of learning. In the same way that it can tell us that we will enjoy playing the guitar once we are in a band, it can feed us thoughts like these:

* **I will feel self-confident when I marry an attractive spouse.**
* **I will no longer struggle with the pain of my childhood when I'm famous.**
* **I will stop worrying about the future when I have a lot of money.**
* **My anxiety and self-doubt will go away when I get a promotion.**

As the Dictator deflects our attention away from the intrinsic value of our current efforts, including the learning we can gain from our stumbles, and focuses our mind on the need for achievement, we can slip into another type of avoidance. Despite their appearances, some forms of persistence are actually forms of avoidance, driven by fear (of failure, for example). Workaholism and perfectionism are examples. These rigid forms of persistence carry with them a strong negative health impact as well as leading people to ignore relationships and recreation.

The Action pivot takes the yearning for competence and directs it toward building habits of values-based actions that are authentically meaningful to us. That undermines both procrastination and workaholism.

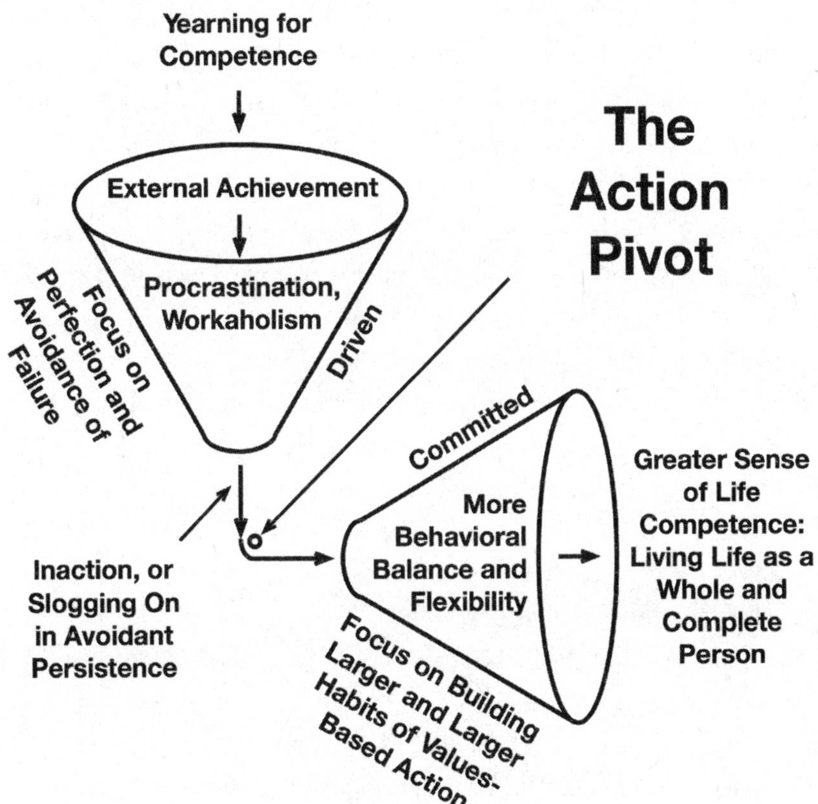

SMART Goals

As we embark on committing to a new plan of action, we should develop SMART goals: specific, measurable, attainable, results-focused, and time-bound. It does not help to set a goal like "I will be better" because it has no increments of progress. It's counterproductive to set unrealistic expectations such as "I will never feel depressed again." And setting a realistic time frame for achievement of a goal helps to tamp down the sense of urgency about achieving it *now*.

If you are committed to helping veterans heal their wounds from war, you might set a goal of obtaining a degree in clinical social work in the next three or four years, so that you can work with them professionally. Once that goal is set, you may need to go through multiple rounds of goal-setting to find the right program, apply for it, and finish the degree. Each of these steps is specific, measurable, attainable, results-focused, and time-bound.

The other flexibility skills help with commitment to the actions that will allow us to achieve these goals. Defusion allows us to distance ourselves from negative thoughts and judgments about our progress. Connecting to our transcendent self keeps our focus on taking action because we care, not to comply with social expectations or avoid guilt. Acceptance helps us maintain our grit when the going gets tough. Presence helps us stay focused on the process rather than the end goal—and how far from it we are. Connecting with our values reminds us that these difficult actions are in the service of living the life we will find meaningful, rather than in service of proving our self-worth or escaping from difficult experiences.

Taking Pleasure in the Process

A great way to think about the process of building new habits of living is embarking on a hero's journey. You may be familiar with the concept. It's the basic plot of the greatest stories told in books, in films, and even before them in the myths of cultures all around the world, as famously shown by the late Joseph Campbell, a renowned expert in comparative mythology.

The basic trajectory is that the hero's normal routine is suddenly interrupted with some great challenge that he or she must face and somehow resolve. In myth, the hero is unfortunately usually a man, but the journey applies just as cogently to women, so let's adopt that language here. As she embarks on her quest, she discovers that doing so involves internal challenges as well: fears, pain, false beliefs, or limited perspective. The hero wrestles with self-doubt, mistakes, and setbacks. Then, in the darkest of dark hours, the hero comes to a pivotal moment in which she discovers inner resources she did not know she had. Often these are spiritual in quality, but they may be supported by external resources, or by the help of companions. The hero finds a way to face her fears, self-doubts, or delusion, and to persist. Often a more limited conceptualized self drops away and a broader and more open or interconnected sense of self emerges. Finally, the hero turns her attention wholeheartedly toward commitment to values such as honor, love, kindness, courage, and community, and through committed action the quest is accomplished. As the journey resolves, she returns to her daily routine as a transformed person.

Whether it's *Star Wars* or *Snow White, Hunger Games* or *Alice in Wonderland,* this fundamental story arc applies. Think about it.

I expect that in reading that description of the hero's journey, you saw how the flexibility skills are involved. It is, in essence, the arc of acquiring greater psychological flexibility: facing difficult emotions and thoughts with greater openness; letting go of limiting self-stories; finding resources within that allow us to see ourselves and our situation in a new way; connecting with a deeper and more authentic sense of self; connecting with a chosen purpose and discovering the actions that help us to fulfill it; and finally committing to those actions with perseverance.

So, as you commit to take the actions that will align your life with your values, consider this: would these still be great stories if the hero didn't have to cope with internal struggles and scary, disheartening setbacks? What if the accomplishment didn't require perseverance? A story featuring a hero who never doubted herself or never made a wrong step would quickly become boring—oh, surprise, surprise, she just shot that dragon right out of the sky before it could cause any havoc. Just as the joy of becoming involved in a great story in a film or book comes from the vicarious experience of facing challenges, so too the richness of meaning and purpose in life comes from persevering through difficulties as we acquire flexibility skills. Passion without perseverance is a tragedy; persistence without purpose is a mockery of human potential.

Making the Pivot

As you set forth on your journey, make the Action pivot by answering this question:

> Based on a distinction between you as a conscious being and the story the mind tells of who you are, in this time and situation are you willing to experience your experiences as they are, not as what they say they are, fully and without needless defense, and direct your attention and effort to creating larger and larger habits of behavior that reflect your chosen values? YES or NO?

It reads a little like a marriage vow, and no wonder. It is a commitment. Every flexibility process is in that question. Life asks it of you over and over and over—without end, so far as I know. Each time you answer "yes," your life expands. Each time you answer "no," it contracts. A habit of answering "yes" will likely make your life more difficult at times in the days and years ahead; it will also make your life more vital and meaningful, even in times of doubt and pain.

It's OK if you're not ready to answer "yes." Just keep your eyes wide open. If you find yourself stuck on "no," commit to noticing how that plays out in your life. And then come back to the question.

Actually, you can't really avoid coming back to it. That's not because there is some cosmic imperative that you eventually "get it right," but because life affords us the potential to take committed action in every moment of every day. That is how it is. Just as we have within us the knowledge about the value of the other flexibility skills, so too we have within us the awareness that we have the power to take the actions to change our lives. We sense the possibility of our own agency.

So, here is life, asking you the question once again.

> Based on a distinction between you as a conscious being and the story the mind tells of who you are, in this time and situation are you

willing to experience your experiences as they are, not as what they say they are, fully and without needless defense, and direct your attention and effort to creating larger and larger habits of behavior that reflect your chosen values? YES or NO?

If your answer is "yes," then it is time to move on to your action steps.

In the introduction to Part Two I pointed out that ACT complements the utility of other evidence-based behavior change methods. It is impossible to put every change method in this chapter, or to cover them all in Part Three. Thus, the best way to think of what follows is as a general guide that needs to be tailored to the specifics of the challenges you are working on. The skills can be applied to any endeavor, whether that is a class, your work, a sport, a diet, a mental health issue, physical health challenges, an exercise program, or your relationships. You can feel free to pick any of the methods for building habits of action that I present here as they fit with the particular kind of habit change you're undertaking, After all, ACT is all about flexibility!

Also, feel free to draw on other behavior change science. There is a vast sea of knowledge about behavior change, including methods for developing social skills, learning to communicate with your spouse, acquiring management abilities, overcoming procrastination, and managing your time better. The flexibility skills will complement those approaches. One word of caution if you do plunge into the literature: focus on evidence-based methods for which multiple studies in major journals have been published that attest to their positive effects. Advice without that rigorous scientific foundation is often misleading.

If you are in treatment, or you plan to go into it, your therapist or doctor may know something about the methods that would be most helpful in behavioral change of the specific kinds you are targeting. If you are engaged in a behavior change program of some kind, use your flexibility skills to help you take whatever actions are required.

A Starter Set of Methods

In previous chapters I offered a handful of initial exercises to do before moving on to the next chapter. Here, because building new habits of behavior is best done incrementally over time, I am giving just two methods for you to use initially, perhaps for a couple of weeks at least, as you go back to the additional exercises in the prior chapters to keep building the other flexibility skills. As I said, behavior change is hard, and it's generally best to start small. Continuing to build your other flexibility skills will be of great help in tackling progressively more difficult commitments.

Sometimes an initial experience with ACT exercises leads people to make big changes in their behavior quickly, as was the case with Alice Lindquist, whose story I told in Chapter Five. She went back to work after years of suffering the life of a shut-in because of her grief about her son's death. If such a dramatic change becomes possible for you after reading this book and doing the exercises, that is marvelous. But it's crucial not to think you *should* be able to accomplish that. *Do not* beat yourself up with that unhelpful rule!

I advise that you start your behavior change efforts by applying these first two methods to a couple or a few of the actions you'd like to commit to that you wrote down in the values writing exercise in the last chapter. Keep working on those until the behaviors become easy for you and you are fully committed to them. Then progress to incorporating the additional methods offered here into your behavior change efforts.

Once you have worked through all of the exercises in each Part Two chapter, create your ACT toolkit of your favorite exercises and then continue to practice those regularly. I discuss how to create your toolkit and build a routine of practice in the introduction to Part Three. The chapters in that part then offer guidance about how to keep applying the skills to new areas of challenge in your life.

OK, time to get started with committing to some new actions!

1. Make Small Adjustments

The wonderful (and terrible) thing about human behavior is that it tends to support itself. Lives fall into behavioral patterns. We do what we do, because it's what we've always done. This can become problematic for all the reasons described: we can fall into psychologically rigid habits. But small behavioral direction changes can build to create a huge change in direction over time. The trick is to calibrate your efforts.

Initially it's best to make changes that are simple and quick. If you want to read more and watch television less, start with no television after work until you've read for thirty minutes. Even if the commitment you've decided on is small, it can help to make it smaller still. Make it fifteen minutes of reading, or cut out a single show you think is mindless but you find yourself watching anyway (do you really need to see more back episodes of *Cupcake Wars*?).

It does not matter how small it is. You're making progress.

There are exceptions to every rule. You cannot leap across a canyon in two steps. For example, if you've tried the well-established harm reduction approach to dealing with an addiction and it did not work, it may be time to make a full-stop commitment to sobriety. That's a case of tailoring which methods you practice to suit your challenge. The good news is that psychological flexibility skills help with such challenging leaps.

2. Work New Habits into Established Routines

It is wise to create new behavioral habits that are initially anchored to your regular activities so that they can cue the new behavior. It is far easier to combine habits than to swap them out cold. For example, suppose you want to eat more fruit and less refined sugar but you find that you are regularly eating a cookie soon after you wake up. If you have a morning coffee, you might focus on creating a habit of grabbing an apple as you grab your coffee, taking it to your favorite chair, and taking a small bite before your first sip.

Or suppose you want to be more effective in managing your work habits. You might set a goal of answering all e-mails each day so your inbox doesn't get overstuffed. Soon you'll likely have some tough days and not get them all answered, and you might then just give up. If instead you established a habit of answering e-mails for, say, thirty minutes over your morning coffee (with an apple!), that e-mail habit would be easier to establish.

Additional Methods

3. Develop Reverse Compass Habits

In an earlier chapter I talked about how to build habits that are the opposite of what your mind is pushing you to do. You can also apply this practice to committing to new actions. For example, I seem to have inherited from my mother a tendency toward obsessive thoughts of contamination, and I've developed a "reverse compass" strategy for countering it. Suppose I am leaving the restroom at school and the thought comes to mind that "that door handle might be contaminated." If I sense that the thought is dominating me, after grabbing the handle to leave the bathroom, I will rub my hand on my face, or even put a finger that touched the handle in my mouth. It generally does not take more than a few reverse compass actions like that before the thought stops being a bother.

Mind you, if I were in a public restroom that appeared to be genuinely dodgy, I'd have no problem avoiding the handle. Reverse compass actions should not themselves become compulsive. It just helps to have little habits that give a needed poke to the Dictator Within.

You can devise reverse compass habits for all sorts of behavior you want to change. For example, I've found that when I'm tempted to procrastinate, even a few minutes of work on the avoided task will help me get into full gear again later that day or the next day, rather than falling down the rabbit hole of putting things off for extended periods. If you need *not* do something, like biting your nails, you can try habit reversal—deliberately creating a better habit that interferes with the habit you want to reduce. This is a case of applying ACT to established methods from other domains. Habit reversal is a behavioral psychology method. It involves awareness training (noticing that you are about to bite your nails), followed by practicing a new habit that interferes with the old, such as picking up and holding a pen or pencil. Recent research has shown that habit reversal is even more powerful when combined with ACT methods.

4. Practice "Just Because I Choose To"

Another great way to strengthen your commitment skills is always to have at least one slightly difficult thing you are doing "just cuz." When we commit to values, our minds sometimes e-value-ate those choices in ways that miss their deeper point. The mind can easily turn a value into another cudgel for beating ourselves about the head and ears.

A playful way to get around this is to practice commitment behaviors that are established "just because I choose to" without any possible reason to give. Again, start small with these. The following are some examples:

* **Go a week without a preferred food, just cuz.**
* **For a month go to bed an hour earlier than usual and get up an hour earlier, just cuz.**
* **Deliberately embarrass yourself by wearing something slightly off (e.g., a loud and unattractive shirt, mismatched socks) each week, just cuz.**

When I was walking out of panic disorder, I did longer and longer exercises of this kind: first hours, then days, then months. One of the final commitments was to go for a year without dessert—not because that was important, but precisely because it wasn't! I slipped once (I put a spoonful of ice cream in my mouth before remembering and spitting it out), but with that exception I met the goal. I began to trust that I could do what I said I would do and that, in and of itself, was a huge benefit to me.

Why does this help? It undercuts the tendency to slip into the judgmental frame of mind that we must keep our commitments because doing so *is important*, rather than because it's our choice and habit. Suddenly, the judgmental voice of the Dictator begins to speak, telling us "I *have to* be someone who keeps my commitment" or "I am bad if I don't keep my commitment" (conceptualized self) or "I will feel guilty if I don't keep my commitment" (experiential avoidance). Before we know it, we're "committing" based on the usual robbers' den lineup of guilt, shame, self-loathing, self-criticism, compliance, and emotional avoidance. By committing to some actions "just cuz," we stay more aware when these other motivators are raising their ugly heads.

5. No One Is an Island

Shared or public commitments are more likely to be maintained, as long as we don't shift the responsibility for our behavior to others. That is likely why certain important life commitments (e.g., marriages) include rituals asking for the community to witness the commitment and to support it. It's tricky, of course: the mind can begin to claim that it is others who must now do the heavy lifting, but flexibility skills can help keep that process reined in.

There is another reason it is useful to think of others when making commitments: our behavioral patterns don't only affect us as individuals. They touch the people around us. All parents experience this challenge as they watch their children respond to—even replicate—their most desired and most abhorrent behavioral traits. Societies and communities respond in kind. If you change your behavior, a similar behavior change is now more likely in your friends, the friends of your friends, and the friends of your friends of your friends. That could mean that thousands of people have a stake in your success (perhaps thousands are looking over your shoulder as you read this book right now!).

When you share a commitment, your friends need to see that this is part of your larger mission, and defending against criticism or needing external control is not the point. It is sharing and caring. It helps if your friends know about flexibility pivots and can see when you get hooked, avoidant, or wrapped up in a self-story, helping you with gentle nudges to stay on course. Those are the benefits you're looking for.

Part Three

INTRODUCTION: USING YOUR ACT TOOLKIT TO EVOLVE YOUR LIFE

Knowing the moves and how to make them happen is not the dance of psychological flexibility. In actual dancing, we really start having fun when we creatively combine moves, fitting them to those of our dance partners in the moment. So too, the true joy of learning the flexibility skills comes from combining them in an ongoing way to rise to the daily challenges of our lives—to pivot toward what matters . . . to *us*. That is the dance of flexibility.

The exercises in the preceding chapters have given you some personal experience with how the skills help contend with certain challenges. If you've applied the exercises to one pressing issue, you can keep that up now, continuing to practice the skills. You may have also already begun applying them to other challenges and found yourself calling on them in a daily way as issues arise. Encouraging you to continue building the skills and applying them to more areas of your life is the purpose of this part of the book.

Sometimes psychological flexibility training leads to major progress, and because people feel they have "solved" the problem that inspired them to try ACT, they stop working on the skills. That's a great shame because if you keep practicing the skills and consciously applying them to new domains of your life, you can keep evolving your life in accordance with your chosen values.

You have to keep practicing because rigid ways of thinking and acting will always keep sneaking up on us. I experienced an example this morning. I have a coffeemaker I used to love that makes fresh coffee one cup at a time. After a few years of great coffee, in the last six or eight months it had not been working well. The coffee was too weak for my taste, even if I filled the coffee strainer to the brim and pushed the "bold" button. I tried different types of coffee; I packed it in tighter. Nothing worked.

My wife heard my complaining and kindly bought me a new one. The instruction book was right there as I unpacked the box, so even though I knew how to use the coffeemaker, I decided to skim it. I soon discovered something I'd forgotten (if I'd ever read about it before). The pamphlet cautioned, *Do not fill the strainer with coffee! If you do, the coffee will be weak because the water will not go through the coffee but will flow out of the overflow tube. Especially do not pack the coffee.*

Aaagh! The coffeemaker was fine! I'd let the commonsense rule "for more, use more" take over my behavior, and it never even *occurred* to me that maybe the right rule was "for more, use less."

That's fusion. That's a lack of variation. That's weak coffee and the unnecessary purchase of a shiny new coffeemaker! Not exactly a tragedy, but a good example of how the skills can help with all of our endeavors, whether big or small.

Assembling Your ACT Toolkit

To make practicing your skill-building a habit, it's helpful to create a set of your own preferred exercises. Here is an example, comprising some of my favorite metaphors and exercises selected from those I've presented. Don't be thinking this is *the* best set—this is just an example of a sensible initial set. Fill in a grid like this with your own favorites.

A SIMPLE ACT TOOLKIT

DEFUSION	Sing Your Thoughts	Give Your Mind a Name	Write Thoughts on Cards and Carry Them in Your Pocket
ACCEPTANCE	Practice the Opposite	Give Difficult Feelings a Color, Weight, Speed, Shape	Practice Dropping the Rope
PRESENCE	Do a Scan of Your Bodily Sensations	Notice Single and Multiple Attention Targets	Open Your Focus
SELF	Rewrite Your Story	Notice Who Is Noticing	Remember I'm Not That
VALUES	Write Out Your Values	Play "I've Got a Secret"	Do a Values Card Sort
ACTION	Hook New Habits to Established Routines	Share Your Commitment with a Good Friend	Link Values to SMART Goals

For the next few months at least, largely limit your practice to playing around with your initial set until they are so familiar that they come naturally to you as you need to call on them day to day. At that point, begin adding one more method at a time. There is no need for you ever to get bored with any given exercise, as a huge number of alternatives are available online and in the scores of ACT books available. See how what you added works, and if it's not helpful, jettison it and move on to something else.

Applying the Skills Broadly

Research has evaluated the effects of ACT in contending with a vast array of difficulties. In addition to those already discussed, these include recovering from eating disorders; coping with performance pressures, whether in school, at work, in the arts, or in sports; dealing with stress; facing the fear of cancer; dealing with prejudice, and many more. ACT training has helped people win Olympic gold medals, manage *Fortune* 100 companies, play a better game of chess, and foster artistic talent.

The mind says that what you learn in one area transfers to others. Well, that can be true, but it is not automatic. You have to consciously work on applying the skills to more and more areas of your life. The chapters in Part Three share insights gained through both research and ACT work with clients about why the flexibility skills are so helpful for specific types of challenges. I explore aspects of the challenges covered that make them so difficult and show how certain of the flexibility skills are especially useful in coping with those. An example is that in trying to recover from substance abuse, shame is a difficult issue, and defusion and self exercises undercut its grip. I also provide some additional exercises that have been effective for certain types of challenges.

As you choose new challenges and life domains to apply your skills to, follow a basic process like that used in the workshop conducted with people who have chronic pain described in Chapter Eight. Recall that the first step was for people to write about what they wanted their life to be like in each of the domains in the Life Compass, and then to identify the barriers they felt were getting in their way and the difficult emotions and unhelpful thoughts holding them back. We can add to that process now by doing a deeper dive into the yearnings that motivate human life before culling the steps you might take.

The domains we covered in Chapter Eight were work, intimate relationships, parenting and children (you don't have to be a parent or have kids to care about those issues), education, the environment, friends, physical well-being, family, spirituality, aesthetics (such as art or beauty), community, and recreation. Once you pick a new domain or specific challenge, remind yourself of what might be at stake there by considering this diagram. These are the six yearnings. Keep each in mind as you unpack what is going on, watching for barriers that pop up when you touch the deeper needs and yearnings that show up in this area.

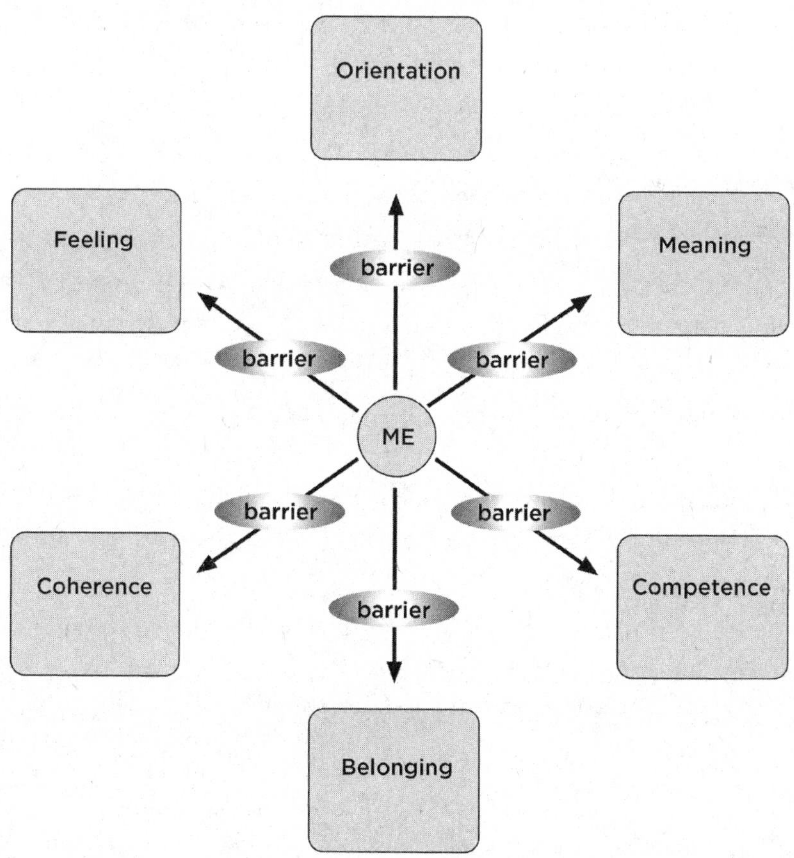

Let's say that you are feeling unhappy at work. Some of the reasons may be obvious, such as if you have a highly critical boss or you've got too much work assigned to you. But you might also be having trouble putting your finger on what is wrong. Catch what reactions you can. Suppose you feel like a cog in a machine, unseen and uncared for. Maybe you feel stuck, and the work you are doing is empty.

See if the issues contain within them some or all of the six basic yearnings we all have. Feeling unseen and uncared for probably reflects a yearning for belonging. A sense of emptiness or feeling stuck suggests a lack of self-directed meaning. Feeling like a cog in a machine suggests a lack of freedom to create your own areas of competence.

As you consider what you yearn for, allow the barriers that stand between you and satisfying those yearnings at work to come to the fore. Some of the issues may be internal, psychological ones, but some may be external. This mix of external and internal barriers is true of most of our difficulties in life, so it's vital to always consider both. Write down all of the barriers you identify, and for those where the reason why you're having difficulty isn't clear, think about what might be underlying your dissatisfaction.

An example of an internal barrier about work might be that you have thoughts like *I'm not good enough* that stop you from reaching out and connecting with others, undermining your sense of belonging. If you're feeling stuck, for example, that may be because you don't feel the work you're doing is meaningful. It's not in line with the values-based way of living you aspire to. But maybe that feeling of being stuck also leads to daydreaming that takes you away from what you are doing. If so, you might want to add to the yearnings that are involved in this problem because perhaps you are also losing a sense of orientation at work.

For those where the reasons for your discomfort seem obvious, such as that critical boss, dig deeper and think about why the criticism is so hard for you to take. You might realize that it's in part because your mother or father also often criticized you when you were growing up and it kicks off an old critical voice within. Add that to your list of barriers.

Now write down the set of solutions you've been trying for coping with the barriers. The list might be quite long, but I'll just give a few examples here:

* **Skipping a weekly staff meeting that is likely to feel too critical**
* **Being silent in meetings to keep the attention elsewhere**
* **Working hard to make sure you get all high marks on your next performance evaluation**
* **Forging a relationship with a co-worker who also likes to talk about the problems and problematic people at work**

Now it's time to use your flexibility skills to see if the solutions you've been trying are likely to work. The first two solutions in the preceding list are clearly avoidant. They offer short-term relief from negative feelings and thoughts, but at the cost of being able to participate, which likely only amplifies a sense of invisibility and lack of belonging or competence and may be undermining your reputation with your boss and colleagues. Trying to ensure a perfect performance evaluation may be fine, but it's important to consider whether the motivation is in part a fear of criticism, rather than intrinsic motivation to achieve. If avoiding criticism is a driver, it's important to realize that this may be self-defeating, since the process generally requires managers to offer at least some critical feedback. What about the friendship with a co-worker? Having work friends is awesome, but constantly discussing with those friends how unhappy you are may be a form of rumination, especially if the co-worker now reciprocates with all of the reasons why the work environment is awful, leading you to do more of the same. You think it's helpful to vent, and it does soothe the yearning for belonging, but it could intensify your unhappiness by creating a work-related echo chamber full of judgment. Not a good idea. Even dogs don't pee in their own beds.

It is worth noting the thoughts and feelings you're having as you consider your problem. What negative messages has your Dictator been berating you with? What emotions are you trying to escape? What memories come up that are haunting you? These may include painful thoughts such as *My colleagues don't respect me*, or *I can't do anything I care about in this job*, and a deep-down core of *Maybe I'm not good enough*. You may also be feeling anger linked to the sense of invisibility.

OK, you're ready to start applying your toolkit. Maybe start with a presence exercise or two to get into a mindful perspective. You could next do some defusion work to distance from those negative thoughts. Do a values exercise to clarify how the way you're working is out of alignment with your chosen values. You might realize that all of that commiserating with your colleague is in conflict with a value of being forthright, and that you would be better served by discussing issues with your boss. As difficult emotions are triggered while you do this work, apply acceptance practices to them. Do a self exercise to soften the self-story and to touch on the part of you that knows how to connect with others. Maybe you'll find that you've been accusing yourself of being incompetent, or spinning the tale that no one really cares about you at work because you're not interesting or charismatic. Maybe finish this deep dive by committing to a small action you'll take the next day. Let's say you commit to speaking up and sharing a suggestion in a meeting that's scheduled. That's all six skills applied!

Now begin applying the learning you've done to more and more experiences at work as they're happening. If you're in a meeting and you start feeling that no one is interested in your input, do a quick defusion exercise in your mind. If your boss makes a nasty comment to you, when you're alone for a moment, do an acceptance exercise, and if your Dictator is assailing you with some negative message because of that criticism, apply your defusion talent to that.

In a focused session at home, perhaps after a week, you could continue with some presence, defusion, self, values, and acceptance work, and then take some time to look carefully at what concrete steps you might take to improve the situation, setting forth more small SMART goals that comport with your values. Maybe those would include talking to friends about how best to carry the criticism; asking the boss if you can take on an additional responsibility that would be meaningful to you and inviting him to give you guidance and critical feedback (essentially defusing from the punches a critical boss will likely deliver, while allowing you greater self-determination); exploring the possibility of a transfer within the company; or beginning to research getting a new job by visiting a job recruitment website.

As you work through this process, you may discover that for this challenge, you need more work with some of the skills than others. For example, you might notice that you can apply defusion very well to thoughts like *I'm not good enough*, but that negative emotions, such as the reemergence of the pain of criticism you felt as a child, knock you over sideways. In that case, you ought to work on relatively more intensive practice with acceptance skills. You might attribute that to being afraid of what might happen. But you should also look again at whether the goals are truly in alignment with your values. You might realize that you've become quite disconnected from a sense of what your authentic values regarding work are, and in that case, you'd want to do more intensive values exercises. It's important, though, to also continue applying all of the skills to the challenge.

Progress with some challenges may take more time than with others. That's perfectly fine; don't get discouraged. You've started dancing. You are moving with increasing flexibility. Always keep in mind that value-based living is not about reaching goalposts, it's about moving in your new chosen direction.

Actively Look for More Challenges

In Chapter Twenty, I discuss my experience with tinnitus. I'd never faced an acceptance problem like that before. It took just days to solve once I saw the connection, but it took me years to see that I should apply my skills to the condition. You can do better than I did by continuously looking for new ways to challenge your skills. If your life has become quite problem-free, fantastic! You can begin applying the skills to making life even more fulfilling. How?

Give yourself a new problem! I mean it. Look at all of the things we do for fun and think of how many are new ways to create problems. Jigsaw puzzles, game shows, sports, competition of all kinds, building a business, learning a language or a musical instrument. And yes, learning to dance.

Once you've applied your skills to some key challenges in the focused way just described, building them into habits, you can keep working with them in smaller doses, as an ongoing life enhancement. A great way to pick new problems is to think of the yearnings that are redirected by the flexibility pivots: feeling, belonging, competence, meaningful self-direction, coherence, orientation. In each of the values domains explored in Chapter Thirteen, consider each of these yearnings and how you can do an even better job of fulfilling them.

Say the domain is family.

How could you do a better job of feeling in your family? You might deepen your emotional connection by listening more or by exploring hard issues with family members. You could work on compassion and deliberately feeling the feelings of others in your family. You could share your feelings more.

You might strengthen your sense of connection with some more distant family members by writing them and calling more or by doing them some favors or responsibly asking for their help. You might write letters of appreciation or gratitude.

You might work on competence by taking a communication workshop or reading about how to foster a healthy family life. You might say "yes" more often to activities your family likes that you don't, or don't know whether or not you like them.

You might share your values and vulnerabilities more openly with your family and invite them to do the same with you.

You might let go of being "right" about some past event or trouble spot and focus on what is functionally most helpful right now in your relationships with your family.

You might practice being attentive and "here" when you are with your family. Look them in the eye; be more interested in being interested and less interested in being interesting. Validate, listen, and be present—let go of giving easy advice.

I just visited our yearnings for feeling, belonging, competence, meaningful self-direction, coherence, and orientation. I used them to create a fresh, exciting, progressive new set of problems.

There is no reason to stop applying the flexibility skills to new possibilities. My advice is to *do one new thing every day*—something that requires you to be open and present and that engages your values. To make sure your focus is broad, I suggest cycling through each of the values domains, perhaps focusing on each for a week or two at a time.

Share the Enrichment with Others

Many of us have been taught the economic theory that people are fundamentally selfish, and that is how the "invisible hand" of the market works. *Homo economicus*, they call humans. That vision of human nature is demonstrably false. Evolution science has discovered that, in fact, we are deeply prosocial beings, naturally given to helping others. We're *Homo prosocialis*, as my colleague Paul Atkins has said. Yes, we can be selfish, when the mind gets in the way and psychological inflexibility takes over. But 99 percent of the values people have are prosocial. As you keep pushing to evolve your life, a great project is to do *one kind thing every day for someone*, whether a friend, family member, colleague, or stranger—something that is compassionate and nonjudgmental and that matters to you and to the person you reach out to. In doing that, you are practicing how to support flexibility with flexibility, which is key to extending flexibility processes to others (which will be covered more in Chapter Nineteen). If you are not sure how to start, start small and play I've Got a Secret (see Chapter Thirteen) with what you do: kind anonymous acts are incredibly powerful. The Dictator doesn't know what to make of them!

As before, cycle through each of the values domains and each of the yearnings. Maybe for citizenship, you could help someone get to the polling place, or for work, you could take on part of a project a colleague is struggling with. You can always find new ways to live more in accord with your values, and your life and the lives of others will be ever more enriched as you do.

Reading the Part Three Chapters

Feel free to turn right to whichever chapter most interests you. Some of them, or sections of them, may pertain to issues neither you nor your loved ones are facing at the moment, and you can safely give them a pass. They may become helpful to you at some point, however, so keep them in mind. This book is designed as an ongoing life resource.

I do advise that minimally you read Chapter Fifteen, on adopting healthy behaviors; Chapter Seventeen, on nurturing relationships; and Chapter Twenty-One, on how ACT can support social transformation. I would venture that all of us could benefit from using the skills to adopt some behaviors that would be good for our physical health. I've also never known anyone who couldn't use some help in coping better with relationship stresses.

Chapter Twenty-One shows how ACT can be applied on the larger social scale, such as to a whole school or community. I think you will be moved by the story I tell there of how ACT training helped a city in Sierra Leone effectively combat an Ebola outbreak as well as cope with the grief of the death of their loved ones. That effort is only one way ACT is being used to address large-scale social problems. WHO has created an ACT self-help program and has successfully tested it in a program for refugees in Africa, for example. I'm asking that you read the chapter because I hope it will lead you to share my enthusiasm that psychological flexibility training offers great promise for helping to address the many social, behavioral, economic, and environmental ills that plague communities, whole countries, and indeed the world. Perhaps you will be inspired to help spread the word and build support for ACT teaching in whatever way you can—maybe providing ACT training for your team at work or guiding your family through it. With the pace of life today and all of its pressures, everyone has so much to gain from learning about psychological flexibility.

Chapter Fifteen

ADOPTING HEALTHY BEHAVIORS

A large study that analyzed the effects of all the known risk factors for poor health, such as exposure to pollution, an absence of clean water, and high blood pressure, recently produced a shocking finding. Nearly two-thirds of all poor health is due to behavior. Not infections, toxins, or genetic predisposition. What kinds of behavior? Smoking, drinking, eating an unhealthy diet, failing to exercise, not taking care of your teeth, and not getting good sleep, just to name a few.

Meanwhile, for every dollar spent on healthcare, less than a dime is spent on helping people change their unhealthy behaviors. Physical interventions, such as medications or surgery, are the go-to method for health problems in Western medicine, even though they usually carry their own risks and for some problems have limited effects. Proven psychological interventions are vastly underprescribed. But we as individuals can take charge. Let's face it, we pretty much know what we should be doing. The problem is that adopting new routines, and especially sticking with them, can be daunting.

ACT Skills Are Proven to Help

Let me give you just two quick examples. A recent study asked over one hundred self-declared chocolate cravers to carry around a bag of chocolates for a week and not eat them (if you are a chocoholic like me, you know this is almost cruel!). Some participants were given training specifically in ACT defusion and how it can free us from the grip of unhelpful thoughts and feelings, like cravings. Others were taught to directly challenge their cravings with cognitive restructuring techniques, such as telling themselves, "If I don't give in to this craving for chocolate, it will eventually fade." Guess how much more likely those who had been taught defusion were to not eat any chocolates? A whopping 326 percent!

Another study assessed the effects of ACT training on committing to exercise more often. One group of participants was given two short training sessions of exercise advice based on the guidelines of the American College of Sports Medicine. The other group was given two sessions of ACT training. Before the training sessions, the members of both groups were going to the gym about once a week. Afterward, those who received the ACT training went 65 percent more often over the next month, tailing off to an increase of 30 percent at a seven-week follow-up. Those in the other group actually *decreased* their amount of exercise by 24 percent over the same time.

Aaagh!

The fact is that just getting advice, and even tough-love messages about how important it is that we change our behavior, simply isn't very motivating—it may even be demotivating. Few of us need a lecture. Really. We don't. What we do need is help in freeing ourselves from the grip of unhelpful thoughts and emotions that get in our way of change. Here I'll discuss how the flexibility skills help with dieting and exercise, as well as with coping with stress—a major culprit in bad health—and with getting better sleep.

Dieting and Exercise

If you're struggling to stay on a diet and develop long-term healthier eating habits, you are in good company. About one in seven adults has gone on a diet in a given year. Unfortunately, much of the information offered in the vast supply of books, tapes, and online programs and by food supply services is not very well founded in science. Even the best and most extensive science-based programs have been found to lead to only about a 5 to 10 percent loss of body mass over two years of follow-up.

Consider one of the most effective programs, the Lifestyle, Exercise, Attitudes, Relationships and Nutrition (LEARN) Program for Weight Management. It was developed by Duke University psychologist Kelly Brownell, who is perhaps the world's leading expert on the psychology of weight loss (and who also happens to be one of my best and oldest friends). The program teaches various strategies for reducing unhealthy eating, such as keeping unhealthy foods out of your home; avoiding periods of abstinence, which can result in binge eating; counting calories; and committing to specific exercise goals. The program also advises that people distract themselves from food-related thoughts by deliberately thinking of other things and also coach themselves with helpful thoughts like *If I don't eat that cookie, this urge will eventually pass.* The approach can be quite helpful, but ACT was found to be more effective. In another study requiring people to refrain from eating chocolates, people given thirty minutes of ACT training were 30 percent less likely to eat them, and they were far less likely to experience their food urges as being aversive and overwhelming than people given thirty minutes of LEARN training, as above. This is because ACT helps so much with the psychological challenges that are such strong factors in unhealthy eating and failing to exercise for so many people.

As we've investigated why ACT training is effective in helping people change their eating and exercise behavior, we've found that one reason is that the flexibility skills help people cope with the difficult emotions and negative self-talk that are at the root of so much bad eating and exercise avoidance. So many of us fall into the habit of emotional eating, such as when we're lonely, sad, or stressed, as a way to self-soothe.

Shame is also a common problem for people working on their weight. It is easy to become hooked by toxic shame and self-stigma about being overweight and out of shape. And no wonder. The ridicule that is directed at people struggling with weight problems is appalling. While it has thankfully become taboo to tell racist or sexist jokes, or jokes about disabled people or gay people, telling jokes about people with weight problems is still often tolerated. There is *nothing* funny about them. A quarter to a third of all adults are dissatisfied with their body. Even physicians, who should know better, often shame patients about their excess weight.

I know that sense of shame very well from my own experience. Years ago, I weighed 235 pounds, which was a good 40 to 50 pounds more than was healthy, and I had to use all of my ACT skills to get down into the 180s or 190s, where I've remained ever since. I watched as my mind tried to "motivate" me with shame and blame, which did not help one bit. I couldn't make *any* progress until I really let go of that.

To precisely measure the role of shame and self-stigma in the battle with weight issues, my students and I developed a questionnaire for people to take that measures their level of weight-related shame. The amount of shame and the intensity of self-negative thoughts we have found is horrifying. So many agree to statements like *I became overweight because I'm a weak person*, *Others will think I lack self-control because of my weight problems*, or even *Others are ashamed to be around me because of my weight.*

Ouch.

People tend to fuse with thoughts like that, hoping they will motivate change. That is like cutting yourself off at the knees before running a race.

Our research team conducted a study to evaluate the impact of a single day of ACT training for overweight and obese people that was *entirely* focused on shame and self-stigma. All eighty-four of the participants had participated recently for at least six months in an organized weight loss program, and about a third were still in such a program. Half of the participants were randomly assigned to learn how to apply ACT skills to their negative emotions and thoughts, and nary a word was said about how they should work at losing weight. Helping them lose weight wasn't actually our goal; helping them to feel better about themselves and enhance the quality of their lives was our goal. Compared to a control group, those who got the ACT training reported a large reduction in both psychological distress and weight-related shame, and a large increase in quality of life. The big surprise was that many of them also did lose weight, on average at least five pounds by the time of a three-month follow-up we did with them. Their binge eating decreased by nearly 50 percent by that time, while the control group's binges had *increased* by about the same amount. Equally important, those in the ACT group reported that their distress about their weight decreased considerably *even if they did not lose weight.*

The physical distress of exercise is another major impediment, which acceptance also helps with. Even competitive athletes can do better work by focusing on their willingness to experience unpleasant sensations. But ironically, compulsive overexercise is also driven by avoidance of even more difficult emotions, such as appearance fears.

ACT values work helps with motivating us to keep up our efforts. The typical approach to motivating people to push themselves to exercise is "just do it" messages like "Keep going!" That may actually be *unhelpful* for many people. In a study we conducted with participants of a spin class, we gave all of them cards to read as they cycled. Some of the cards had command-style messages like *Keep your back straight and spin hard!* while others took an ACT approach, reminding them of a goal or life value from exercising they'd told us was important to them, such as *Exercise will improve my respiratory system* or *Exercise will make my clothes fit better.* The typical coaching advice actually *decreased* the effort people put into the class, while the values messages increased it.

One of the most problematic aspects of so many people's efforts to trim down and get in shape is that they're doing it so much *for others*. They're not finding intrinsic value in the process. Eating well and exercising can indeed be enormously fulfilling in themselves: we feel more vital when we care for our bodies. Be careful of values like "looking good," which can be self-objectifying and lead you down the path of judging yourself harshly. Focus instead on the advantages of a healthy lifestyle, such as imparting a devotion to healthy living to your children and living longer.

Values work also helps with shame. For example, for one of my clients, Susan, who was a hundred pounds overweight, shame about how her body looked when she was exercising was the key stumbling block to exercising. She was embarrassed by the way her fat jiggled when she ran. The turning point for her was the onset of early signs of diabetes. When I helped her look closely at her values around exercise, she was surprised to find that what she most wanted was not to look good, but to be back inside her body, as she put it, so she could dance, hug, bowl, ski, swim, and play. In other words, she wanted to feel comfortable being herself and live as she desired without inflicting all sorts of negative messaging on herself. When she realized that, she saw how shaking a finger at herself about how she looked was a values violation. As she learned to embrace a positive vision for her health, an increase in exercise came along for the ride. She lost about fifty pounds over the next year, and her psychological and physical health improved rapidly.

Negative self-talk is another major impediment to sticking with diet and exercise routines. People berate themselves with messages like *Who are you kidding, you don't have the strength!* or unhelpful defensiveness like *I need some comfort ice cream, so sue me!* Defusion exercises help break the spell of this messaging.

What about self skills? Many people who are locked in unhealthy behavior have been weaving an entangling negative self-story like *I'm just fat; I was born that way and I'm always going to be that way* or *I just have a low threshold for pain; I'm a wimp.* The self skills will bring that to the surface and help to break free.

How can presence practices help? One of the great frustrations in trying to stick with healthier eating and exercising is that results take time. The end goal seems so far away. Whenever you find yourself thinking about how much more progress you've got to make, do some presence work to bring your focus back to the moment and to the recognition that habit building happens in small steps. You can continually redirect your attention to the progress you're making right now.

Finally, your action exercises will help you set SMART goals and stick to them. So many of the diets hyped in the media are extreme, and sometimes actually unhealthy. Many exercise classes and recommendations about how much exercise to do are overtaxing for people embarking on the journey. Use your action practices to devise your own game plan and discover what works best for you.

You might want to start by taking the assessment that measures the amount of shame you may be feeling about your weight or being out of shape, which you can find at my website (http://www.stevenchayes.com). Next, write down all of the negative emotions you've been feeling and unhelpful messages you've been berating yourself with. Then systematically go through the exercises in your toolkit using these thoughts and emotions as the target. After you've applied the exercises you've put in your toolkit, you might want to keep going by doing all of the other exercises presented in the Part Two chapters. You can also consult more advice to be found in entire books devoted to applying ACT to eating and exercise. Here are just a few special pieces of additional advice that I have found helpful in improving physical fitness in an ACT way.

Read Your Own Body and Do What Works

The range of advice on diet and exercise is overwhelming. While it makes sense to try to keep up with the latest information, and to try things that are well supported by research, much dieting advice in particular is not established by science. So much advice is also contradictory. Fat is awful; no, it depends. Sugar is terrible, but wait, artificial sweeteners are poison.

Choose rational things you'd like to try and experiment with them. Remember: variation, selection, retention. Keep only what you find helpful. What works for others may not be good for you. For example, lots of programs tell you to eat a big breakfast. But I like a very light and very late breakfast of a few walnuts and an apple. I settled on that because I can sense in my body that for me light is better, and even that walnuts are better than, say pecans. I call it *body knowledge*.

I've been watching and tweaking these patterns for years (other examples from my own body knowledge are cutting down on flour or decreasing the total time window for eating to under eight hours), and I'm not usually surprised to read studies that back up *what I've seen with my own body.* But a few months ago, I was startled to see a large new study that actually *tested* ACT plus (wait for it) walnuts! Lo and behold, while ACT alone was better than usual care, they saw even better outcomes by adding walnuts. Apparently, my body is not the only one reacting this way!

You might be different. Don't follow my pattern: watch the science and try things out. Pay attention to your body and let it educate you. You are evolving your life *as you choose.*

Make Friends with Your Cravings

The next time you feel a craving come on, try this. Instead of fighting it, take a step back and notice it for what it is. You might even label it "craving." Don't fight it. Just look at it. Then ask yourself the following questions:

1. **If your craving had a shape, what would it be?**
2. **If it had a color, what would it be?**
3. **If it had a size, how big or small would it be?**
4. **Does it seem solid, like an object, or does it shimmer, flutter, shake, or move?**
5. **Where does it live in your body? Do you experience it in your head? Your belly? Somewhere else?**
6. **Are there any emotions that are connected to this craving? Do you feel anxious, stressed out, sad, angry, or something else?**

Now, imagine you can reach out and touch your craving. At first, you might give it a sympathetic pat on the back, so to speak. See if eventually you can actually embrace the craving, figuratively cradling it in your arms like you would a child. Feel empathy for it, noticing how much it wants, how hungry it is for attention.

You can do all of this without acting on the craving. In fact, you can take this craving with you while you engage in any action of your choosing. In time, the craving may fade. But if it doesn't, you can carry it as long as it needs. It's not you—it's a part of you.

Build in Tiny Amounts of Exercise Everywhere You Go

The demand for quick, big success has produced more failure than any other verbal rule. In the area of exercise, *small and now* will beat *big and then* any day. Pick small exercises you can do during the day and link them to your regular activities. Then build small habits of doing them. If your mind complains that these exercises are too small to matter, agree enthusiastically and go right on doing them.

Here are some ways to begin.

* **While in line anywhere, slowly do toe raises.**
* **Always take the stairs if you have time and it is safe. Always.**
* **When grocery shopping, grab a gallon of milk in a plastic jug with a handle and, while you shop, *slowly* do curls or triceps presses to the point of muscle exhaustion (a count of eight up and four down is about right—yes, there has actually been research on this!). If you ever see me in an airport, chances are you will see me doing this with my briefcase. People will look at you funny, but do you care?**
* **While waiting for your coffee to brew in the morning, do squats.**

* **Do push-ups every other night before going to bed, having the goal of doing as many as your years on the planet (yes, I can do seventy of them).**

Get a Shame Buddy and Push Your Own Buttons

If your defusion skills allow you to use advanced social defusion methods (see Chapter Eight), exercise together with friends who are willing to put common shame statements out there for all to see. Do this only if you have a gut sense that you are truly ready for this practice. Say you have a friend who is also trying to lose weight and is willing to do vigorous walks with you. Both of you are ashamed of the way your bodies jiggle as you walk. Get T-shirts made with statements like *My Body Jiggles. So Sue Me!* and wear them together during your exercise program.

Timed well, this can be extremely liberating, even fun! Think of it as a mental Declaration of Independence, as if you are underlining that it's OK to be you, *really*.

Coping with Stress

Excessive stress is one of the most widespread and pernicious assaults on general health and well-being. It's been implicated in the suppression of the immune system and in the development of chronic diseases, including diabetes, cancer, and cardiovascular disease. Work is one of the chief sources of stress, often leading to low work satisfaction, emotional exhaustion, and burnout. Numerous studies done with workers in a number of high-stress professions, including nursing, social work, and teaching, have shown that learning flexibility skills helps significantly in lowering stress levels and mitigating their negative effects.

The ACT skills are so helpful in coping with stress because its harmful effects come more from our *reactivity* to stress than from stress itself. There is bad stress and good stress. Stress-producing tasks include positive challenges, such as developing new relationships, pursuing job opportunities, competing in athletics, and raising children. We should not seek to eliminate stress by opting out of desired challenges. Of course, there is also the stress caused by undue pressures put on us, particularly at work, and impediments of all sorts, like being stuck in bad traffic on a regular morning work commute, or wading through time-sucking bureaucratic processes.

With some sources of stress, seeking to eliminate it is the right way to go, and many methods of tamping it down are great. If you can move to a better location that would not have a horrific commute, that might be a smart choice. If you have a hostile boss, changing jobs may be well advised. If you can find ways to bring your workload down while still meeting performance requirements and carrying your work life in a valued direction, you should absolutely do that. If you sense that exercising helps reduce stress, that's another fantastic reason to commit to regular workouts. Spending more restorative time with friends and family is also important.

But if you find that you are focusing on your stress and mentally trying to fight it, you may be caught in the grip of a negative thought network that is actually intensifying the impact of stress. Frank Bond, who conducted pioneering research on applying ACT to work, developed a metaphor I like: Think of yourself as being a sink and the sources of stress as the taps pouring stress into you. One way to reduce your stress level would be to shut off the taps, but just as effective would be to unplug the drain, letting the stress flow through you.

Research has shown that flexibility skills help with *both* tasks: confronting the stressful situation and changing it, as well as learning how to reduce stress reactivity. That was shown years ago in the first ACT study done on worksite stress: ACT reduced stress reactivity in call center workers. In addition, even though the study had not encouraged them to, the workers then began to fight for healthy changes in their work environment.

Acceptance is especially helpful in dealing with stress because so much stress is caused by factors in our lives we can't change. Say you have a nasty boss. You may be feeling intense stress because you're focusing on how unfair his behavior is and you want to be able to change it. But you most likely can't. Or maybe you're facing a debilitating disease, or family members hate your political views. Accepting unchangeables is the first step in pursuing more constructive approaches to coping with them.

The other flexibility skills assist in dealing with stress for a number of key reasons. One is that some of our stress is caused by overidentification with our work and achievements. Our sense of self becomes too wrapped up in our job title—"I'm a doctor"—or in the need to be seen as a certain kind of worker—"I'm a high performer." Many companies reinforce this by administering employee evaluations that imply that we are defined by our performance, with little to no accounting for whether the company is providing the support needed for good performance. Lots of bosses also cause us to engage in excessive self-monitoring and harmful self-criticism by overemphasizing problems they see in our performance while offering nary a word of praise. Workplaces are cauldrons of social compliance pressure and judgment. They can provoke our Dictator to raise its ugly head with a steady stream of self-rebuke, which often undermines our effectiveness at tasks, in turn leading to further self-criticism and more stress.

Defusion helps us distance from this negative self-talk, "opening the drain." Self skills remind us that we are not the roles we play, or the perceptions others have of us; we are the "I" deep within. Maybe your boss characterizes you as disorganized. Connecting with your transcendent self will help you see that even though she sees you that way, it is not *who you are*. By not identifying with such characterizations, we're able to listen to criticism in a constructive way. That in turn helps us make changes in our behavior that relieve stress, such as no longer procrastinating. Self perspective-taking also helps us put ourselves in the shoes of those whose behavior causes us stress and see that a spouse's nasty comment or a boss's eruption at us often has more to do with them and the stress they're feeling than with us.

Developing presence helps us focus on the tasks at hand rather than on our worries about how we'll perform them. When we're deeply absorbed in the moment, we often find that even the most potentially stress-inducing tasks are actually hugely enjoyable. Values work will help us throw ourselves into meaningful challenges despite the stress we know they'll cause us.

Action skills help us reduce stress by crafting goals that are manageable and then getting going rather than stalling because of anxiety, which only increases our stress.

To begin applying ACT to whatever stresses you're struggling with, write down your list of barriers and the ways in which you've been trying to contend with them. These are your stress buttons—the people, challenges, worries, or thoughts and emotions of any kind that cause you stress. If you are feeling stress due to illness, the situations might be going for a medical procedure or sitting in the waiting room worrying about what the doctor will tell you. For those experiencing work stress, perhaps they include meeting with your boss or giving presentations, while stress at home might be provoked by trying to get a child to go to bed. You get the drill.

A good way to do this is to write each situation on a slip of paper. Now go through that pile and sort them into a "change the situation" pile, meaning that there are actions you can take to relieve the stress, and a "change the relationship to the situation" pile for the unchangeables. Now, for each of the changeables, use the flexibility skills to think through why you're not taking the actions that could improve things and commit to a set of SMART goals.

For the unchangeables, focus on accepting and learning from the situation as it is. Say that you're feeling lots of stress in your role as a parent, but you are confident that you are doing all of the right things. Even so, you are plagued by negative self-judgments about your adequacy. Your stress is not going to go down by working even harder to be a good parent; in fact, that's likely to lead to more stress. Your task is to become less *reactive* to the unavoidable stress you're feeling. Do lots of defusion work to distance from the voice of criticism. Say "I'm a bad parent" rapidly (shorten it as you go to simply "bad parent"—that makes it easier to say repeatedly) until it sounds like mere gibberish. Write down all of your self-recriminations on pieces of paper and carry them around with you. If you are truly ready to let go of this self-criticism, you might even write *Bad Parent* in bold letters on a sticky note and wear it during family outings.

Apply your self-learning to recraft the story you're telling yourself about the kind of parent you are and to stop comparing yourself to society's fairy-tale notions of what raising children should be like. Parenting is messy and frustrating; it involves lots of anger and upset along with the good times. How could that not be stressful? Make a practice of reminding yourself that you're feeling stress because you're a good parent who cares about parenting well.

Here are a couple of additional practices that are especially helpful in dealing with stress.

Practice a Flexibility Habit Linked to a Stressor

Pick something that you often do that is not itself that stressful but is reliably linked to a stressor. Suppose a stressor for you is facing your boss in the morning. The thing linked to it might be driving to work. Let's say you realize that facing your boss is stressful partly because of thoughts about how your boss judges you, such as *He thinks I'm not very smart.* In the car each day as you drive to work, take a few minutes to practice defusion from those thoughts. Maybe you like to sing in the car. Sing *She's not smart* to your favorite tune. After a few days of this, drives to work may be both more fun and helpful in dialing down stress reactivity.

Stress-Inducing Passengers on the Bus

One of the most commonly used ACT metaphors is "the passengers on the bus." Imagine that you are driving a bus called "your life." Like any bus, as you move along you pick up passengers. Your passengers are your memories, bodily sensations, conditioned emotions, and networked thoughts. With stressful passengers, like anxiety about being criticized, if you pay attention to them, you'll be taking your eyes off the road. It's natural to want to boot them off the bus, but that requires you to stop the bus, interfering with getting where you want to go. Meanwhile some passengers are so obnoxious that they simply refuse to leave. Then you're engaged in a mighty struggle. The healthy alternative is to keep driving and keep your focus on the road.

To turn this metaphor into an exercise, list some of your stress passengers on small cards, and carry them with you during the next week. Whenever you remember the exercise, pat where you are carrying the cards, as if to welcome them all on that bus of life called you, and notice again that you are the driver here. You may not choose your passengers . . . but as the driver you do choose the journey.

Sleep

A great irony of having insomnia is that some of the difficulty comes from awareness of how important getting good sleep is. One of the biggest predictors of poor sleep is entanglement with repetitive negative thoughts and worries, including worry about getting to sleep. I'm sure poor sleepers know the problem well. You find yourself lying in bed worrying about some event you've got coming up, or caught up in problem solving or planning, and then, because you're failing to fall asleep, you begin worrying about that too.

Trying to make ourselves go to sleep is one of the most frustrating things we can ever experience. And we're not wrong to make the effort. The toll from lack of sleep is atrocious.

A wealth of research has revealed a wide range of unhealthy effects. People with poor sleep patterns incur healthcare costs that are 10 to 20 percent higher than those who get good sleep. Inadequate sleep also impairs cognitive functioning, such as working memory and problem solving, and it can cause or worsen depression and anxiety and lead to irritability, which can all undermine the quality of our relationships. On top of these consequences, there are the costs to individuals, companies, and society at large in terms of missed workdays and poor decisions that may have costs for others as well, such as bad medical decisions by sleepy healthcare providers.

ACT studies in chronic pain and depression have documented that better sleep can come along as a kind of good side effect of flexibility processes, and pilot studies of ACT for insomnia are producing good outcomes. But this is an area where large controlled scientific studies of ACT have not yet been done. The best-supported treatment approach is cognitive behavioral therapy for insomnia, or CBTi, and most consumers should start there but with an eye toward using flexibility skills as well. Let me explain.

CBTi is generally administered in a series of therapist-guided sessions, usually between five and eight, that focus on good sleep hygiene, such as avoiding smoking, consuming caffeine or alcohol late in the day, or exercising right before bed; establishing a regular sleep schedule; using the bed only for sleep and sex (no reading, texting, or watching TV); and strictly limiting the time spent lying awake in bed, so we don't come to associate being in bed with insomnia. For example, often people are advised that if they still can't go to sleep after twenty minutes, they should get out of bed. The treatment also involves restructuring of catastrophizing thoughts (for example, "I have to go to sleep or else I'll blow that meeting and get fired" might be changed to "It would be nice to go to sleep, but either way I can handle it"). Often relaxation techniques are also taught, and people are cautioned to avoid consciously *trying* to sleep.

While the approach works well for many, for some it's ineffective. One reason may be the problem with cognitive restructuring we've considered before. Changing your thoughts in a given direction means taking their content seriously. You have to notice them and evaluate them in order to try to change them, which may actually strengthen their hold over your mind and wake you up.

To address this problem, researchers tested a combination of ACT training and a modified form of CBTi with a patient who had initially seen good effects from CBTi but had relapsed into insomnia. He was first put through three new sessions of CBTi, which was modified by instructing him not to do cognitive restructuring of the thoughts that were keeping him up. He was also given six sessions of ACT training, in which he was taught to accept those thoughts as well as the feeling of fatigue his lack of sleep was causing. This included doing the "leaves on the stream" exercise with the thoughts and imagining that his fatigue was an object, describing its shape, color, and size, as well a defusion exercise, like those given in Chapter Nine. He also did values work, committing to activities he had avoided but loved such as nighttime reading (he'd been afraid it would make his mind active) or scheduling weekend activities with his family (he'd been afraid he would be too tired to do them). By the end of the therapy he reported feeling more energy as well as coping better when he was fatigued, and he said his relationship with his family was improving. So while I do not advise using ACT as a first treatment instead of CBTi, if CBTi isn't having good enough effects for you, try adding ACT methods to it this way and not doing the cognitive restructuring.

One ACT-based exercise to try that I've found helpful when I'm struggling to get to sleep is a variation of the "open focus" presence exercise discussed in Chapter Twelve. Purposefully put your mind into a mode of broad and dim attention. It may help to think of this as a slow, fuzzy, dispassionate form of mindful observation, gently noting any mental activity that stands out but without excessive interest. Just passively be with whatever shows up in your mind, the way you can "be with" hot water when you sit in a soaking tub. Don't focus as much on your thoughts and other experiences as in the typical presence exercises; more gently notice what shows up, notice the empty spaces between them, and then do nothing with these experiences and spaces. It may help to think of this as putting your mind on a kind of temporary unemployment status; it has no work to do. While your body knows how to sleep, your problem-solving mind does not, and this helps to convince it that it doesn't have any work to do for you.

Finally, you may also want to consult *The Sleep Book*, by Dr. Guy Meadows, a psychologist in England who runs an "all ACT" sleep clinic. He has developed a detailed ACT approach to sleep therapy, which is presented there.

Chapter Sixteen

MENTAL HEALTH

Mental health conditions have been characterized in the popular media and even in the loose talk of researchers as *diseases*, as though depression, OCD, and addiction are comparable to cancer or diabetes. They are not. To qualify as a disease, a condition has to have a known originating cause (an *etiology*), be expressed through known processes (a *course*), and respond in particular ways to treatment. Mental health conditions don't meet those criteria. The medical community actually refers to them as syndromes, and they are rather roughly diagnosed through lists of symptoms. People are said to have a condition if they display a little more than half of the list.

The group of psychiatrists and psychologists tasked with creating the latest set of names for syndromes know that full well. An article from the developers noted that treating syndromes as if they are equivalent to diseases "is more likely to obscure than to elucidate research findings" because research based on them may "never be successful in uncovering their underlying etiologies. For that to happen, an as yet unknown paradigm shift may need to occur." I and my colleagues agree and have been attempting to create a shift to a more process-oriented approach to an understanding of mental health conditions.

The popular understanding of mental health has been pushed too far in a medical direction. An example is the idea that mental health conditions and addiction are fundamentally determined by genes. Now that we can map the entire genome of hundreds of thousands of people, we know that entire gene systems account for only a small fraction of any given mental health or addiction condition. Environment and behavior are big influences. Indeed, no clear biological marker has been found for any common mental health condition.

An example of how genes and environment interact is provided by family risk studies that show that depression, anxiety, and substance abuse tend to "hang out together." So, if your father had alcoholism, as mine did, you might be vulnerable not only to alcoholism but also to depression and anxiety. Some of that is due to genetically determined differences in how readily the nervous system links previous events to psychological pain. If you are "high strung" and can easily connect neutral experiences to later bad events, you are genetically prepared to be hit harder by psychologically painful events. If you have that tendency but are raised in a family with a high level of nurturance and secure attachments (solid and safe relationships), all may be well. Even when bad things happen, if your parents do not model experiential avoidance, problems may not result. But take a person who is genetically primed to react to negative events; mix in painful or abusive experiences, especially in the absence of security and nurturance; and add a dollop of family traditions of avoidance and inflexibility, and voilà, you have the formula for mental health problems.

A wealth of studies show that learning psychological skills can lead to notable improvements in coping with mental health challenges, often with better long-term outcomes and fewer side effects than with medications. Mental health conditions are often characterized by excessive amounts of behavior that may be adaptive in some contexts. For example, thinking through how to learn from past mistakes is not a bad thing—but allowing that pattern to cycle into outright rumination predicts depression. Flexibility skills motivate us to consider thoughts and behaviors that break the hold of a narrow repertoire of unhealthy ones and to focus on what works. That naturally leads to better balance, which is essential to evolving on purpose.

If you are struggling with mental health conditions, you should view reading books like this one as a supplement to professional help, not a replacement. Getting treatment when you are struggling is vital, and too many people fail to go for it. A major reason for this omission is, unfortunately, stigma. Research indicates that across the world, as many as one in five people will experience a common mental health condition during a given year, and that as many as one in three people will experience some form of mental health challenge during their lifetime. Nonetheless, many people hold judgmental views about these conditions. Many see mental struggles as a weakness of character. People with mental illness are tagged as incompetent, dangerous, or irreparably "broken," leading to discrimination in hiring and social distancing.

The result is that people with such conditions often hide their symptoms, even from loved ones, and avoid treatment or support. In fact, only about one in five will seek assistance from a mental health provider. That is a tragedy, especially because scientifically well-established treatment is available. In other words, there is help.

Stigmatization can also be internalized in the form of self-blame and even self-loathing. Misguided cultural messages like "just think positive thoughts" only encourage more avoidance and make it worse. ACT helps people cope with the pain of stigma and defuse from unhelpful messages.

If you do seek treatment, ACT skills will complement those efforts. ACT is familiar enough to the professional therapeutic community that you may be able to engage your therapist in a conversation about how best to do so, and you could supplement that by online searches of your own about how ACT and flexibility processes are in accord with the concepts and approaches your provider is using. Or see if any ACT therapists are nearby: http://bit.ly/FindanACTtherapist.

At this point in the book you likely appreciate why ACT is helpful with mental challenges: it strengthens a different mode of mind that is more observant, appreciative, and empowering, and less critical and mindless. Flexibility skills lessen the impact of unhealthy self messages and help people come into the present; opening up, noticing, and naming difficult emotions that echo forward from our history. That lays the foundation to focus instead on our authentic values and to take steps to make them central to our lives.

The action exercises provide assistance in following prescribed steps, whether those are SMART goals you set for yourself or ones recommended by a therapist or a program. ACT practices can support other established programs for coping with mental health issues, such as AA, peer support groups, or online programs.

A good general approach to applying ACT to mental health struggles is to once again start by considering the internal barriers that are contributing to the difficulty you're experiencing and making a list of the strategies you've been trying for coping with them. Often you will see obvious ways to begin practicing the exercises in your toolkit with these barriers as your targets.

All of the flexibility skills are relevant, but some will be especially helpful for some conditions. For example, because of the prominent role of rumination in depression, the power of defusion exercises to free you from its grip can be especially helpful. For anxiety, exposure exercises are helpful, and acceptance and values work will help make exposure both more possible and more useful. For substance abuse, acceptance helps greatly in dealing with the psychological and physical discomfort of cravings as well as with the emotional pain people are so often trying to numb out. Experience itself will help you focus more on the skills that you find most helpful, but it is best to work with the other tools in your toolkit too because they'll reinforce your progress.

Now, here is more specific guidance about common conditions.

Depression

If you have depression, you probably know that it's quite common. But you may not know just how common. Depression is now the leading cause of disability in the world—about 350 million people around the globe are wrestling with it, including one in twenty Americans over age twelve.

Antidepressant medication is helpful for severely depressed people over the short term, but many fail to respond. The effects for most are not large, and long-term or high-dose use carries the risk of a long list of side effects, including sexual dysfunction and an increased risk of relapse. Psychotherapy has been found comparably effective for depression over the short term, with notably lower side effects and more benefits after treatment is stopped. Researchers are still trying to figure out if there is an advantage to combining therapy with medication for truly major depression, but the combination for lesser depression is not significantly more effective. As long as the jury is still out, it's important to check out the current research as best you can before agreeing to any course of treatment.

You may already be in therapy, or may be considering what sort of therapy to go for, so let me offer some guidance about ACT vis-à-vis other options. The leading form of therapy prescribed for depression for many years has been traditional CBT, and many studies have shown that it can lead to good outcomes. But why traditional CBT works is still confusing. As discussed earlier, many studies have indicated that the benefits of CBT are largely due to the behavioral elements, not just restructuring thoughts. Meanwhile, dozens of randomized trials have measured ACT's effects on depression, and so far ACT has been found just as effective as CBT. In addition, we know more about why it works—because it develops psychological flexibility, which gives people a clearer focus on the immediate targets of change.

For example, as noted, rumination is a leading contributor to depression. ACT research has uncovered part of the reason. Researchers studied people who had experienced a major loss to see if rumination led them to become depressed; the answer was yes, but only if they were ruminating to avoid difficult emotions. If your mind simply returns to the loss repeatedly, without efforts to avoid the pain, the rumination will eventually diminish and not cause much, if any, harm.

Suppose you have experienced a major loss such as the suicide of a close friend. All of us will wonder, "Is there something I missed?" or "Why didn't

I call her and ask how she was doing?" If you are reliving the past to avoid the pain of the loss, however, you will be unable to connect fully with the love you felt toward your friend; you will be less likely to reach out to other friends for support. You are risking getting "stuck" in that state we call depression.

ACT is linked to the CBT tradition, so many CBT therapists are willing to draw on ACT to complement the elements of CBT we know are helpful, especially the behavioral elements. Flexibility pivots can easily be combined with virtually any well-validated method. An example is provided by one of the best types of therapy for depression, Behavioral Activation (BA). Great results have been found in research that combines it with ACT.

BA was developed by the late Neil Jacobson, a good friend who overlapped with me as an intern. He combined acceptance practices with methods for helping patients do more of what they care about, focusing on replacement behaviors. If someone is sleeping late in an effort to escape depressive feelings, a replacement behavior of going for an early-morning walk might be recommended. A schedule of positive replacement activities is generally created to help move toward goals. Emotional avoidance is discouraged.

BA and ACT agree about the futility of trying to directly change the content of thoughts that are contributing to depression, and also about helping people see the negative effects of avoidance strategies. ACT adds defusion, self, and presence practices and emphasizes that actions should be in the service of valued living. These skills help people commit to replacement behaviors. If you're in BA therapy, talk to your provider about how to add ACT into it.

I can't let this section close without a brief shout-out to Neil, since he was one of the early supporters of ACT. Neil called me as his second large study on BA, which showed that BA was better than traditional CBT, was winding down. He told me it was time to stage a "contextual revolution" combining my early ACT methods with BA and other new CBT methods that had recently been developed. I excitedly agreed and booked a flight to Seattle for a few weeks later to plot the revolution. But Neil tragically died of a heart attack days before that flight. I eventually declared the arrival of the Third Wave of CBT (with ACT as a foremost example) on my own, but the Third Wave would surely have benefited greatly had this science warrior lived!

Anxiety

About 12 percent of people around the world will experience some form of anxiety challenge during any given year, and as many as 30 percent of us can expect to grapple with an anxiety condition during the course of our lives. The good news is that research has shown ACT to be highly effective across the many different kinds. Here I'll introduce some of the results and highlight a few specific guidelines about tailoring ACT to coping with anxiety.

The standard of care for anxiety, as for depression, is CBT, and ACT has proven either comparable or somewhat more effective for anxiety than traditional CBT in many studies. One well-done study comes from a research team at UCLA supervised by psychology professor Michelle Craske—one of the best CBT researchers on the planet. Participants were given twelve hour-long sessions of individual counseling, one session a week, which was either ACT-based or CBT-based. Both groups showed great improvement by the end of the sessions, but in a follow-up with them twelve months later, the ACT group showed much greater improvement. They were moving on in their lives and engaging in significantly less avoidant behavior and negative thinking. The defusion and acceptance skills were found to account for the difference.

The ACT community has discovered some key ways the flexibility practices can be tailored to anxiety. These concern how one engages in exposure to triggers of anxiety, which is a main component of traditional treatment for phobias, social anxiety disorder, and OCD. ACT therapists have learned that rather than starting right away with some exposure work, it's best to begin by building defusion and acceptance skills and doing values work and then start doing exposure. For example, in one study that produced strong results, exposure exercises weren't introduced until the sixth session out of twelve. The first five sessions were devoted entirely to the flexibility skills. This was so that participants could draw on their ACT learning as they began facing the discomfort of exposure. Defusion and acceptance help with difficult thoughts and feelings, and several studies have shown that it is easier to do exposure if the activities are meaningful to people. Say that you have social anxiety and an activity recommended to you is attending a cocktail party. That kind of socializing may not be of interest to you. Instead you could use values work to identify activities that you've been avoiding that you'd really like to be doing. Maybe that would be attending an exercise class.

Another modification to traditional exposure is that patients are instructed to start with activities that are relatively easy to manage and work up to the most challenging ones. ACT doesn't put a premium on the amount of discomfort the activity provokes. The ACT approach is that you are free to choose whichever activities you prefer, because they're of value to you, whether they are easy or challenging.

If you discover that you weren't as ready for exposure as you had thought, and you have to stop, or maybe you even had a panic attack, don't let your Dictator beat you up. Walking out of an anxiety struggle is a journey that will inevitably involve some trying times. Since my last panic attack twenty-three years ago I have sometimes been very anxious, but I have been able to keep doing anxiety-inducing activities, such as giving lectures to large crowds, by using my skills whenever anxiety starts creeping up on me. To be honest, writing this book is an example. If it is hugely successful, who knows? Maybe Oprah will call.

Aaagh!!!

One exercise that I've found helpful as a regular practice is the reverse compass trick I wrote about earlier. I used the example of assigning myself the task of rubbing my hands over my face if I have an obsessive thought about cleanliness when leaving a restroom. To apply this to your own anxiety, make a list of activities that can be anxiety-provoking that you avoid and start picking them off, one by one. For example, perhaps you've noticed your mind telling you that it is too scary to ride a roller coaster, take a dance lesson, take a trip by yourself, agree to talk to a church group, sing at a karaoke bar, ride a zip line, tell a friend how much they mean to you, or any of a hundred such things. Try to do at least one new anxiety-provoking thing from your list every week, and during the exercise itself, work on your mindfulness skills, including presence, acceptance, defusion, and self.

I've learned never to say never about anxiety, and about life. I hope and pray I will stand with myself even if Oprah dials me up!

Substance Abuse

Flexibility skills will complement whatever approach to recovering from substance abuse and addiction one pursues, whether that's a twelve-step program, residential treatment, individual counseling, use of agonists and antagonists (e.g., methadone for opiate addiction), motivational interviewing, contingency management, or any of several others. Controlled studies have verified that ACT training enhances outcomes during treatment programs and in staying abstinent after treatment. The skills will also help with seeking treatment, which is a huge barrier for so many people who are experiencing any problem.

One of our earliest large studies on ACT for substance abuse assessed the effects of the skills used in conjunction with methadone maintenance for people struggling with opiate addiction. At a six-month follow-up assessment, 50 percent of those in the ACT group were clean, as measured by urine tests, as compared to 12 percent of those getting methadone and standard drug counseling alone.

In the years since, there have been over a dozen decent quality studies on ACT for substance abuse, and they have shown that it appears to help across a wide range of specific types. We've learned a lot about why. For one thing, substance use is often motivated by avoidance. While some people just stumble into it because initially it's fun, or because all their friends are using and then their use escalates, many people are drawn to taking harmful drugs and drinking excessively because they're seeking to numb difficult thoughts and feelings, whether they're fully aware of that or not. By stressing the power of acceptance and the harm caused by avoidance, ACT training helps undermine the power of substances to fool the person using them. We have a phrase we like to use: "ACT—we take the fun out of addiction!" Yes, it's a joke, but the point is serious. Real avoidance works 100 percent *only if you do not know you are doing it*. At the point that you *know* that you are using substances as an avoidance mechanism, you have a chance to choose a different direction. Of course, the process is challenging.

Recovery involves both the physical challenges of withdrawal and the psychological challenges of abandoning deeply ingrained habits. In addition, substance abuse is one of the most stigmatized problems anyone can develop, and internalizing that sense of stigma is a powerful predictor of poor outcomes. That internalization is pushed deeper by psychological inflexibility but can be alleviated by learning flexibility skills.

Acceptance skills help in coping with the physical and psychological distress of withdrawal. The many ways in which the body and mind inveigh against efforts to stop are a challenging aspect of substance abuse, with cravings and other withdrawal symptoms often motivating relapse. Acceptance can help stay the course of abstinence and break the negative feedback loop.

ACT skills can also help people move beyond compulsive thoughts about using and tamp down the effects of deeply embedded psychological triggers. Recall that RFT explains that dense networks of relations become fixed in our minds, and that thoughts embedded in them can be triggered at any moment. Neuroscientific research on addiction has shown that precisely this process is at play. All sorts of cues that have been related to substance use can trigger thoughts of using. Some are obvious, like seeing a beer commercial or catching a whiff of marijuana, but others may be totally outside our awareness.

Therapists know this, which is why a standard component of most substance abuse treatment programs is avoiding triggers. The problem is that the degree to which we can control our exposure to them is limited because the networks of relations in our minds are so elaborate. For example, a relative we don't see often might be related in our minds to drinking, because on occasions when we do see him, there is always some drinking going on. Maybe we hear someone say something this relative once said. Our brain may immediately call drinking to mind. Even our efforts to abstain become related in our minds to using, as when I noticed that having the thought *I'm calm and relaxed* kicked off my anxiety. Likewise, thoughts about using can themselves trigger a physical reaction similar to actual using—albeit a more moderate one. For example, people with a history of using cocaine respond to videos of people using cocaine by experiencing a release of dopamine into their brains similar to the one they'd get if they were using themselves.

ACT gives us another route forward: reduce the impact of triggers when they occur. Eradicating all subconscious cues and cravings is unrealistic, but building up acceptance and commitment skills creates room for those unwanted thoughts and impulses to roam through our minds without compelling us to act on them, gradually reducing their impact. They assist with what a friend and colleague, the late alcoholism researcher Alan Marlatt, referred to as "surfing the urge."

ACT learning also disempowers the harmful negative self-talk that those who struggle with substance abuse so often inflict on themselves. Intense self-recrimination contributes to the pain of addiction, further fueling the impulse to avoid by using. Recrimination after relapse can be especially brutal. In addition, the pain of stigma and the shame it induces are powerful impediments to seeking assistance. So many people delay until the problem is acute or they've hit bottom. Learning to distance oneself from the inner voice of shame and blame and to see oneself again as a whole person who is so much more than the sum of addictive behaviors makes room for self-compassion.

Values work helps by reconnecting people with their aspirations for their lives, enabling them to see past the powerful allure of the transitory relief of numbing the pain and commit to behavior change.

Finally, substance abuse is a common companion to other mental health challenges, such as depression and anxiety, which ACT is also so helpful with. So strong is the link to mood disorders that people who have one are twice as likely to be substance abusers, and the link is especially powerful if people are psychologically inflexible.

If you are in treatment or want to pursue it, which I strongly advise if substance use is a problem, you can include ACT exercises to complement those efforts. Indeed, ACT is largely in sympathy with the twelve-step treatment process popularized by AA and incorporated into the approaches of so many treatment centers. The twelve-step approach shares the ACT emphasis on accepting what we can't change and bringing one's life into alignment with one's values through committing to specific actions. The famous Serenity Prayer, which is featured in slightly modified form in the AA program, asks for the serenity to accept what we can't change, the courage to change what we can—our behavior and the situations influenced by it—and the wisdom to know the difference. ACT has used science to help guide that wise distinction.

We recently tested applying ACT training specifically to shame for people in treatment for substance use, compared it to a standard twelve-step program, and verified that it enhanced the effects of the in-patient treatment. What's more, while initially both groups improved comparably, in follow-up the clients exposed to ACT kept improving, doing better than those in the twelve-step facilitation alone.

Because ACT is evidence-based, combining it with a traditional twelve-step program also addresses the objection some raise about the AA approach: that it is not scientific. In addition, for those who are drawn to the twelve-step approach but are turned off by some of its features, such as its strong emphasis on spirituality, my former student Kelly Wilson, who is in long-term recovery from heroin addiction, has written a book, *The Wisdom to Know the Difference*, which walks the reader through a twelve-step approach that is written entirely from the ACT perspective.

The bottom line is that whatever prior or current approaches you or a loved one may have been taking to beat substance abuse, building psychological flexibility skills will help.

To start the process, I advise focusing on values work and revisiting that work regularly as you work on the other skills. This is because when one sees clearly how substance use is preventing one from living in accord with one's true values and life aspirations, that is a powerful motivation to persist through the pain of the process.

To gauge how much of a role avoidant inflexibililty may be playing in your substance use, you can take the assessment designed for measuring flexibility regarding substance abuse available at my website (http://www.stevenchayes.com).

Kelly Wilson distills the ACT message for addiction down to a single question: *In this very moment, will you accept the sad and the sweet, hold lightly stories about what is possible, and be the author of a life that has meaning and purpose for you, turning in kindness back to that life when you find yourself moving away from it?* It is a courageous journey, a hero's journey, to walk out of an addiction. That question is like a map for how to do so: at each choice point it will help those in recovery find their way home.

Eating Disorders

Perhaps the first thing to say about eating disorders (EDs) is that some of them are extremely serious medical conditions and that professional treatment should be sought out immediately once signs of a disorder are detected. EDs are among the most difficult mental health conditions to treat, with high rates of failure and of relapse after initially successful treatment. While EDs have tended to be viewed as a female issue—they are more common in females than males—the diagnosis of EDs in males has been on the rise. About twenty million women and ten million men in the United States will experience a clinical ED during their lives, and the first decade of this century saw a 66 percent increase in diagnosis of EDs in men. As is true with all mental health conditions, the causes are complex and still not well understood, involving what appears to be a wide range of genetic, neurobiological, psychological, and social factors.

One thing known for sure is that emotional avoidance is relatively high in people with EDs. Self-starvation, binging, and purging are motivated, at least in part, by the desire to avoid difficult thoughts and feelings, whether about body image or other life issues, such as fear of intimacy or of failure. People with EDs often actively use thought suppression as a form of experiential avoidance, and the more they do that, the worse their symptoms become. This helps to explain why many people with EDs are also dealing with depression and anxiety, which are both also strongly predicted by avoidance. Rumination, in the form of negative self-talk about body image and obsessive thoughts about eating and weight, has also been found to contribute significantly to the development and persistence of EDs. ACT helps counteract all of these factors.

One of the toughest aspects of treatment is that people with EDs are so often ambivalent about, or outright opposed to, getting treatment. ACT values work helps them see how they have subverted other life aspirations in their pursuit of weight control and then make an authentic commitment of their own to realigning their lives with their values.

In addition, extreme allegiance to elaborate food-related rules is a major feature of ED behavior, and a relatively high number of people with EDs also struggle with OCD. Defusion helps them break the grip of those rules.

Self work can help people with EDs find a place where they are OK even with thoughts like *I'm too fat* or *My body is disgusting.* A transcendent sense of self gives people with EDs a foundation for wholeness.

ACT also helps with the anxiety that is a common problem for people with EDs. Psychiatrist Emmett Bishop, who has developed an ACT-based ED treatment program, explained to me that EDs are so hard to treat in part because food restriction gives people significant relief from negative emotions that have tormented them, with anxiety being core to that turmoil. Research shows that about two-thirds of people with EDs also have an anxiety disorder. Emmett says that they attain "an adaptive peak of experiential avoidance" and compares the effect to that of anti-anxiety medications, known as anxiolytics. ACT, he says, helps people "get off the peak and deal with the resultant anxiety." He says, "Our patients are lost in a tangle of anxious details." Flexibility training helps them create a healthy coherence in their minds focused on their values instead of on preoccupation with moment-to-moment monitoring of how well they're following their elaborate eating rules.

CBT is still the gold standard for psychological treatment of eating disorders, so perhaps the wisest course is to add ACT skills to support traditional CBT approaches. A recent study did just that with an Internet program that combined CBT with ACT. The CBT elements focused on achieving early change and stabilizing healthy eating patterns, noticing overevaluation of body shape and weight, and working on such core issues as interpersonal difficulties or perfectionism. ACT values work was added to motivate change, and acceptance and mindfulness work was used to help let go of perfectionism and rigid thinking. The study found that nearly 40 percent of those who used the website were helped, versus only 7 percent for those who were not given access to the site.

The power of adding ACT training to a program for treating EDs was also empirically assessed in a study at the Renfrew Center in 2013. One group of people with EDs were given the center's standard treatment, which involves common methods like regular weighing, exposure to feared foods, and the normalization of eating habits. Another group was given the standard treatment as well as the choice of attending eight nighttime group training sessions, each of which combined instruction in a number of the ACT skills. Anyone who attended at least three was counted as having completed the training, so engagement with the practices was sometimes limited. Nonetheless, the study showed that those who got some ACT training showed significantly less concern about their weight and greater intake of food—by almost twice as much—as the non-ACT group. At a six-month follow-up, fewer of those in the ACT group had been rehospitalized.

Successes like this have led a number of ED treatment programs around the United States to use ACT as a main approach. Emmett Bishop's program is one example. He founded the Eating Recovery Center, which has locations in a number of states. One of the things I like about Emmett's program is that he carefully collects data from all of the patients he treats, and he periodically publishes it. That is as rare as it is honorable. He recently published results from six hundred of his patients and found that about 60 percent were significantly helped by his largely ACT-based treatment program, and that changes in psychological flexibility strongly predicted the improvement.

The measure of eating-related psychological flexibility Emmett uses is a modification of one that a former student, Jason Lillis, and I published years ago. It asks people to rate statements such as the following:

* **I need to feel better about how I look in order to live the life I want.**
* **Other people make it hard for me to accept myself.**
* **If I feel unattractive, there is no point in trying to be intimate.**
* **If I gain weight, that means I have failed.**
* **My eating urges control me.**
* **I need to get rid of my eating urges to eat better.**
* **If I eat something bad, the whole day is a waste.**
* **I should be ashamed of my body.**
* **I need to avoid social situations where people might judge me.**

You can take the full assessment to determine your own degree of flexibility at http://www.stevenchayes.com.

When I asked Emmett to sum up the wisdom he's learned from his work with thousands of people with EDs, his bottom line resonated deeply with me: "Don't get mired in anxious details of the moment, but identify the overarching values of your life and follow them in an open, curious, and flexible way." Every one of us could benefit from this advice, and if you or a loved one have an ED, I hope it will point the way to healing.

Psychosis

I do not want this chapter to end without mentioning psychosis. The late Albert Ellis, a friend and the developer of rational emotive behavior therapy (REBT), liked ACT but once told me to my face, "Steve, ACT is for—— eggheads" (if you knew Al, you know he threw in several cuss words in the——part). I asked for clarification and he said, for example, it would never work for people with hallucinations or delusions.

We promptly did a study to see.

If you've seen the movie *A Beautiful Mind* about the Nobel Prize–winning mathematician John Nash, you've essentially seen what we tried to teach. In that film, Nash became so entangled in his delusions that he was about to lose his family and his academic job. Instead he learned to watch his symptoms from a bit of a distance psychologically instead of fighting with them or complying with them. That distancing allowed him to focus more on what he really cared about (his family and his work). That is the core of the ACT approach to coping with psychosis.

We now know that even three to four hours of ACT can lead to a significant reduction in rehospitalization over the next year, and we know why: it changes how hallucinations and delusions affect a person. Building flexibility leads to less distress from them, less belief that they are literally true, and lower behavioral impact from them. The depression that commonly sets in following a psychotic break is diminished as well. The work is still young, but it is unfolding nicely to a drumbeat of studies and programs worldwide.

I disagree with my late friend. Flexibility processes are not for eggheads, they are for us all, regardless of the kind or severity of the experiences we are struggling with. People with psychosis experience intense stigmatization. They tend to be seen as having a brain disease or a genetic flaw that makes them seem profoundly "other." It is not true. As with all mental health conditions, we do not yet know why people have these hallucinations or delusions, but hearing voices (for example) is not in and of itself crippling any more than chronic pain, or anxiety, or a painful loss. People are people, pure and simple, and a growing body of research suggests that inflexibility processes increase the impact and perhaps even the emergence of hallucinations and delusions. People who hear voices and others dealing with these experiences are not "other." We all have within us some of what leads to severe mental health issues. Mental health is not a "them" issue, it is an "us" issue, and I hope that over time we can all learn to bring the same compassion that ACT teaches us to direct toward our own mental struggles to those who face the most profound challenges.

Chapter Seventeen

NURTURING RELATIONSHIPS

When I ask my clients or workshop attendees to closely consider their values, I know one thing I will see—the importance of people to people. Our relationships with lovers, spouses, children, parents, friends, and co-workers are central to our well-being. We know it, and our values show it.

We are built to bond with others. Just looking into the eyes of someone you care for releases natural opiates, as if your neurobiology is saying, "This connection is good for you." But, of course, healthy bonding also requires thoughtful nurturing. What pulls you even closer to people is being able to share what you care about, and your thoughts and feelings, in an open and honest way, as well as listening attentively and with openness, rather than judgment or defensiveness, when they do the same. Yet we so often find ourselves hiding our true thoughts and feelings from those we care about, as they do from us.

Consider romantic relationships, and the ways that anger or hurt can encourage us to close down rather than risk losing our composure and provoking conflict. We may worry that our partner will erupt at us if we share that we're angry or hurt by something they've done, or not done. Or we might not want to seem vulnerable or may fear that our partner will defensively distance from us.

That is all understandable. But here is a simple formula about relationships to keep in mind: in a context that maintains a secure connection, intimacy = shared values + shared vulnerabilities. Psychological flexibility allows us to stay focused on nurturing intimacy even when we are angry or hurt. It helps us weather the stresses that are inevitable in any close relationship.

When engineers want to build an earthquake-safe house, they add flexibility to the foundation. Just so, the flexibility skills provide a strong foundation for our relationships. They help us contend better not only with our own difficult thoughts and feelings about relationships but with those of the people we care about, as well as the behavior of theirs we find upsetting. The skills also help us foster flexibility in our loved ones.

Why are they so helpful?

Defusion helps us step back from unhelpful thoughts and feelings about others and how they've treated us and consciously reject negative behavior they can trigger, like lashing out in anger. People appreciate this forbearance, and it tends to inspire them to be less negative and reactive as well. That opens up room for thoughtful, caring communication that does not threaten withdrawal or termination of the relationship.

Attachment to a conceptualized self creates distance between us and others. We often inadvertently pressure our family and friends to support that self-image, even though, because they know us well, they can see it's distorted. Connecting with our transcendent sense of self undercuts this tendency, helping us bring our whole, true selves into relationships and recognize the wholeness of others.

Acceptance helps us be honest with ourselves about pain we're feeling in a relationship, which in turn allows us to articulate those feelings to others, rather than covering them up or acting out in ways that are unhelpful such as threats to withdraw in the service of eliminating pain. Of course there are times to withdraw based on safety or self-care, such as from an abusive relationship, but acceptance of the pain of doing so will help there too.

Presence keeps us from slipping into rehearsing past wrongs in our mind or imagining future pain and disappointment, and instead helps us focus on the potential for connection and healthy attachment in the present. Others perceive that we are looking to make the most of the opportunities of the moment, and that encourages them to do the same.

Doing values work helps reorient us toward how important relationships are to us, and to build our relationships on a basis of shared values, and, as the case may be, acceptance of some differences in values. Research has shown that the ability to choose one's values is related to the capacity for healthy attachment to others, probably because it is easier to own and make real our yearning to attach and belong when it is a choice we make rather than feeling as though it is out of our control.

Caring for others is not only a matter of feelings, of course; we must take actions that nurture relationships, such as initiating needed conversations or committing to constructive changes in our behavior, even if we don't feel like doing so. Commitment practice helps with these actions, which can be quite difficult, such as forgiving, letting go of conflict, and doing small loving things in an active, consistent, and thoughtful way.

Applying flexibility skills to relationships involves not only directing them toward our own behavior, thoughts, and feelings—it means applying them to the behavior, thoughts, and feelings of others. Consider defusion. The focus thus far in the book has mostly been on defusing from our own harsh messages about ourselves. But we can also use defusion to step back from our harsh judgments of others. This allows us to show them more understanding and kindness. In addition, they will sense that we are doing so, and that, in turn, gives them more space to look at their own thoughts and behavior more openly, because they become less defensive. We can also use defusion to step back from harsh judgments others have of us, which we tend to internalize and then inflict on ourselves. That allows us to be less defensive in our interactions with others.

In extending self-work to others, we can apply the same lessons we learned about how unhelpful our self-stories can be to appreciating that we also weave stories about others. We make assumptions about what they are thinking and feeling and why they're behaving as they are, often without asking what's going on for them. We've probably all experienced this being done to us and haven't liked it one bit.

To stop ourselves from doing this, we can use the same I/here/now perspective-taking practices we used in Chapter Ten to gain awareness of our characterizations of others and consider alternative explanations of their behavior, putting ourselves in their shoes and looking through their eyes.

The social extension of acceptance is, in part, showing compassion for others, even when they may be causing us pain. Acknowledging that they are feeling their own pain helps us avoid the traps of lashing out in response or breaking away from them. Extending acceptance also involves being willing to share with them about the pain they're causing us, despite the fear we may have about doing so. All too often, we assume that people understand they're causing us pain, when, in fact, they may be largely unaware. Sharing about it in a nonaccusatory way can be difficult, but it can also lead to breakthroughs.

Extending values work involves sharing our values with others and learning about theirs, discussing values with them in a respectful way rather than making assumptions. We build mutual appreciation of one another's life aspirations and learn how we can help one another fulfill them.

Committed action is extended by cooperating with others to find more effective approaches to solving problems and pursuing goals together. One of the great sources of frustration, and rancor, in relationships is that we tend to want to change some behavior in the other person that annoys or hurts us. They often resist this change, and we become even more irritated. When we connect with others based on shared values and vulnerability it is much easier to set SMART goals and agree on compromises that will work for both parties.

You can apply most of the exercises presented in Part Two to any relationship you want to nurture. Say that you are feeling really resentful toward your spouse. To defuse from the negative thoughts you're having about him or her, you could write them down and then practice the "look at it as an object" exercise from Chapter Nine on them, in which you ask questions such as if the resentment had a shape, what would that be, and if it had a speed, how fast would it go? You could also create a pack of cards with those thoughts written on them, carry them around with you, and apply whichever of the defusion exercises you've found most helpful.

If you've woven the story that your spouse is totally inconsiderate, you could apply the exercise of rewriting your self-story to your story of your spouse. If you go back through the Part Two chapters you will see that applying the exercises this way to relationship issues is really just a small step, and in fact, it's one that many people who learn the skills take quite naturally.

Helping Others Nurture Flexibility

A further step in extending flexibility skills to those we care about is to use them to help others develop their own flexibility. As we learn the value of flexibility skills, we want those we care about to also gain the benefits of being more self-accepting, less entangled in painful thoughts and feelings, and more able to commit to needed behavior change. We can be of great help to them in developing flexibility, but it's important to go about this in a psychologically flexible way.

Suppose an ACT-aware mother was interested in nurturing acceptance in her teenage daughter. She's seen that her daughter is besieged by social fears, which is so common in the adolescent years, and that she's begun trying to avoid that fear by withdrawing from some of her friends and activities she's enjoyed. Mom finds herself saying to her daughter, "You need to learn to accept your feelings" and "You don't need to be so afraid of fear. It will not harm you. Just feel it!"

The goal is laudable, but those statements are not likely to be of much help. Stand back and you can see that Mom's well-meaning advice will likely come across as judgmental, and no wonder: she is dictating rules to her daughter.

Bad idea.

If we are going to increase acceptance, we will need to do so in an *accept-*

ing, nonjudgmental, and values-based way. There is a formula for ensuring that we're doing so:

Instigate, Model, and Reinforce it, From, Toward and With It!

I *love* that formula, and not just because it's so helpful, which it is. I also love the fact that the acronym that it spells out is:

I'm RFT With It!

(I can't help it . . . it still makes me smile.)

What it means, in essence, is that to help others build their flexibility, we should *instigate* open, aware, and values-based interactions with them about the struggles we see them going through in a way that *models* flexibility skills and provides positive *reinforcement* of their tentative steps toward flexibility. We operate *from* a place of flexibility internally, working *toward* them developing it, and doing so *with* flexibility skills.

How can this help our ACT-aware mother? Here is a series of questions for her to consider.

* **If it is painful to see your child's painful struggle, can you start with owning and sharing that fact?**

That is instigating. It is inviting her daughter to notice her own pain in a way that might lead her to have more openness and curiosity about it.

* **Can you ask her some open questions about her feelings without moving quickly to "helping" or to "changing" but instead just listening with openness and curiosity?**
* **Can you have this discussion without the hint of a suggestion that it is your daughter's task to rescue**

you from pain or self-criticism you're feeling about her pain? Can you show her that you are OK with your emotion? For example, would it be OK to tear up?

* **Can you tell her that you will stay with her in her moments of pain, no matter how hard that is for you?**

All of that is modeling; in this case modeling the skill of acceptance, which invites her daughter to let herself feel her own emotions.

The actual dialogue might proceed this way:

> ***Mom:*** It hurts to see you suffer in a struggle against fear. It just stabs me through the heart. I've been in what I think are pretty similar situations and I remember how helpless and hopeless I felt at the time—almost as if it weren't OK to be me. I think I believed I needed to be fixed before others would want to be with me. Is what you're going through anything at all like that?
>
> ***Daughter:*** It's hard even to go there. It's a dark place.
>
> ***Mom:*** I get that. Would you be willing to help me know a bit more what that is like? Maybe just a little? I'm not trying to fix anything—I just want to see you from the inside. What you are feeling matters to me. When those fears really get going, what is it like?

If the daughter then does open up and share, the mother should use the moment to deepen the connection and caring between them. For example, suppose the daughter says she is afraid fear will overwhelm her. Her mother might respond by saying:

> Thank you for sharing that with me, for trusting me with it. I feel closer to you when I know what you feel, even when what you are feeling is hard for you to share and hard for me to hear.

The more you work on this approach to helping others cultivate their own flexibility, the more natural the process will become. This is a powerful way to strengthen the bonds in your relationships, creating more interpersonal flexibility, which becomes mutually reinforcing.

In addition to these general guidelines about applying the skills to relationships, some specific findings about flexibility in particular kinds of relationships are important to know about. Next, I discuss a little more about parenting, then address some special issues about romantic relationships, including the problem of abuse, and I conclude with a discussion of how ACT can be applied to countering prejudice.

It's not my purpose to lay out a detailed program for relationship health in any of these areas. These discussions are meant to open a door to insights from ACT. If you are struggling with serious relationship problems, I encourage you to seek help from a professional. Common therapy approaches for relationships that are easy to integrate with ACT include emotion-focused therapy, the Gottman Method, and integrated behavioral couples therapy.

Parenting

It's hard to be a parent.

I should know. By the time little Stevie goes off to college, I will have been raising children in the developmental period continuously for fifty-five years (*Guinness Book of World Records*—take note).

Parenting involves such a roiling mix of emotions. As with the mother dealing with her daughter's struggle with social fears, it's difficult to watch our children suffer, to be rejected, to make mistakes, to stumble and fall. But it's wonderful to watch them overcome obstacles, to step forward and find the courage to be more fully themselves, and to discover their own sense of purpose in life.

Researchers have found that psychological inflexibility makes it hard to interact with our children in a healthy way, especially when we are feeling vulnerable or stressed. Conversely, psychologically flexible parents are more able to learn good parenting skills and to deploy them when needed.

One of the trickiest aspects of parenting is that we are constantly modeling, instigating, and reinforcing either flexibility *or* inflexibility with our children. We can't avoid that impact. When children see our own flexibility or inflexibility, they internalize it.

That matters.

Parents' inflexibility significantly predicts their *children's* anxiety, their acting out, and whether they will develop actual trauma if bad things happen. For example, if there is a nearby school shooting or a destructive storm rolls through town, you can predict which kids will have an especially hard time. It's not those who were especially anxious; it's those with especially inflexible parents.

A recent study done by ACT researchers in Australia followed 750 children and their parents over a six-year period from middle school to the end of high school. The children of parents who did their parenting in a rigid and authoritarian way, which was low in warmth or emotional sensitivity and high in control, showed decreases in psychological flexibility during the course of the study. Making matters worse, as kids became less flexible, parents tended to respond by becoming yet more authoritarian, plugging into a feedback loop from hell.

Of course, flexibility can be difficult when it comes to parenting, for a couple of key reasons. For one, as parents we must set some rules for our children, and doing that without being overly rigid about them is a delicate balancing act. After all, the rules we give children are aimed at protecting them and helping them become responsible, caring, and competent beings. It's scary, not to mention infuriating, when they disregard our guidance.

The dance of flexibility in parenting is to support your child's autonomy and freedom to make their own discoveries, and their own values choices, while also setting age-appropriate and reasonable limits and monitoring and disciplining them in ways that are consistent and reasonable. This is what parenting experts have called *authoritative* parenting, a term that points to another tricky issue in guiding our children. They tend to want us to be authorities.

When our children are young, they expect that we have all the answers about life (of course, they usually grow out of that before long). We can easily slip into the role of all-knowing advisors rather than nurturing our children's awareness that there is no one "right" answer to many of life's questions, which means they will inevitably face challenges in discovering their own answers. Affording them the latitude to go through those struggles can be difficult. The one thing I ask my twelve-year-old almost every day is "What did you do today that was hard?" I want him thinking of his own skills in doing hard things.

Let me give an example, using one of the most challenging questions a parent can face, to show how ACT learning can help. I've had to field it from all of my children.

Between ages eight and fourteen all four of them have shared somewhat suicidal thoughts with me, asking, each in their own way, what is the purpose of living if you are only going to die anyway? As a psychologist, I benefited from knowing that such thoughts are common even in children and adolescents—most high school students agree with the statement *I have had thoughts about killing myself but did not actually try.* Such thoughts easily lead children to think that they are alone, isolated, and different from other people. Insight from ACT helps us understand that suicidal thoughts reflect the mind trying to "solve the problem" of feeling bad inside—even if it kills us. They're not indications that people are broken, but rather that we need to go beyond that problem-solving mode of mind to begin to learn how to carry emotional distress.

My son Charlie asked me a meaning-of-life question in the most initially provocative way of all of my children. He was almost demanding that I *prove* that life isn't empty and meaningless (with a tone that suggested "and if you can't, then why *shouldn't* I kill myself?").

I knew the idea that life has to *prove* itself to be meaningful is dangerous: our judgmental minds can work around anything we give them. Meaning matters when it comes as a choice, and trying to offer him proof would move choice over to a logical decision. It is a natural impulse but could actually feed a dangerous idea. It was a tricky moment.

What I said stopped Charlie in his tracks. "We all have thoughts like that," I said. "Me too! I still have them." Charlie's eyes widened just a bit.

"So, let's go with it. 'Life is empty and meaningless. That is the secret of life. Whatever you do, in the end it's all meaningless because you are going to die anyway and in the end the sun is a big iceball.' Let's just take that as a given." He looked a bit stunned. He'd been ready for an argument, not for agreement. "And," I added as I leaned closer after a pause, "I love you, and I know you love me. Whatever else our minds have to say, that is also true."

Years later, Charlie told me that conversation was something of a turning point in his young life. He saw that he could choose what was meaningful to him, and he didn't need to win an argument with his mind to validate his choice.

The current data on how best to address suicidality fits well with the insights of ACT: normalize, validate the distress, frame the issue as an effort to deal with pain and purpose, and encourage active steps that will help do that in a healthy way. If it becomes evident that your children are struggling with thoughts that are persistent, highly distressing, entangling, or focused on concrete deadly plans, it is time to seek professional help. You can look for ACT-trained clinicians, who will help you and your child walk through the "normalize, validate, reframe, activate" sequence.

For the more regular, daily stresses of parenting, to keep yourself on your toes about being flexible with your children, whenever you are feeling frustrated with them or have the impulse to harshly lay the law down, take a moment and quickly swoop through these steps in your mind:

1. **Show up and check in.** Start with what's going on for you. Are you angry? Is that because you're afraid? Or insecure? Maybe you're just tired and feeling worn down. Or maybe your child's behavior is reminding you of things in your life that were traumatizing, such as an accident. Take a moment to open up to what you're feeling with curiosity and without harsh judgment. If what you see there is hard, acknowledge that difficulty to yourself before shifting your attention to how to support the flexibility of your child in this situation.

Why is this the first step? Because parenting with flexibility will be only play-acting if you're fused and avoidant. Your kids will see through that in an instant.

2. Take perspective. Spend another moment to see if you can put yourself in your child's shoes with a sense of empathy and compassion. We tend to treat our children's behavior as we would a math problem. Instead, look at your children as you might a beautifully told story—with an attitude of appreciation. You and your children are about to write the next lines in that story. What is your child yearning to write? What is he or she afraid the next lines will be?

3. Check in with your values. Focus on how important it is to you to behave with flexibility toward your child. Remind yourself that we're all on a journey when it comes to values, and progress is more important than perfection. Consider what you can do right then and there to foster greater openness, awareness, and values-based action in your child.

That three-part formula will help carry you through the rocky parts of parenting with your values and your relationship to your children intact. You need to combine these steps with specific skills (consistent and reasonable discipline, good monitoring, positive rewards, and other actual behaviors any good science-based books on parenting skills will walk through), but these three steps will help with the most important parenting feature of all: nurturance.

Relationships with Romantic Partners

The more you practice applying your flexibility skills to your relationship with your partner, the more readily you will be able to remind yourself in the heat of the moment about the insights you've gained, listen to but disregard unhelpful thoughts and emotions, and engage in constructive dialogue and behavior instead of falling back into negative patterns. A special issue to address here is communication in the service of emotional connection, which fosters a more secure attachment.

Research has shown that people who are more able to defuse from their judgments of others tend to be more satisfied with their long-term relationships. It is far easier to love a fantasy than a person. When we use our flexibility skills to stay connected and be understanding even when our mind is telling us to lash out at or create distance from our partners, they sense the love and safety that flexibility provides. That is likely why our partners are more satisfied when we are more accepting of our difficult thoughts and feelings, both about ourselves and about them. The primary reason for improved satisfaction is that psychologically flexible individuals do a better job of identifying and communicating their own emotions and values, which deepens relationships as zones of safety and growth.

To nurture better emotional connection and communication with your partner, I recommend these two exercises that are helpful in fostering better sharing and caring.

> **1.** Take ten minutes for each of you to do some values writing as you did in Chapter Thirteen. Do it about any shared domain, such as raising children, having fun, working together, handling money, or creating a home. Don't write about complaints and what is wrong about your partner or relationship: write about your values. What are they? Why are they important to do? What happens when you forget that?

After you've written for a while, take turns reading what you've written out loud. Listen to your partner using "mindful eyes and ears," and ask that they do the same for you. Be sure that you are fully present, orienting your body toward your partner and looking at your partner rather than listening with head down, for example. Do not comment, or correct, or challenge. Just listen, carefully. After you have heard what your partner wrote, restate it to your partner (who then also adopts "mindful eyes and ears") and see if they think you've got it right. If what you say is not quite what was meant, your partner can clarify. Then you should restate what they've told you until your partner says you really understand. Then it is your turn to share your values, and to go through the same process.

After each person has had the chance to be heard, it is time to share your feelings and thoughts that came up during the exercise. Be careful not to be drawn into a round of criticism. Keep the "I'm RFT With It" formula in the front of your mind, doing this exercise from, toward, and with your skills. Hang on to your purpose: a safe and secure zone in which each of you can be more fully yourself.

2. Do a version of the "Social Sharing and Defusion" exercise in Chapter Nine with your partner (it is the last of the "additional methods" at the end of the chapter). Each of you should write down on a card, in just one or two words, an internal barrier you are ready to let go of, such as a fear of sharing irritation with a partner, or anger about a past hurt. Make sure it is not a secret criticism of your partner. Then each of you can turn over your cards.

Each person should then state in two to three minutes what this barrier feels like; share thoughts about where it originated (e.g., when you were a child, expressing irritation would only provoke a big fight); and consider how avoidance of that barrier, or entanglement in thoughts about it, has been costly. Then commit to actions to move beyond that barrier. Be sure to use all of your defusion and acceptance skills as you go through this (e.g., "I have the thought that . . ."). Then the listener should share (in the following order) an emotional reaction to hearing this, a point of appreciation about how your partner addressed it, and finally at least one area that is similar or overlapping. This is a way to share your vulnerabilities in a context that feels safe, so that you are unlikely to withdraw or threaten abandonment.

Combating Abuse

Across the planet, 30 percent of women age fifteen and over have experienced violence from an intimate partner during their lifetime, either physical, sexual, or both. Men are abused too, but less frequently. Abusive relationships have a strong negative impact on mental and behavioral health, and the flexibility skills can help combat this.

People who are abused often struggle with shame, self-blame, and anxiety, and as we've seen, flexibility skills help us cope with all of these. Flexibility also helps us protect ourselves from future abuse. The risk of becoming a victim again rises considerably if abuse survivors are psychologically inflexible. We need our feelers out to seek out partners who are good for us, which is hard for experiential avoiders.

ACT helps with taking the difficult actions to get out of abusive relationships. All too often people experiencing abuse are simply told "just leave," as if that is easy. It can be a herculean feat, and flexibility skills help survivors acknowledge what is hard even while emphasizing the commitment to change. That is self-validating and empowering.

One study that showed how effective ACT training is in helping people recover from abuse was conducted by colleagues and my wife, Jacqueline Pistorello, using an online program based on a book she and Victoria Follette wrote for trauma survivors. Of the twenty-five participants, 96 percent had been sexually assaulted, 84 percent had been raped, and 60 percent had experienced physical abuse. Intimate partners had inflicted the abuse in half of the cases. The participants were provided six sessions of online video introduction to the flexibility skills, along with exercises. By the end of the study, nearly half were recovered from their trauma according to the magnitude of the changes in symptoms they reported, while another third had improved significantly.

There are other good programs for trauma. Exposure therapy and cognitive processing therapy are among the best, and both of these currently have more data than ACT, so I recommend them. But these programs are helped by openness and connection to one's values too, so flexibility skills will likely assist with whatever approach is chosen.

Reducing Abuse with ACT

If you follow the discourse on this critical issue in the media, you could be forgiven for hoping that positive results will ultimately come from public campaigns or by treating intimate-partner abuse as the crime that it is. That is not likely. WHO concluded that criminal prosecution is not a deterrent, and while public campaigns lead to better support for government action, they do not significantly reduce abuse itself.

Mandatory psychological treatment for abusers has also shown dispiriting results. The two most common interventions are cognitive behavior therapy and a consciousness-raising approach called the Duluth Model. Often they're used in combination. Unfortunately, both have shown only a minor reduction in future abuse and battering (about 5 percent or less overall).

A new approach is needed.

Efforts to use ACT training with perpetrators of domestic violence are in the early stages, but they have so far proved powerful by comparison. In an ACT approach, batterers are never shamed, talked down to, or lectured. Research shows that most of them were themselves victims of abuse as children, and their abuse is often deeply ingrained avoidant behavior to deal with a sense of shame or threat of loss. *That is no justification for their abuse.* Domestic violence is a crime, and that should not be forgotten, but the simple empirical fact is that shaming these men does not reduce their violence, especially since shame is often a trigger. Then why do it?

The ACT approach is to instead work on building men's emotional openness as well as their awareness of their relationship values. The intervention follows the "I'm RFT With It" rule for creating interpersonal flexibility; the process of intervention is compassionate, nonjudgmental, and engaged. Group sessions introduce the flexibility skills, and participants are also given homework about how to apply the skills in challenging relationship moments. Throughout the treatment, clients complete daily monitoring forms on the emotional precipitants of abuse as well as the consequences of their behaviors. The men are taught to recognize that they're being emotionally avoidant and to practice instead engaging in actions consistent with chosen personal values.

The first study testing this approach was a randomized trial conducted by Iowa State psychologist Amie Zarling. It was a well-controlled study done with perpetrators who had volunteered for treatment, and it was published in one of the world's best clinical psychology journals. It found that three months of weekly ACT sessions (as compared to a supportive discussion group) led to a profound effect, based on reports from the participants' partners. Over the six months following treatment, partner reports of physical violence went down by 73 percent, and reports of verbal or psychological aggression decreased by 60 percent. Tests of the men's emotional regulation skills indicated that improvements in flexibility skills accounted for the reductions in abuse.

When I read these results, I was excited but cautious because these were voluntary participants who were apparently motivated to stop their abuse. Most perpetrators do *not* enter treatment voluntarily: the court tells them they have to go. Would it still work in that event?

Apparently, yes.

In the next study Zarling conducted, she worked with men across Iowa who were court-mandated to seek treatment. A large number, nearly 3,500 men, who had been arrested for domestic assault were put through either a Duluth Model plus CBT treatment group or ACT training. The results startled the domestic violence community. Over the next year, arrest records showed that those in the ACT group had 31 percent fewer additional domestic assault charges, and 37 percent had fewer violent charges of any kind. That is a far larger effect than the few percentage point drops the field has come to expect.

Again, it's early going for this research, and a one-year follow-up is only a beginning. I will not be convinced until the results are replicated and follow-ups show they are long-lasting. But certainly, the work so far is very hopeful. Meanwhile the state of Iowa is so impressed that they have implemented the program statewide.

Overcoming Prejudice

Prejudice is hard to talk about; we tend to think of it as something other people—bad people—have in their hearts and minds. The sad truth is that it is inside us all. The good news is that ACT provides a powerful new way to combat this deeply entrenched social plague.

Prejudice is due in part to cultural learning, from our parents, our schools, and pervasive prejudicial messages and depictions in the media. But prejudice is ingrained in us so easily because of our evolutionary heritage. Human beings evolved in small groups that formed strong social identities. Unfortunately, while that group identification was good for bonding and cooperation within groups, it also resulted in competition with other small groups. We divided ourselves into *ingroups* and *outgroups*, and as we developed distinctive cultures, we created "otherizing" stories about outgroups.

We have come a long way from living in small tribal groups crowded around campfires on open savannas, in danger of attack at any moment by competing groups. But our minds still think in terms of "us versus them." Researchers have shown how strong this drive is by dividing people into two groups according to the flip of a coin. Even though the participants were aware their division into groups was random, they still readily began to consider their group as better than the other group.

This instinctive otherizing is horribly outmoded. We are all one people, and that is not a matter of mere moralizing. Genetics research has shown how deeply and completely the same in our biology all humans are. Think of it this way: we all had the same parents not so very long ago. If only that knowledge were enough to stop us from otherizing, but alas, research has shown that the tendency is built deep into us.

Many social scientists have argued that continuing social diversification will inexorably combat prejudice, but the change process is more complex than that. We should have known that, even without research, since gender bias is ingrained in all of us, and men and women have been closely interacting ever since humans have existed or we wouldn't be here.

In 2007, Harvard political scientist Robert Putnam published a major study of the impact of diversity on community life. He found that the more diverse a community was, the less people trusted others, even within "their own" groups. Fewer people voted, volunteered, gave to charity, and worked on community projects. In other words, he concluded, as diversity grew, people withdrew from many of the processes of community formation. It's not enough to live in a diverse world—to take advantage of that diversity we need also to live in the space provided by flexible minds.

That is because the core of the problem is that prejudice is deeply embedded into our thought networks. Voluminous studies have been done on *implicit bias*—negative stereotyping and otherizing that we are not consciously aware of. If you ask people their views regarding stereotyped groups, they tend to give answers that fit with what they want to believe they believe. RFT methods currently provide the world's best tests of people's implicit biases, and the results show that most people do harbor negative stereotypes of those they see as being in outgroups.

Prejudice easily digs into us, whether we like it or not, so if we're going to combat bias more effectively, we need to change how our minds deal with it. We need to create modern minds for this modern world we're living in. I have been deeply gratified to find that ACT can help. Since I was a young child, I've been pained by the brutality of prejudice and how it impacts us all, including myself. I've also learned how profoundly it shaped the fortunes of my Jewish ancestors, and I've witnessed it directed at my children.

I knew I had witnessed something important the day I sat next to my mother as a kindergartner watching our small black-and-white television set as a funny-looking man with a small mustache barked out incomprehensible staccato German words, pausing only for the roars of an unseen crowd. My mother suddenly leapt forward, spit on the television screen, turned it off, and ran from the room.

I did not know then that the funny little man had started a brutal war that had ended less than a decade earlier. I also did not know that my mother had been told by her own German father, as he became swept up in fervor over the fatherland, never to tell anyone that she had "tainted blood." I did not even know my mother's name. It was actually not Ruth Eileen Dreyer, as she had always claimed—it was the telltale Ruth Esther. It was several more years before I learned that truth and discovered that half of my mother's maternal aunts and uncles had died while crowded into "shower rooms" meant not to cleanse them, but to cleanse the world of them.

I first encountered raw prejudice in my childhood friend Tom. He constantly spewed venom about "niggers," and "spics," and "kikes," which he learned from his dad, who was even worse. It bothered me. I even got into a fistfight with him once trying to make him stop. It just felt wrong.

At the time about all I could have said was that my mother would not like it. His slurs didn't land on me personally. Or so I thought. I didn't know yet that I myself was a "kike," nor that I would go on to marry two Latinas, nor that I would adopt an African American daughter. I didn't know I would eventually be connected to all three of his favorite groups to hate.

Most frustrating of all, his slurs sank into my mind regardless of my contempt for them. I learned that by seeing how my mind could leapfrog decades of family experience and instead give voice instead to a cruel moment when we were kids.

Tom, another friend Joe, and I had ridden our bikes to the bowling alley. As we set up for our game, Tom strangely commented, "It looks like rain." He and Joe smirked at each other and giggled. I had no idea what was going on. You couldn't even see outside from the lanes, and it had been cloudless when we rode there. "It looks like raaaain," Tom repeated loudly as they both tried to repress laughter. Finally, I noticed a black man within earshot walking toward us. It clicked. A black cloud was rolling in. Rain. Get it?

I was horrified and felt slightly sick to my stomach. But then the thought also flittered into my mind that I was damn glad it was not me they were making fun of.

Flash forward a decade. My Hispanic first wife and our three-year-old African-Hispanic-American daughter (Camille was born to my wife before we were married, and I adopted her later) were at a private club pool in Salem, Virginia, in the summer of 1973. Our host, a member of the club, had gone home early, leaving us to swim a little more. Not long after he left, a prim woman with puffed blond hair walked gingerly toward us wearing the kind of pressed cotton dresses Southern women wore back then. She was smiling, but it looked forced. After glancing back and forth at all three of us, she announced that she was the social secretary of the club, adding, "Your baby is rather brown." At first I thought she was concerned about Camille getting sunburned, but a rictus on her face that Batman's Joker would be proud to display quickly made me realize what was happening. We were being thrown out of that pool because of our mixed-race daughter. We, or at least she, was not welcome here.

I remember no sense of anger—only shock and disgust, and then an anxious feeling that I would not be able to fully protect my sweet little girl from things like *this*.

Jump ahead another dozen years. My then teenaged daughter is dressed to the nines for a school dance, looking absolutely wonderful. As I watch her approach from across the room, and I see her beautiful brown face, a voice bubbles up inside my head, unbidden and unwelcome. The auditory equivalent of a smirk, it's Tom's voice, saying very clearly, *It looks like raaaain*.

Tom was in my head, now smirking and sneering *at my own family through my own mind*. It did not matter that I had repeatedly seen and loathed racial injustice, up close and personal. I would not be given a pass on that basis. The casual cruelty of those racist slurs were *in me*.

Just last year I told the story of Tom's voice popping into my head that day to my daughter. Camille was so sweet and pure in her response: "I love you, Daddy," she said. "We all have burdens like that to carry."

Yes, we do.

Prejudicial cultural messages have been embedded in all of our minds. Perhaps we've heard an AIDS joke, or witnessed gender bias. Negative ethnic stereotypes pervade the media. Even if you hate them, or are the victim of them, you know them; they are in your cognitive network. And that means they are perpetually available to do mischief even when you are not looking.

If we are brutally honest with ourselves, we know that in some of the thousand forms that funny little man with the mustache knows to take, he lurks inside us. Every one of us. If you look closely you can see him leering back from the mirror. If you go to the rigid, defended, frightened, angry, judgmental parts of your own heart, you will see that he resides there.

But you can learn to use that recognition and apply it to shrivel down the harmful *impact* of that part of you, and thus to reduce just a bit the likelihood that your own invisible privilege will hide the ways you pass it to others despite your best intentions. By applying the ACT practices to an investigation of your implicit biases, you can become more aware of them and bring your actions more in line with your conscious beliefs. Whereas if you try to suppress prejudiced thoughts, you actually *foster* implicit bias, because mindful defused awareness allows prejudicial thoughts to become less dominant. Research shows that it helps us do more as well, committing to positive actions to combat prejudice.

Why exactly does psychological flexibility help?

My lab researched this. We studied the many forms of prejudice: gender bias, bias against people who are overweight, bias based on sexual orientation, ethnic bias, and many more. We expected that underneath the superficial differences we'd find a common core, and our research confirmed this. We found that all forms of prejudice can be largely explained by *authoritarian distancing*. This is "otherizing" due to the belief that we are different from some group of "others," and because they are different, they represent a threat to us that we need to control. Said another way, prejudice involves interpersonal inflexibility.

When my lab examined what psychological factors lead some people to settle into authoritarian distancing more than others, we found three key characteristics: the relative inability to take the perspective of other people; the inability to feel the pain of others when you do take their perspective; and the inability to be emotionally open to the pain of others when you do feel it—in other words, experiential avoidance. If these three processes are flipped in a positive direction (called *flexible connectedness*), not only does prejudice go down, but enjoyment of others goes up.

Drawing on these findings, we developed ACT interventions that have been found to significantly reduce prejudice, with successful studies done regarding biases about weight; sexual orientation; HIV/AIDS; racial prejudice; and people with mental health problems, substance abuse problems, and physical health problems. Doing something about it within yourself always requires a first step: looking and listening.

In some ways the most costly and difficult-to-eradicate forms of bias are invisible because they are based on privilege. A man can believe he is absolutely without gender bias and still talk more in meetings, or readily assume that he should lead the group because of his abilities, not being aware that these very actions are a form of gender bias. The white person who honestly and somewhat pridefully says "I don't think about race" may not be aware of how much that models privilege when a black neighbor has to send her teenaged son out into the world every morning knowing he is more likely to be arrested or shot at because he is black, and thus *has* to think about race.

It is unfair and irresponsible to ask those who bear the costs of privilege to do all the heavy lifting to correct it, so the first step has to be to dig in. You can safely assume that you host bias you cannot see in most or even all of the major areas (why *wouldn't* you?), so learn more about the indirect indicators of bias that will help you catch it in yourself (I just gave you two in the area of gender, for example). Indirect indicators will help you begin to catch bias in all of its forms—even in forms that are initially invisible.

Once you are doing that, it is time to ask people who are close to you and have experienced bias to help you note your own invisible forms. For example, when I start mansplaining, my wife gives me a little look. Do not expect this to feel good. Personally, I feel like putting a paper bag over my head when I leave the house because as I turn up the mental lights, I see more bias in me, not less. No matter. It's a worthy journey and it helps me take steps to change.

After you've done that work, you are ready for a simple exercise that we've found is powerful:

1. ***Own.*** Stand back and notice your own tendencies to judge others (or yourself), or to enact bias based on privilege, and bring as much self-compassion and emotional openness to that awareness as you can. When do prejudicial thoughts or biased actions like this pop up? Let go of any tendency either to buy into them or to make them more important by avoiding awareness of them or by criticizing yourself for hosting them. These are thoughts, feelings, and invisible habits. They are yours. You are not to blame, but you are responsible. Just note their existence, consciously increasing your awareness of the heavy negative cultural programming we all carry.

2. ***Connect.*** Deliberately take the perspective of those your mind judges, feeling what it's like to be subjected to stigma and enacted bias, sometimes even without any conscious awareness by the person doing harm. Do not run from the pain of seeing that cost or allow it to slip into guilt or shame. The goal is connection and ownership. Allow the pain of being judged or being hurt without awareness by the person doing harm to penetrate you. As you do so, bring your awareness to how causing anyone that pain goes against your values.

3. ***Commit.*** Channel the discomfort of ownership and the pain of connection into motivation to act. Make a commitment to concrete steps you can take that will alleviate the impact of stigma and prejudice on others, including the invisible forms. That could mean learning to listen more; it could mean speaking out when jokes make light of prejudice; it may mean responsibly sharing what you are owning; it could mean stepping back so that others can step forward; it could mean joining an advocacy group; it could mean making friends who are members of groups

your mind judges. Make a plan to take some of the actions you come up with, and follow through thoughtfully and mindfully, not to erase what you are carrying, but to channel the pain inside it toward compassion and human values.

You can practice this exercise regularly. As you undercut the grip of your implicit biases with flexible connectedness, you will find that your enjoyment of being with people of all sorts increases, no matter how different they may have seemed to you before.

The sad fact is that if we're not helping to solve the problem of prejudice, we are helping to perpetuate it. If we do not learn how to catch our invisible privilege or the subtly prejudicial thoughts as they course through our minds, we will inevitably be somewhat complicit in stereotyping and dehumanizing others based on them, unwittingly supporting underlying bias and passing it on to yet another generation. It is hard to admit to ourselves how complicit we have been, and it's hard to diminish the impact of implicit biases. But with work, we can do it.

Yes, my beloved Ruth Esther with her "tainted blood"; yes, my hate-spewing childhood friend Tom; yes, my beautiful brown daughter; yes, Steve in the mirror; yes, yes, we can.

Chapter Eighteen

BRINGING FLEXIBILITY TO PERFORMANCE

Human beings naturally yearn for competence. Good thing. From infancy forward we have things to learn, mountains to move, games to play, and races to win. The flexibility skills are of great assistance in all these endeavors. Here I'll first discuss how they help with general performance challenges, whether in school, at work, in the arts, or in sports. Then I'll take a special look at how the skills can be applied to our work lives, including how they can make managers better leaders and how companies can tap the power of flexibility. Finally, I'll address how the skills help with a set of typical problems with sports training.

Let's begin with the role of values work. One of the ways that ACT training helps with performance in any of our undertakings is reminding us to be values-focused in our pursuits. When it comes to performance, this can be quite difficult. For one thing, we're under intense social pressure to achieve. We've probably all heard the old maxim "It's not whether you win or lose, but how you play the game." And we've probably all rolled our eyes about it. Oh, yeah? Tell that to my boss (or coach or parents)!

We've discussed how important intrinsic motivation is in values-based living. A problem in staying intrinsically motivated when it comes to performance is that so many extrinsic motivators are thrust at us, and crude or improper use of them can interfere with the development of values-based motivation. In school, a healthy desire to do well can turn into the feeling that we *need* to score high or else. Avoidance of mental threats soon overwhelms intrinsically positive motivations to learn. In addition, in many schools, children face testing regimens that push aside time for creative and effective forms of exploratory learning.

At work, many of us are given specific goals, and our performance is measured through annual evaluations tied to bonuses and pay increases. We're often incentivized in a crude transactional way, with the carrot of monetary rewards or the stick of the threat of admonishment or being let go. In professional sports, there is the imperative to please fans, as well as the reward of large salaries. Even in amateur athletics competitions, music performance, theater, or dance, medals and trophies send the message loud and clear that participating is all about achieving.

External rewards are fine—few of us would work for a job that paid us nothing. The trick is to use your flexibility skills to direct your focus to the intrinsic benefits of performance, allowing concrete rewards to facilitate rather than to substitute for values-based actions.

Start by taking some time to consider the negative self-talk you've been engaging in about whatever performance issue you're struggling with. The Dictator can become an absolute demon in driving us to achieve the outward signs of success. "*If you don't get an* A *in this class, you're a total loser.*" "*You haven't had a promotion in three years; what is* wrong *with you?*" Write down any such messages and practice your defusion exercises on them. That will help you be aware of them whenever they start jabbering at you, and you can say, "Thanks, but I've got this covered" to them. Maybe write them on a pack of cards that you carry with you and touch the cards whenever you hear one of them jabbering at you. You'll get better and better at catching them and letting go of an interest in them.

There is nothing wrong with wanting to succeed, as long as the achievements you're pursuing are in line with your chosen values and not in the service of avoiding fears and doubts. Values and self work will help greatly with staying focused on the intrinsic rewards of achievement. Taking some time to reflect on how your hard work is serving your life aspirations can help you see course corrections you should make. Maybe you should leave work earlier to spend more time with loved ones or to pursue other passions. Or perhaps you've let achieving some goal in a sport undermine the joy of playing and refining your skills.

With any given performance challenge, write down the values that your devotion to it is serving. Hopefully you will find that some of them are authentically meaningful to you, like supporting your family and bringing joy to others. But you may also find that some of them are primarily about social compliance and propping up an image of yourself, like impressing co-workers or making enough money that others have to treat you with deference. Use your toolkit exercises to explore whether your self-story might be too tied up with certain outward indicators of achievement.

The flexibility skills also help with the many emotional stresses involved with performance. These include performance anxiety, the fear of failure—and fear of success—and the pain of the disappointment and shame that comes with inevitable failures. There is also the sting of self-recrimination about missteps; the pain of criticism from a teacher or boss; the anger over impediments put in our way, such as needless bureaucratic paperwork; and the stress from being tested constantly in school or being assigned too much to do at work.

Practice acceptance exercises to cope with these emotional challenges. You can systematically apply your toolkit acceptance practices to them. For example, pick out a specific performance area or situation that's difficult for you and write down the difficult emotions it provokes. Then do the Say "Yes" and Caring exercises introduced in Chapter Eleven with them.

In the heat of the moment, as these emotions and negative thoughts flare up, call on your defusion practices. Presence exercises will also help, redirecting your attention from your inner battle to the task at hand. If you can get some privacy, do the Simple Meditation exercise introduced in Chapter Twelve. In any situation, you can quickly go through the practice also presented there of shifting your attention to the soles of your feet. By regularly practicing these and other presence methods, you'll find you can call on them even in the most intense moments.

Presence and defusion practices are also helpful with one of the most pernicious effects of our worries about performance, the phenomenon known as choking. It is common in sports. We're so distracted by worries about how we're doing that we flub a shot or take our eye off the ball. Choking occurs in school and work too, such as in taking a test we're anxious about or giving a presentation. If this is a problem for you, start calling on your favorite defusion and presence drills whenever you're feeling the heat, and over time, you will become better and better at returning your focus to the action of the moment.

The ACT message about performance can be summarized in a sentence. High-level performance is best pursued not out of fear, judgment, and avoidance, but with mindfulness, commitment, and love.

Tackling Procrastination

A common impediment to performance is procrastination, which is a form of emotional avoidance, and for this reason, ACT skills help counteract it. ACT research has shown that procrastination is predicted by psychological inflexibility. The stress and anxiety of an assignment is diminished briefly by delay, but that smaller, sooner reward can lead to major performance failures. Even if you're able to pull off a good job with a project once you do finally dive in, developing a reputation as a procrastinator can hold you back, especially in work.

ACT programs for procrastination have been developed. They teach people to follow three steps when they become aware that they're stalling on a task: (1) insert a mindful pause and recognize current thoughts and feelings, (2) accept and defuse, and (3) choose to act based on values.

If you want to try this approach, for the next week, every time you become aware you're procrastinating, in that very moment practice a presence exercise or two for a few minutes. This is like dropping an anchor of attention into your body. A good strategy is to envision touching the pull to procrastinate and then observe the sensations in your body. As you identify each one, breathe into it as if to embrace it consciously. If you are feeling your stomach tighten, for example, direct your breath there. Then do the same for thirty seconds or so with the emotions and thoughts you become aware of.

If any unhelpful thoughts and feelings show up, use your defusion and acceptance methods to observe them.

Next, review which of your values you will be acting on by doing the task. Then consider this: what has it been costing you not to live up to that value?

Finally, with that inspiration to break free from your procrastination, craft a small set of SMART goals that will get you moving. Begin with some behavior, no matter how small.

Learning and Creativity

A special type of flexibility—cognitive flexibility, which we discussed in Chapter Nine—is also a powerful tool for performance. In the earlier discussion, the focus was on not being enslaved by the unhelpful rules the Dictator wants us to follow. Here I want to emphasize that cognitive flexibility is a great aid to learning and creativity, which are both so important in performance. The results seen in research on cognitive flexibility are so striking that the topic merits special focus here.

Performance in any of our undertakings is significantly enhanced by being able to fluidly consider many alternatives for tackling a challenge, keeping them in our minds all at once and playing around with them. Our problem-solving ability is more creative when we are able to let ideas ping off one another in our minds, including contradictory ones, allowing room for unexpected possibilities, or even seemingly absurd notions, to gain some traction. In creativity research this is called *lateral thinking*, and studies have shown that many of the most important innovations have resulted from it because of the novel connections made. Why does a phone have to be just a phone? Why can't it also be a music player? Better yet, why can't it be a computer?

ACT and RFT researchers have created training programs for developing cognitive flexibility based on the speed, accuracy, and context sensitivity of relational framing, and the results in tests of the effects on intellectual problem solving are astonishing. Several studies have shown that this cognitive skill correlates greatly with traditional IQ scores. More exciting is the finding that *training* cognitive flexibility until relations are fluent can raise IQ scores significantly. Some studies have shown a rise over several months of nine to twenty-two points in children—far beyond the two- or three-point improvement that IQ training programs more commonly produce. No published studies have yet tested what happens with adults regarding IQ scores. Some hopeful results have been found, though, in a small randomized study with elderly people (average age seventy-eight) with mild to moderate Alzheimer's disease when given RFT-based cognitive flexibility training. The control group received only medications commonly prescribed for Alzheimer's disease—over three months they deteriorated slightly (as might be expected given that Alzheimer's is a progressive disease). The experimental group received one hour a week of relational framing flexibility training in addition to the medications. Their cognitive functioning improved moderately—a statistically significant difference. We do not yet know what would happen with longer training—more research will be needed to find out.

In Chapter Ten, I introduced some perspective-taking exercises that ask you to answer questions like "I have a cup, and you have a pen; if I were you and you were me, what would you have?" or, more complicated, "Now I have a cup and you have a pen; but yesterday I had a book and you had a phone; if today were yesterday and yesterday were today, and if I were you and you were me, what would you have here today?" Those were cognitive flexibility questions. Answering them required that you use the perspective-taking relations of person and time in unusual ways. Cognitive flexibility training uses many such exercises, but across a wider variety of relations and with the goal of greater speed while retaining accuracy. I've played many hours of these games with my children, mostly while in the car, and I've seen how powerful the results are.

See how quickly you can answer this question:

If inside were outside, top were bottom, pretty were ugly, and I put a pretty rabbit inside a box and closed the door, what would I see?

Quick! Answer! Quick!

I asked that exact question of about two hundred psychologists in an RFT demonstration some years ago. My then six-year-old daughter Esther was sitting in the front row. After three or four seconds of awkward silence while this room full of PhDs practically drooled on themselves trying to get the right answer, I said "Essie?" She immediately and somewhat disdainfully answered (as if this were too easy even to respond to), "You'd see an ugly rabbit on the top of the box."

Exactly right.

Esther had developed great dexterity with such thinking because of our car practice. For years we'd passed the time when driving by playing cognitive games I made up on the fly that required relational framing to be fast, accurate, and flexible to get the right answer. As she got a little older we'd take turns, each of us thinking up an item and then challenging the other to answer it accurately and quickly (more than once she stopped me dead in my tracks). Once you get the principle, you can come up with a good item in less than a minute. You might try this with child passengers (I've played it with adults too). It looks like this:

Drive Time

> ***Q:*** [When coming up on a red light] If red were green and green were red, what should I do now?"
>
> **A:** Go
>
> ***Q:*** If I were you and you were me, who'd be driving?
>
> **A:** [child answering] "I would."
>
> ***Q:*** If corrugated were bumpy, and smarmy were the opposite, which road would you choose? Smarmy or corrugated?

> *A:* Smarmy
>
> *Q:* [When coming up on a green light] If red were green and green were red, and in front was in back and in back was in front, what should I do now?
>
> *A:* Go—the red light is behind you.

Here are some other exercises that you can do to increase your cognitive flexibility and to begin to see useful options that might otherwise be missed.

Uses for an Object

Take any object . . . say a paper cup. Quick, say out loud all of the things you could do with it. Give yourself thirty seconds and note the total number of ideas and the number of different categories or functions (e.g., if you say you could use it to hold jewelry, or make an ear protector, or make a clown nose, that's three ideas and two different functions).

Opposite Day

Write a series of sentences that express an opinion of yours, but use words that are opposite to your views. For example, to state the opinion that you love nature and it should be preserved, you could write, *I hate artificial things and they should not despoil nature.*

Turn Thoughts into Metaphors

Take a negative thought you have about a performance problem and create a metaphoric way of expressing it that reveals its negativity and suggests other ways of acting when the thought occurs. For example, if the thought is an escapist version of *I should just quit*, you might turn it into *I should quit . . . like a person going to sleep on the couch.* If it is a self-defeating thought that leads to workaholism, like *I should work even harder and just forget about how tired I am*, it might be changed to *I should work even harder . . . like a tired and poor ditch digger getting paid the same no matter how deep the ditch he digs.* Next, transform the metaphor into a positive approach to the problem.

For example, *What if I get up off the couch, take a good stretch and get going?* Or *What if I get out of the ditch, hang up my shovel for the day, and head home and give my kids some time?*

Dealing with Constraints at Work

If you sleep eight hours a day (and I hope you do), each year gives you 5,840 hours of awake time to spend. If you work full time, even before you count bringing work home, over a third of those hours will likely be spent working.

For far too many of us, that time is much less rewarding than it should be, or is outright dispiriting and even psychologically punishing. That's due in part to the internal pressures and fears we inflict on ourselves, but much of it is due to the nature of management and workplace environments. Gallup polls show that most people are not engaged by their work or suffer under bad bosses who are ineffective leaders.

The problem is that as right as we may be about what's wrong at the office, there is usually little we can do to change the way our managers lead us or to improve bureaucratic processes that frustrate us. In essence, most workplaces are quite rigid environments, full of all sorts of rules and constraints on how we pursue our work. Fortunately, there's a great deal we can do to change how we respond to the slings and arrows of work life. I offered a basic description for how to apply the skills to becoming happier and more fulfilled at work in the introduction to this part.

Here are some additional ways that we can pivot the energy inside our frustrations about what we can't change at work to focus on the things we *can* do.

Sculpt Your Work to Your Values

The term *job sculpting* was coined by career experts Timothy Butler and James Waldroop. It means finding ways to tailor your work better to your interests and skills so that it is more satisfying to you. While that may require the big step of making a career change, which the flexibility skills can help with, you can also find smaller ways to make changes that can have big payoffs.

The simplest form is reexamining your work and reconnecting with how fulfilling some aspects of the job actually are. The satisfaction of some parts of our work is often overshadowed by our displeasures. We can consciously redirect our attention. We can also often find ways to spend more of our time on those fulfilling tasks. Sometimes that's a matter of scrutinizing closely how we're spending our time and finding ways to be more efficient with some tasks, making room for time spent as we prefer. It may also require the bigger step of discussing our interest in a different mix of responsibilities with our boss. We can use our committed action learning to help with that. Just as we should craft SMART goals—ones that are specific, measurable, attainable, results-focused, and time-bound—in the other areas of our lives, requests we make for some modification of our job description should be SMART, not only for us but for the organization.

Here's where I'll make my plea to any of you who are managers and corporate executives. You will be a better leader if you give your people this kind of latitude to do some job sculpting, and if you model flexibility with them in other ways, which will foster it in them. If you're skeptical about the benefits, let me share the results of the first large study that looked at the relation of psychological flexibility to work performance. It was conducted in 2003 by a team headed by psychologist Frank Bond. At two intervals, a year apart, they measured each of four hundred workers' perceived amount of job control, as well as their psychological flexibility and their mental health, using questionnaires. During that year, every error each worker made on the computer was automatically recorded.

Workers who felt they had very little control over their job made more errors per hour and had poor mental health over the entire year. The same was true for inflexible workers. The best work results were seen with those who both felt they had a flexible work environment *and* had good psychological flexibility. Several studies have confirmed these results.

The bottom line: flexibility is good for business. Both employees looking to boost their own performance and managers and company leaders seeking to assist employees in doing so should take note of this formula: flexible workers + flexible work environments = success.

What's the best way to foster flexibility in one's team? Modeling it. Research shows that leaders who manage with psychological flexibility help workers strengthen their own flexibility skills. What does that comprise? Helping workers satisfy their core yearnings at work for competence, chosen meaning, and belonging. Inspiring people to work for more than short-term self-gain—establish a team mission, vision, and group identity that stimulates workers to be more engaged and collaborate better. Attending to the emotional needs of team members and giving them the thoughtful feedback and resources they need to prosper. Sharing openly with employees about difficulties a team is facing, and even about their own mistakes, which both empowers employees with vital information, so that they can be more helpful in devising solutions, and builds trust. When leaders use individual rewards as incentives, they make sure it doesn't feel like a crude transaction and is instead an expression of authentic appreciation as part of a long-term commitment.

Keep Learning

One of the leading causes of job dissatisfaction is feeling stuck in the same old routines; we feel that we're not learning and growing. We can all take the initiative to teach ourselves new skills. This can seem like a daunting prospect, but we can direct our flexibility skills to committing to it. And a plethora of online courses and training programs are available.

This proactive skill building can also help with the widespread anxiety these days about the future of jobs. Specialists on the future of work have warned that automation will be taking the place of many employees and that learning how to work with the new technologies, such as artificial intelligence and machine learning, or how to move from office and factory work into human services work, are ways to "future-proof" one's career. Applying flexibility skills to continuous learning is a great way to prepare for this brave new world of work.

Consult the Matrix

In a work environment, we often can't take much of a "time-out" to practice flexibility skills; we've got to be very quick. The ACT community has developed several mental tools you can use to remind yourself of your ACT learning in a flash. One that I especially like and have used successfully in organizational settings is called the Matrix, developed initially by Kevin Polk. The heart and head of these walking figures represent your thoughts and feelings, which no one else can see, and the hands and feet represent your overt actions.

You first write down answers to the four questions that follow, putting short versions into the boxes in the Matrix figure beginning with the upper right quadrant and moving counterclockwise:

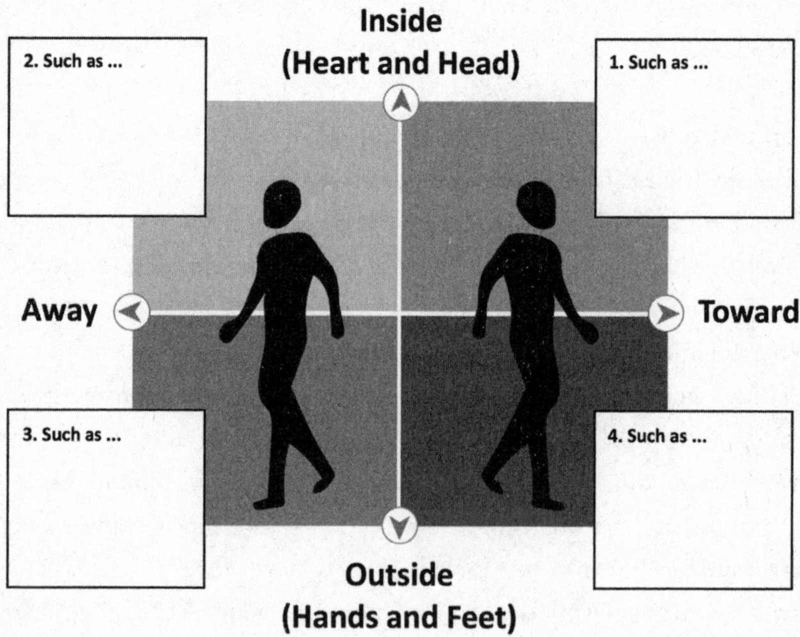

These are the questions:

1. *In the area of work, what are the things inside you that you would most want to walk toward?* I'm thinking of things like the joy you get from being helpful to customers and being kind to co-workers, the satisfaction of being honest and genuine, and the thought that you are making a positive difference in the world.

2. *What are the things inside you that most move you in the opposite direction at work?* I'm thinking of things like the resentment you feel about being overlooked, fear of being shown to be stupid, and uncertainty about your own abilities.

3. *When you are moving away from the things you want to walk toward, what are you doing?* I'm thinking of things like being silent in meetings, gossiping, and deliberately avoiding responsibilities.

4. *When you are moving in your chosen direction, what are you doing?* I'm thinking of things like coming to meetings prepared, making suggestions, and actively listening to the ideas of others.

5. *The final step is not a question. Look at the figure and where the two lines intersect and notice who is noticing the answers you've written. Think of that connection as linking your transcendent observing self to the "now" of these pulls toward and away. Remind yourself that you can choose which direction you're going.*

Once you've filled this figure in, revisit it regularly until you've planted it solidly in your memory. Then, in the trying moments at work when you want to call on your skills, quickly bring it to mind and swoop your way mentally around the quadrants, updating it as you go with tweaks that fit the current situation. Then notice who is noticing, and see if this swoop around the Matrix provides you some support and guidance.

Sports Performance

Everyone who has played a sport knows how the voice of the Dictator can hobble performance. We get entangled in thoughts about what we should be doing. Psychological flexibility helps with quieting all that messaging so you can put your focus where it should be—being in the flow of the game. This approach not only leads to lower levels of distress among athletes, it leads to better performance as compared to traditional sport psychology interventions such as psychological skills training, consisting of goal setting, relaxation training, attention training, and anxiety management.

Research has shown that ACT helps not only for physical sports, but other types of sporting competition or performance situations. For example, the ranking of internationally visible chess players was improved in randomized trials of ACT training. The benefit appears to come from tamping down the emotional effects of mistakes and reducing impulsive moves. Likewise, musicians, actors, and others have used ACT successfully to deal with performance anxiety that interferes with their art.

ACT helps to correct for a good deal of advice given to athletes, even by professional coaches and consultants, that is badly misguided. For example, athletes are often taught to do mental training in which they envision their competitor's moves in order to plan for them. But what you imagined may not be what your competitor does. The better mental preparation is presence practice, to build up one's acuity of observation about what a competitor is actually doing, in the moment of play.

Similarly, athletes are commonly taught to distract themselves from pain, thinking of something pleasant instead, or to focus just on their form. Both of these common forms of coaching have notable limits. A student of mine, Emily Leeming, recently studied competitive CrossFit athletes as part of her dissertation. CrossFit is a program of constantly varied functional movements performed at high intensity. Think of it as boot camp for Olympic athletes who are training for several sports at once. At the competitive level, these folks exercise so hard they practically sweat blood. She had them hold a two-pound weight away from their body at a ninety-degree angle until they couldn't do it anymore. (It just takes a few minutes. Try it. Hold a quart of milk out there and see what happens.) In one group, she had them focus on their form, keeping their arm at ninety degrees; in another she told them to think of something pleasant so as to distract themselves from distressing feelings; and in a third group she advised them to focus on their acceptance of discomfort. Even in this elite exercise group, coaching about acceptance significantly increased their ability to persist (up nearly 25 percent in some comparisons), while the other two approaches produced no benefits. It's important for athletes to be mindful of the degree of pain they're feeling and respond in a well-calibrated way. Otherwise they are at risk of injury. Flexibility processes foster such openness. Research has also shown that if athletes do suffer injury, they are more likely to go through rehabilitation successfully if they are psychologically flexible. The effect appears to be due to better adherence to rehabilitation requirements.

If you want to apply your ACT skills to your sports performance, a good place to start is with any training exercises that are difficult, boring, or painful. Cycle through applying the flexibility skills to your practice of them, maybe one skill per day of your exercise sessions, such as the following:

Defusion day. As you're working out, watch for thoughts that are intruding on your engagement with the work, such as *This machine is killing me* or *I* hate *sit-ups*, and sic your favorite defusion methods on them.

Acceptance day. When you feel difficult sensations that you know are not dangerous but that are urging you to stop, bring your attention to the sensation and tell yourself, *I am willing to feel this, it's OK*. Imagine that you've created the sensation on purpose, which is a way to get out of your defensive posture about it and be the author of your experience.

Now day. Practice attentional flexibility as you work out and see if you can sense which attentional strategies most empower your training. For example, if you ride a bike for exercise, bring your attention to all of the sensations in your body, and then move it to the scenery around you. Then bring it back to your body, focusing on the feeling of pushing down the pedals and then noticing your breath. Try to pay attention to things you do not usually notice while you're working out, like sounds around the room or the air drying the sweat on your skin.

Perspective day. As you start to feel discomfort or are getting bored, ask yourself: What would you say to yourself if you were watching from across the room? What advice would you give yourself from a distant, wiser future?

Values day. Call to mind the qualities you most want to show in the way you engage with your training. For example, maybe you want to be friendly to the other people working out around you rather than closed in and just focusing on yourself. Or maybe you want to show gratitude to your trainer. Find ways to act accordingly.

Commitment day. Try making some modification to your routine that will enhance your training, such as adding even a few more of those dreaded sit-ups, or doing some work on a machine you've been avoiding.

Performance in sports inevitably involves some pain and failure. But just as developing your physical flexibility helps you optimize your performance while also minimizing the toll it takes, so too will cultivating your psychological flexibility.

Chapter Nineteen

CULTIVATING SPIRITUAL WELL-BEING

Spiritual well-being is an important contributor to mental and physical health; a large research literature attests to that. This is true whether one is religious and believes in God or not. While for much of recorded history, spirituality has been promoted primarily through religious traditions and practices, such as prayer and contemplation of scripture, more recently, cultivation of spirituality has been encouraged through methods such as yoga and mindfulness meditation that have been part of religious traditions but can be engaged in as secular practices. Whichever ways you seek to nurture your own spiritual well-being, the ACT skills will be helpful. A little consideration of the nature of spiritual well-being will illuminate why. At the end of this chapter I will address how compatible ACT is with all of the faith traditions and how it can enhance one's engagement with specific religious practices.

While there is no one universally agreed upon definition of spiritual wellness, a wide range of sources describe these essential characteristics: a feeling of peace of mind, being in harmony with oneself and others, a deep sense of connection with others, compassion toward oneself and others, the sense of a domain of life that transcends the bounds of the material world and the confines of self, a feeling of living with meaning and purpose, being able to trust oneself, reverence for life, and having faith or hope in life. This helpful statement from the National Wellness Institute sums up the quest for spiritual well-being as "the search for meaning and purpose in human existence, leading one to strive for a state of harmony with oneself and others while working to balance inner needs with the rest of the world." Clearly these qualities of living are entirely resonant with the aims of ACT.

Defusion helps develop peace of mind and a hopeful perspective by freeing us from negativity. It also helps us keep our focus outward, on helping others with their needs, rather than inward on rumination about our own needs and difficulties. Acceptance helps us let go of anger and resentment, which work against compassion and trust. It's also of great assistance when we face major life challenges, such as a diagnosis of illness, being fired, or the breakup of a marriage, which can shake our faith in life. Values work helps us focus on what we find full of meaning and purpose, and action tools help us commit to a steady schedule of activities that build spiritual well-being. In addition to activities that reach out to others and build community, such as signing up for volunteer work we've long thought of doing, these should include ones that are internally directed, such as prayer and meditation.

Which brings me to the presence and self skills. They contribute to spiritual wellness in ways that are fundamental but a little trickier to appreciate, and I focus on them here. They help with what I'll call purposeful connection with transcendence.

The belief in a spiritual dimension of life is solidified for many people by having an intense experience of transcendence of the normal state of life. This has been described as a profound sense of boundlessness, of oneness with a realm of life beyond physical constraints of time and place, and beyond self as an individual person with particular attributes. The experience usually involves a different sense of self. This can include the feeling that one's very being is becoming one with the universe—which has been called a state of *cosmic consciousness*. Many spiritual guides and authors of popular books about spirituality, such as Eckhart Tolle, have described such experiences as being pivotal in their life, as of course have many religious teachers over the millennia.

Such experiences were once characterized as extremely rare. Psychiatrist

Richard Bucke, who studied the phenomenon and published the influential book *Cosmic Consciousness* in 1901, estimated that only one in a million people experience them. That conjecture was widely accepted for many years. But a few decades ago researchers began to discover that these experiences are actually far more common. Studies have found that between a third and four-fifths of all adults report having had them. That considerable range in numbers is partly explained by the fact that many people who have these experiences are reluctant to talk about them. Some worry that they'll sound crazy; others find the experience difficult to describe, or they sense that it is so special and personal that, like a sweet kiss from someone you love, it almost seems wrong to characterize it using words.

I have confidence that these experiences are not uncommon, in part because I experienced one myself that night on the carpet when I made my first pivots in coping with my anxiety. I felt a powerful sense of transcendence, as if I were leaving my own body and looking back at myself, and from there I made life-altering choices that are still with me almost four decades later. As I stood up from that carpet, I immediately realized I'd had a spiritual experience, and the first article I wrote as I began developing ACT, published a year later, was titled "Making Sense of Spirituality."

Although these experiences are not uncommon, they are not universal, and in their most profound form they are rarely repeated. One of my aims in developing ACT has been to help people foster a more enduring sense of connection to this place of transcendence. We can experience small day-to-day connections to transcendence, which offer inspiration and guidance, much in the way even a tiny crack of light in a darkened room keeps you from running into the furniture. The presence and self exercises are relevant in providing that crack of light. Let me explain why and offer some exercises that I've found powerful.

Practicing Perspective-Taking

Recall that we develop our sense of self when we learn the three perspective-taking relations: I—you; here—there; now—then. I've already introduced a number of exercises for heightening our awareness of our observing self. I've asked you to look back at yourself from a wiser future; to mentally cross the room and look back at yourself; and to view yourself through the eyes of an admired friend or advisor. In each case I asked you to slide your focus from one end of the three perspective-taking continuums—now/then; here/there; I/them—to the opposite. Imagining a wiser future moves awareness from *now* to *then*. Mentally going across the room and looking back moves consciousness from *here* to *there*. Imagining an advisor looking at you from their perspective moves awareness from *I* to *you*. In other words, the first of these exercises fosters a transcendent sense of time. The second cultivates a transcendent sense of space. And the last builds the sense of transcending the boundaries of self and connecting with others in that realm of spiritual oneness.

In my first article about ACT I speculated why. I speculated that a characteristic of intense experiences of transcendence is that we are able to experience perceiving from *both* ends of all three of these perspective-taking continuums, all at once. It's as if we are seeing through the eyes of both *I* and *you*, are in both the *now* and the *then*, and are both *here* and *there* all at once. We have entered a mental realm that is not characterized by those divisions. We feel as though we are participating in a larger, all-encompassing consciousness, a consciousness of "everyone, everywhere, always," because our minds have somehow been opened to a *both/and* way of perceiving, rather than the conventional *either/or.* Research on transformational experiences of many kinds backs this up, having found that divergent *both/and* thinking is central to these experiences.

In a sense, consciousness itself provides the seeds for spiritual experience. Understanding the cognitive foundation of consciousness leads to methods of intentionally investing our day-to-day life with this feature of spirituality. Here are two exercises to practice on a regular basis.

The first exercise combines perspective-taking and acceptance to foster compassion toward oneself and others. Compassion is a hallmark of spiritual well-being; if we are interested in expanding consciousness it's a great place to start.

It's best if you record yourself reading this exercise slowly, out loud, and then go through it from the recording, so that you can do it with your eyes closed. Insert a short pause after each sentence, and where I've put ellipses, you should pause for a handful of seconds.

Get yourself in a quiet and comfortable place where you will not be disturbed. Begin by noticing your senses with your eyes open—notice something you can see and look at it, seeing your seeing. Then notice something you can touch, and reach out and touch it, noticing how it feels. Then allow your eyes to close and notice something you can hear. As you notice yourself noticing these things, touch just for an instant that you are the one noticing. Sit inside that awareness for a few moments.

. . . .

Then gently bring your attention to a painful emotion you've felt in the last day. As you open up to that experience, see if you can do so with a sense of warmth and wisdom, as if you are expanding your awareness, your simple ability to notice, so that it totally surrounds the emotion. Notice your breath and with each breath out, expand that sense of kindness and strength a little more, as if gently wrapping this emotion in compassionate awareness. Expand until you are feeling every nook and cranny of that feeling on purpose: gently, kindly, compassionately.

. . . .

Now realize that there are other people in other places and at other times who are feeling difficult emotions exactly like that. Imagine that you can reach across space and time and bring your expanding sense of compassion to them, as if to guide their awareness to do what you were just doing. Others are hurting, often through no fault of their own. Imagine a person who is suffering in that way—they have a difficult emotion to feel and they do not know how. You do not have to know them personally. In your mind, guide this other person to expand their sense of self-kindness and awareness, much like guiding another person's hands to hold something gently. Notice your breath, and with each breath out, mentally reach out and imagine that both of you are gradually wrapping this emotion of theirs in compassionate awareness, together. Keep expanding around the emotion until the two of you are feeling every nook and cranny of that feeling on purpose: gently, kindly, compassionately. It does not matter if your mind says you do not have these qualities . . . simply imagine them and be aware gently, kindly, and compassionately.

■ ■ ■ ■

Finally, imagine that as both of you find that place of self-kindness and awareness, *your* painful emotion can be added to the mix. Both of you are gradually wrapping each other's difficult emotions in compassionate awareness, together. See if you can allow yourself to be a *receiver* of compassion, as well as a giver. Set down your needless defenses against receiving the compassion of others. Allow your awareness to wrap the pain—yours and that of the suffering person you imagined, and of everyone who is suffering anywhere—in the power of human kindness.

■ ■ ■ ■

Sit inside that space quietly until you decide to come back to the room and then open your eyes.

The second exercise helps with developing your *both/and* perspective. It may seem a bit odd, but stay with it and just see what shows up.

Doing this exercise requires that you record yourself and then listen to the recording. Read the script slowly and in a gentle, relaxed voice; pause for a moment at the end of each sentence, and add a handful of seconds at each ellipse.

Begin with an open scan of your sensory experiences. What are you touching right now? What are you hearing?

Now notice who's noticing those things. Catch, just for a moment, that you are here and aware. There is a person behind those eyes of yours.

■ ■ ■ ■

Now remember looking into the eyes of somebody you know very well. It could be a good friend, a spouse, a lover, anyone. Perhaps in real life you did not look into their eyes for very long, but in this exercise we will imagine that it is OK to do so. Picture those eyes and look at them.

As you remember looking into those eyes, notice that not only were you seeing someone else's eyes, but also you could see them as they were seeing you.

To experience what *that* is like, just for a moment imagine moving over into their awareness and looking back at yourself from the *other* person's eyes. Take a moment to notice what your face looks like, and then see *your* eyes looking.

But those eyes you are now looking at, your eyes, are aware too. Your eyes are seeing the other person looking at them. See if you can actually see that awareness in your eyes. The eyes you are imagining are not just *objects* called "eyes." You are seeing eyes that see. See if you can see that. And when you see that, move back over to where you started. Now you are "yourself" again, looking at someone else's eyes looking back at you.

■ ■ ■ ■

Finally, for the next minute or so, keep shifting perspective in the same way you just did. Each time you can become clear that you (or in imagination, they) were being seen, breathe into that experience as if to note it gently and then shift perspective. Slowly and calmly move back and forth between these two perspectives. As you do so, watch for a sense that the two of you are not entirely separate. In consciousness, the two of you are interconnected . . . as if the boundaries between the two of you are softening and there is a *both/and* or a *we* quality to awareness, not just an *either/or* or a *me* quality to awareness.

This exercise is deeply spiritual because it develops our sense of cosmic connection with others. I've done variants of it many times and whenever I have, I touch a sense of *we*. Recall that RFT argues that developing this sense of *we* was essential to creating the two-way street of symbolic relations that led to our advanced consciousness. We are the social primates. Connection with others is good for us and is part of what makes us human.

Once you've practiced this exercise a bit, I think you will find that you begin carrying this sense of *we* into your daily life, becoming more aware of the consciousness interconnection we all have with one another with just a second's glance or a moment's consideration. You will more keenly see people seeing you and you will see them more keenly, feeling the bonds of consciousness that interconnect us all in our humanity.

Cultivating Forgiveness

Combining perspective-taking with defusion helps you foster another aspect of intense spiritual experiences—the desire to forgive. Forgiveness is a powerful force for connection, allowing us to cast away all past grievances and forge ahead on a new path of life without that debilitating baggage. You don't need to record yourself doing this exercise, so I haven't included ellipses for pauses. Be sure not to race through this, however. Pause at each step and proceed only when you feel you've completed that part, which requires some reflection.

Allow your mind to settle on someone in your life whom you tend to judge. They may irritate you. You may disapprove of them. Perhaps they hurt you in some way. You may hold them to account for a wrong.

Whatever it is, just for a moment allow your judgments of that person to float to the surface. Don't buy into them and justify them, but don't try to get rid of them either. See the judgments as something *you* are *doing*—not as something being done to you. Be careful not to judge your judging. The goal is just to take responsibility (you could write it *response-ability*) for the judgments. Let them be there as they are and treat yourself kindly. Even if there are facts behind the judgment, see if you can notice that the judging goes beyond those facts—this is something you are doing.

When you are clear on the kinds of judgments this person pulls from you, let your mind settle on other people you have judged in similar ways. Who else irritates you for the same reasons? How old is this pattern? When do you first remember making judgments of that kind? Were they present in childhood? Were they in your family? Again, don't judge the judging: just notice it and notice that you are doing it.

Now see if you can find something about *your* behavior that you judge others for. If you are quite critical of someone because they seem manipulative, look to see if there are times *you* seem manipulative, perhaps even manipulating yourself. If you are quite critical because someone seems full of themself, look to see if there are times *you* seem to be full of yourself.

Be careful if shame shows up, with its hidden message of *I am bad*. Defuse from that self-judgment by looking at your own experience with dispassionate curiosity: *Look at that, I did* X and *my mind judged me.*

Now comes a choice point. Are you willing to give yourself the gift called forgiveness? Would you be willing to move ahead from here as a whole person without having to either invalidate that judgment of yourself or cling to it? Could you instead allow yourself a fresh start? Could you take yourself off the hook?

Finally, come back to the person whom you tend to judge. Could you give that same gift to them? Do not answer right away—just sit inside the question.

This does *not* mean that you will no longer see the other person's harmful actions as wrong. It's vital that you not invalidate yourself or change facts to forgive. What forgiving *does* mean is that while you still see the actions as wrong, at the same time you are willing to take the person "off the hook." You will no longer seek to keep proving the point that they've wronged you. This is the gift of a fresh start, not based on any kind of denial of truth, but on the choice to let go of anger and pain. You can defuse from your judgments, and their effects on you, by just allowing them to be there as judgments. Put them on leaves and let them float by.

It's also helpful to say the following statement, ideally out loud, though if that's not possible because you're not in private while you read this, say it to yourself in your mind.

"I choose to forgive, even though I will not forget. I am willing to let go of entanglement with my judgments . . . both of myself and of others. I am ready to give myself more of what was there before these experiences led me to judge myself and others. I am ready to fore-give."

I put these exercises in the order I chose for a reason: we tend to have a hard time forgiving others until we've done so with ourselves. The word *forgiveness* derives from the Old English word *forgiefan*—which itself was a combination of the Proto-Germanic *fur* meaning "before, in" and *giefan* meaning "to give." I find that this helps me keep in mind that forgiving is a gift we also give ourselves—a gift of some of what was there before. As we take others "off the hook," we can slide off that hook as well, leaving behind not ignorant innocence but experienced innocence, the aware and knowledgeable choice to begin anew.

ACT and Religion

Some people who practice a religious faith may be concerned about whether ACT is compatible with its teachings. I am certainly not the arbiter of that, but I do think it's valuable to point out that ACT has been embraced by many religious leaders, across faiths. For example, when the chaplains in the U.S. military recently decided to train chaplains in psychological care, ACT was one of three methods selected to be taught (in addition to motivational interviewing and problem-solving therapy). The chaplains are of every kind of religious faith, and ACT was chosen in part because all of these different scriptural traditions are compatible with developing the flexibility skills. I've co-edited a book on ACT for use by clergy and pastoral counselors. In writing it we examined the scriptures of Christianity, Judaism, Hinduism, Buddhism, and Islam, and we found a wealth of passages that advise that people live in accordance with flexibility processes.

Why is it that the religious traditions and ACT share common ground? All of the world's great religions emerged after the origin of written language enormously accelerated the development of our symbolic thinking abilities and the emergence of the Dictator Within. Perhaps that is why every major religious tradition includes ancient ways of reducing the automatic dominance of analytic, judgmental thought, such as through chanting, silent contemplation, meditation, dancing, davening, consideration of koans, and other questions that cannot be answered purely analytically, and repeated prayer.

If you are interested in reading more about how you can combine your ACT learning with your religious practice, you can consult the books that have been written for counselors about how to tailor ACT to working with clients from particular religious traditions.

I found a recent case study illuminating. A devotedly Christian Greek-Cypriot woman dealing with breast cancer applied ACT to her religious practice. She deeply feared death, having watched her own older brother succumb to cancer. During chemotherapy following a mastectomy, she spent her days in bed, crying and fearing for her life. She sank into depression and anxiety. An ACT-based values assessment (see Chapter Thirteen) revealed that she wanted to be "a good Christian who is close to God and shows this belief with her actions" but also that she felt she was not living by this value even though it was deeply important to her.

As she moved through a course of ACT, she began directing her religious rituals differently—in a way that was not just more consistent with ACT and with behavioral science but was also more deeply connected with the underlying meaning of her own religious tradition. For example, she began to pray for God to help her accept her fear and live more in accordance with her values, instead of praying for God to remove her fears. That simple change helped channel the energy inside her fear of death and loss back toward engagement and participation instead of suppression and social withdrawal. As a result, she became much more active in her church group and found ways to link even minor tasks to her values. After eight sessions, she said she was her old self again. Her life-threatening illness had become a source of strength.

That story is a moving testament to the role of spirituality in promoting both physical and mental health. Spirituality is a natural feature of human life that we would all do well to foster. We are all on a spiritual journey in the broadest sense of that term. I have been delighted to find that the flexibility skills can help people progress in that journey, nurturing their ability to commit to living a life of awareness, meaning, and compassionate connection.

Chapter Twenty

COPING WITH ILLNESS AND DISABILITY

If you or a family member have faced a serious disease or chronic condition, you know how psychologically difficult they can be, not only for the person who is sick but for caregivers and friends and family witnessing a loved one struggle. Yet many healthcare providers attend only minimally if at all to the psychological side of these challenges. Worse, the information provided about how to cope is often misguided, encouraging people simply to think positively, or to try harder to comply with medical advice.

My wife and I encountered this when she was diagnosed with gestational diabetes while carrying little Stevie. The regime of diet and exercise initially prescribed proved insufficient to control the problem, and insulin shots were required. We were given a wealth of information about the condition and how vital it was to manage Jacque's blood sugar levels. The primary approach to motivating us was the ominous warning that if we didn't carefully follow the instructions, our baby could be harmed. To help us cope with the anxiety about our son's health, a small set of materials encouraged not only positive thinking but also "by the book" cognitive reappraisal—we were advised to try to think rationally, and to detect, challenge, and change negative thoughts.

Even in expert hands (never mind from a pamphlet!) this kind of classical cognitive restructuring and reappraisal is difficult to implement properly, and, perhaps because of that, it has limited benefits when the results of all of the relevant studies are combined. Cognitive flexibility? Yes. That is helpful, and encouragement to explore other thoughts can be useful. Detect, challenge, dispute, and change? Not so much. It is too risky and too likely to lead to poor outcomes.

Had we not known that, we might have followed the classic cognitive challenge advice and blamed ourselves if it was not helpful. Instead, we drew on flexibility skills. They helped us stay focused and persist in taking the glucose readings, accepting the fear when the meter kicked out poor numbers and channeling that fear into finding just the right combination of medication, diet, and exercise to keep the numbers where they needed to be. It was not emotionally easy, but we stuck with it and Little Stevie was born happy and healthy; then Jacque's gestational diabetes rapidly resolved on its own.

Jacque and I were horrified that the advice and informational materials we received were so limited psychologically speaking, and yet entirely in line with the standard of care for diabetes generally. We had been given materials approved by the American Diabetes Association (ADA), as are most patients with diabetes. Had Jacque continued to be diabetic postpartum, we would probably also have been referred to an educational group for several hours of training in how to manage the disease, conducted by a certified diabetes educator. In other words, the healthcare system would have given us all of the *medical* information we needed to know. I agree—that is vital. But that is not *nearly* enough; people need to be given effective psychological tools as well.

That is why ACT is one of the most widely used models in primary care. My good friend Kirk Strosahl, a co-developer of ACT, and his wife, Patti Robinson, have developed the Primary Care Behavioral Health Model to put psychological flexibility and related methods into normal healthcare systems. In part as a result, much of the research on the value of ACT training has been focused on helping people contend with illness and disability, with impressive results overall.

Consider, for example, a study conducted with over four hundred survivors of colorectal cancer. In order to prevent recurrence, these patients needed to increase physical activity and make major dietary changes. One group of patients received the usual education about what they needed to do, including brochures and newsletters, while the other group received ACT training in the form of eleven telephone calls over six months along with written materials and a newsletter. At a one-year follow-up, those receiving ACT training were 44 percent more able to meet their exercise goals than those in the usual care group and had made better improvements in their eating habits.

That is to be expected, perhaps, but more surprising was that significant improvement was also seen in the ACT group with what is called *post-traumatic growth*—the positive psychological change that sometimes follows adversity. This was measured by asking the patients to respond to a series of quality-of-life statements, such as about their relationships (e.g., *I have a new sense of closeness with others*), seeing new life possibilities (e.g., *I developed new interests*), improving their view of their personal strengths (e.g., *I know I can handle difficulties*), positive spiritual change (e.g., *I have a stronger religious faith*), and greater sense of meaning (e.g., *I have a greater appreciation for the value of my own life*). People in the care-as-usual group saw no significant change in any of these areas, but on average, the patients who received ACT training saw significant post-traumatic growth in all of them—about a 15 percent improvement at six months, which was maintained at one year.

Studies have shown similarly promising results in post-traumatic growth with people who have multiple sclerosis, cardiac disease, pediatric cerebral palsy, brain injury, epilepsy, HIV/AIDS, and a number of other conditions. Flexibility skills also help people become more resistant to the development of health problems in the first place.

A study showing this was done in Switzerland with over one thousand participants in a rare *representative sample*, meaning that the results can be reliably generalized to the entire country. The researchers confirmed the well-known fact that daily stress and poor social support predict a wide range of physical and mental health problems. They also found that the degree to which these factors affect health is strongly related to psychological inflexibility. For example, for people who scored low in tests of flexibility, their depression levels increased by 60 percent as daily stressors intensified to a high level. But for people with high flexibility scores, depression increased less than a *tenth* of that as stressors went up!

Flexibility skills also help with the inevitable emotional and physical difficulties of aging. In modern Western culture, we receive little training in how to age in a psychologically healthy way. The culture is rife with ageism. As a result, aging is often feared, and many people work furiously to try to fend it off with untold billions of products and services. Staying *healthy* as we age is a wonderful mission, but trying to *deny* aging and the inevitability of losing roles, friends, or functions is unhealthy. We are all going to be old if we live long enough.

Research has shown that elderly people who have great flexibility skills experience less depression and anxiety in long-term care as well as at the end of life when they are in palliative care. They experience less anticipatory grief about facing death. Flexibility also improves people's acceptance of help from caregivers and the ability to compensate as they lose areas of functioning.

These and a host of additional research results leave no doubt that learning flexibility skills should be seen as a key component of healthcare for everyone. You can apply them to the management of virtually any physical ailment you may experience, and as a complement to virtually any treatment protocol you've been prescribed. Let's examine a few examples.

Chronic Pain

Across the world, an epidemic of chronic pain has baffled medical researchers. It is not just that chronic pain is increasing enormously, it is that countries with some of the best healthcare systems and most ergonomically sensible worker protection laws spend a staggering amount of their gross national product on disability, mostly linked to chronic pain. Scandinavia is an example. On average from 1980 to 2015, Scandinavian countries spent 4.3 percent of their gross domestic product (GDP) on the cost of disability and incapacity, most of it work-related.

Actual disability claims have not reached those levels in the United States (the United States spends 1.1 percent of GDP on disability and incapacity), but it is still not cheap. The medical cost of chronic pain is between one-half and two-thirds of a *trillion* dollars. In 2012, over half of the U.S. population experienced pain over the prior three months—a largely silent epidemic that affects more people than cancer, diabetes, heart attack, and stroke *combined*. Meanwhile, the United States has led the world in trying (unsuccessfully) to treat chronic pain with opiates. That approach may indeed have kept down costs but not because it has solved the problem—it has shifted the burden to patients and their families and has led to the public health crisis of widespread opioid addiction.

Why has this happened all of a sudden? Is the modern world now much more likely to visit physical harm on people than before? Hardly. The change is in part due to how we talk about and treat pain itself.

In the United States about twenty years ago, physicians were encouraged by the hospital accreditation body and others to start treating pain as "the fifth vital sign," as important in assessing a patient's health as measuring temperature, blood pressure, respiratory rate, and heart rate. The intention was to provide people with more assistance in coping with pain, which was long overdue. The problem is that the primary means of assisting them has been the prescription of pills in order to *eliminate* pain, not to manage its psychosocial impact in the short and long term. Psychological approaches have received *much* less support from the medical system, in part because pain treatment is stuck in the wrong model. That is a terrible shame, because research shows that ACT training (and other psychosocial approaches) can help people considerably in coping with the distress of chronic pain and in avoiding the development of chronic pain in the first place.

The great challenge with chronic pain is that unlike acute pain from an injury or surgery, it appears to be deeply ingrained in a neurobiological system called a *persisting aversive memory network*. It is pain, but it is not pain coming from acute sensory processes in injured body tissue. Consider the experience of people with chronic pain in their limbs, such as their hands. Sometimes people beg to have their hands or limbs removed to stop the pain. That is logical but a very bad idea: fully 85 percent of those who have a limb removed still feel pain in the limb even though it's gone! This is not because the removal of the limb damaged nerves—it is because the pain was no longer primarily in the limb in the first place. It had moved to the central nervous system, embedded in our brains, much the way our memories are.

If pain has persisted for three months (the usual criterion in considering it to be "chronic"), there is nearly an 80 percent chance it will persist four years later, and if the criterion for "chronic" is raised to six months or a year, the statistics get even worse. In adults, at least, ACT for chronic pain does not work primarily by eliminating pain (nor does any other evidence-based psychological intervention, such as traditional CBT). Where ACT is powerful is in lowering the level of distress felt about chronic pain, thus reducing its life interference. That helps people continue with their regular life activities *with* the pain, not in opposition to the pain.

If an ACT message were part of the general approach to pain, would it reduce the development of chronic pain? It is still early, but some work with children who have chronic pain has suggested that ACT training can help prevent pain from becoming permanently ingrained. Several world-class pain centers, such as the Karolinska Institute in Stockholm (where the Nobel Prizes are given), use ACT extensively with children. That work has shown that ACT appears to reduce felt pain more noticeably with children than adults, perhaps because pain is less dug in neurobiologically and psychologically with children. New evidence suggests that the same might happen with adults if we deploy ACT at the right time in acute pain situations, before they become chronic (e.g., using ACT before back surgery).

Encouraging people to develop acceptance skills for coping with their pain should in no way be construed as, in effect, telling them to "buck up and deal with it." *Acceptance* can be a loaded word for people who have chronic pain. Telling people they should accept their pain can sound like a way of saying, "Please don't talk about your pain—it is too disturbing to me." That is not humane, and it is not helpful.

ACT acceptance is in no way a denial, or belittling, of pain. It helps create the flexibility to go from living with pain, to *LIVING* with pain by combining acceptance with defusion and committed action. One learns to take pain along for the ride in getting back to the business of living in alignment with chosen values.

In Chapter Eight, I described an ACT intervention for people with chronic pain, and you can follow that approach using your favorite exercises. Then you can keep adding more exercises to your practice. You should also try the following one, which I've found helpful when dealing with pain if there is nothing to be done about it. I use it with one of the most frustrating effects of pain—interfering with sleep.

After doing some presence work—I usually do some mindfulness meditation, focusing on my breath, for two to three minutes—I turn my attention to the part of me that is noticing my breath. In other words, I touch base with me as an "observing self." From there I gently direct my attention to where I feel the pain. As I do this, I try to "drop the rope" on the urge to control the pain, or distract myself from it—no flinching, controlling, distracting, just observing. With each sensation I notice, I try to get to "yes," meaning that I can open myself to feeling what I feel with a sense of equanimity. If negative thoughts intrude, I practice defusion on them until they fade. Then I return my attention to my breath, notice the observing part of me again, and go back to focusing on the pain and finding my way to "yes." When the sensation has lost its punch, I look to see if there are other sensations elsewhere I'm struggling with, and if so, I do the same thing there.

Diabetes

The limits of the standard approach to the treatment of diabetes are clear in the data about outcomes for patients. Over 8 percent of the population worldwide will develop diabetes, most of it type 2, which is an acquired resistance to insulin. In the United States, the figure rises to more than 10 percent, and that is an underestimate, as it's known that many cases of type 2 diabetes are not diagnosed. It is a huge and rising world health problem, driven in part by the spectacular rise of obesity.

Fortunately, in most cases the disease can be managed through changes in diet and exercise, along with medications, but much too often, patients do not stick rigorously to the appropriate regimes. The complications that result from unregulated diabetes are severe, including cardiovascular disease, loss of limbs, and blindness.

In the hope that ACT training could help patients manage their disease better, a student of mine, Jennifer Gregg, conducted a study with me and other colleagues in which she tested the results of six hours of ADA-approved education against a program that cut the ADA curriculum almost in half and replaced it with three and a half hours of ACT training. The ACT sessions involved walking patients through how to defuse from frightening thoughts about their condition and the anxiety involved in properly managing it, as well as working on values to help them commit to the necessary behavior changes.

Jennifer and I developed an assessment of psychological flexibility specific to thoughts and feelings about diabetes. We had all of the participants fill it out before the training, and then again afterward. We found that the psychological flexibility scores of those who got diabetes education alone actually decreased by about 3 percent, while the scores of those who also got ACT training improved by nearly 20 percent. The result was that the number of patients in the ACT group who were in diabetic control by the end of a three-month follow-up was significantly higher than the number in the education-only group. Being in diabetic control means that you're keeping your blood glucose levels low enough for long enough that most complications of the disease can be avoided (it's measured by hemoglobin A1c—a biomarker for average blood glucose levels). For patients in the education group, the percentage in diabetic control actually decreased slightly, from 26 percent to 24 percent, while in the ACT-trained group, it nearly doubled, from 26 percent to 49 percent. If that degree of change were maintained, it would predict nearly an 80 percent reduction in loss of limb and blindness over the years.

When these results were published in 2007, they caused a stir in the field of diabetes research and care, and some researchers questioned the study. But the results were fully replicated in 2016 by an independent research team in an even larger study. I'm sure there will be some hits and misses in the future as we learn how to dial in on this problem, and I'm not saying ACT is a cure-all for diabetes management. But it seems that a focus on psychological flexibility can add an important component.

If you are dealing with diabetes, you should apply your full toolkit of exercises to your difficult thoughts and emotions regarding your condition and to committing to the behavior changes you and your doctor have agreed are needed. Write down all of the barriers you're struggling with in making these changes. Drop the rope on them and get to work applying your ACT toolkit.

Here is an additional exercise you could try, which I've seen is very helpful for people in our diabetes work. We have them do it in a group workshop. You can do it with friends you trust, or family members.

Commit to an action or set of actions and the chosen values or purpose they reflect. Then with your group assembled, stand up and state how you want to be in relation to your diabetes. What do you want your actions to reflect? Why and how is that important to you? What has happened when you've forgotten that? Next, state your commitment to the actions you're going to take. Be specific enough that you're sure they know what you are going to do. We use the phrase *taking a stand* for expressing a strong commitment to something; well, this exercise is taking a stand for your health.

Cancer

Nearly 40 percent of the population will be diagnosed with cancer at some point. While the medical community has made great strides in developing more effective detection and treatment methods, even the National Academy of Medicine worries that attention to the psychological challenge of cancer has lagged. About 30 percent of patients with cancer experience depression, anxiety, and stress, but often they're prescribed little or no therapy.

People with cancer commonly blame themselves for contracting the disease (especially smokers with lung cancer) or for failing to promptly seek medical diagnosis despite experiencing symptoms. Social messaging that they should stay positive makes it hard for patients to talk about the stress of their diagnosis. Friends and family can feel awkward discussing the fear and pain of their loved ones. Withdrawal from life activities is common—some due to the fatigue that is a pervasive symptom of cancer (as well as its treatment), but also because patients do not want their loved ones to see them doing badly.

What's more, the challenge of battling cancer is by no means over once treatment is completed—even if treatment is successful. Fear of recurrence can persist for many years. Many survivors experience long-term disabilities, and some may not be able to return to their jobs, which can not only cause economic stress but contribute to a widely reported feeling of a lack of meaning and purpose in their lives.

Training in the ACT skills has been shown to significantly improve people's ability to cope with these myriad challenges. This is especially true for coping with the common symptoms of depression, anxiety, and fear of recurrence.

A helpful description of tailoring ACT practices to the specific challenges of cancer was provided by psychologists Julie Angiola and Anne Bowen, who wrote in detail about one patient's experience. This fifty-three-year-old woman had stage IIIC epithelial ovarian cancer, which had recurred twice after her initial treatment. Her sessions with an ACT counselor began two months after the second recurrence, and she had told her oncologist that she would have to think about whether to have additional chemotherapy, as was suggested. She reported to her ACT counselor that she vacillated between feeling numb and engaging in "nonstop worrying," and that she was so fatigued that she was having trouble getting out of bed. She also said that she was ashamed about how she was behaving, and that although she would have liked to spend more time with her husband, she didn't want to be a burden to him and had moved into a guest bedroom.

The counselor began by asking her what type of life she wanted to be living, helping her consider what valued living meant to her, and then had her identify the barriers stopping her from living accordingly. She also took psychological flexibility and values assessments, which showed that she scored high in avoidance but also in values, specifically valuing spending time with family, socializing with friends, engaging in recreation, and experiencing physical well-being. As the assessment helped her see, she was not, however, acting in accord with them. Given her strong values score, the counselor had her first do a good amount of work linking values to actions she could commit to. The therapy then progressed to helping her with acceptance, walking her through many of the defusion, self, acceptance, and presence exercises that were introduced in the Part Two chapters. She was able to significantly improve her quality of life and reengage in the activities she valued.

You can tailor your work with flexibility skills to the discoveries you're making about the problems you're having. For example, if anxiety or ruminative thoughts are problems for you, then it might be best to begin with defusion and presence work. If self-blame and shame are difficult issues, then self would be a good beginning.

Tinnitus

I learned the value of the flexibility skills in coping with chronic health conditions from personal experience. Tinnitus is a name for incessant ringing in the ears. It can be quite disabling. The most common treatment is tinnitus retraining therapy (TRT), which uses counseling to interpret noise benignly (as a neutral signal) and noise machines or other sound devices to habituate people with tinnitus to the ringing. The idea behind TRT is that the brain falsely perceives subtle neural stimulation in the ear as noise but would not do that if the general set point for sound were higher. It is sort of like how the noise of an air conditioner would be awful in a quiet room, but in a noisy bar it would hardly be noticed.

I used to love to listen to punk rock and those tatted bare-chested singers roaring like aircraft engines. Now, decades later, tinnitus is the result. I was not impressed with the studies on TRT (the effects are weak), so I opted just to ignore the noise, hoping it would go away. I wore earplugs to prevent further damage. But it steadily grew louder. And louder. And louder! This gradual slide into more and more distress took about three years. It was not until I caught a thought in my mind that the sound would stop if I shot myself that it even *occurred* to me to apply ACT.

I went on a long walk and fully applied my acceptance, defusion, and attention skills. By the time I got home I knew it would work. The effect was virtually immediate. Within two days, I felt no distress about the ringing at all. None. And it has never returned.

The noise did not go away. But it became like the noise of the ventilation system in a hotel—who is interested in that? Now several years later the ringing is still there (louder!), but it *never* bothers me. I rarely even hear it, unless I am talking about it or (as in this moment) when I'm writing about it. No matter: I have respectfully declined my mind's invitation to care about it one way or the other.

Such quick acceptance was only possible because I'd been practicing flexibility skills for decades, and I'm not suggesting that such immediate effects will come right away for new practitioners of ACT. But given my positive outcome, I reached out to Swedish researcher Gerhard Andersson, perhaps the world's leading expert on psychological approaches to tinnitus. Together we created the Tinnitus Acceptance Questionnaire, a twelve-item measure of psychological flexibility regarding tinnitus, and sure enough it strongly predicted tinnitus distress. We now know that psychological inflexibility turns the loudness of the ringing into the negative life impact of tinnitus, even after anxiety and depression symptoms are taken into account.

Gerhard and his team then conducted a trial with sixty-four patients who were divided randomly into two groups assigned to receive either TRT or ten approximately one-hour sessions of ACT training. At a six-month follow-up, 55 percent of the patients who received ACT training were significantly improved in the degree to which their tinnitus was adversely interfering with their lives, such as preventing sound sleep or causing anxiety or depression. That was nearly three times as many as the 20 percent who reported improvement after receiving TRT.

The Swedish team invited me in to help them determine if increased psychological flexibility explained that difference. It did. Furthermore, you could see it happen in how patients began to change the way they talked about their problems after a few sessions of ACT! We tracked the frequency with which patients made statements that suggested they were using flexibility skills when thoughts and emotions came up about their tinnitus. For example, if a person said, "I had the thought that the noise was distressing" instead of a more entangled statement like "The noise was distressing," they were significantly more likely six months later to experience less distress and interference from tinnitus.

There is no leading treatment for tinnitus yet, but this is a great start. My own experience with it suggests that sometimes acceptance should have this form: *I don't care and you can't make me. I have nothing left to learn from the noise.* (Note for my next lifetime: Do not stand near thirty-foot-tall speakers when punk rock is blasting. OK. Got it.)

I think a lot of life events (phantom pain, permanent loss of functioning, and so on) can eventually get to that point. Yes, acceptance means to receive the gift that is offered. But after you explore that thoroughly, the final form may be more like "this is too boring to care about" or like Mark Manson's book *The Subtle Art of Not Giving* A *F*CK*, even "I don't give a f*ck."

Terminal Illness

ACT methods have been shown to help people with a diagnosis of terminal illness cope with the fear and sadness of facing death. The flexibility skills help people feel less distress and direct their energies to more meaningful end-of-life activities. For example, one study was done with women who had late-stage ovarian cancer. Nearly 85 percent of those in this condition will die within a few years. One group of these patients was assigned to a commonly prescribed treatment of twelve therapeutic sessions that included relaxation training, cognitive restructuring, and guidance on how to solve the problem of facing the inevitability of death. The other group was given twelve sessions of ACT skills-building work. The sessions were held wherever they could be arranged given the intensive treatment participants were undergoing, such as in chemotherapy rooms, infusion rooms, and exam rooms.

Those put through ACT training improved significantly more in a number of outcomes. They engaged in less thought suppression and had significantly lower anxiety and depression. In addition, while the patients who got CBT coped with their anxiety in ways that looked more like distraction, such as watching more TV, the ACT group took more meaningful action, such as calling their children, deciding how their possessions might be distributed when they died, making sure their will was in order, and writing letters to friends and family.

Flexibility skills can also help us come to a place of acceptance about the death of loved ones and to spend the time we have left with them more meaningfully. I learned this the hard way.

My family was highly avoidant about facing death. My dad died when I was twenty-four and in graduate school at the other end of the country, and after my sister called me with the news, my mother soon called and actively encouraged me not to come to the funeral. I was poor, she reminded me. She could not help much financially, she said.

I was only too happy to take that guidance, using the expense as my excuse. I've deeply regretted that decision ever since.

When my sister, Suzanne, called me a couple of years ago and told me my ninety-two-year-old mother's pneumonia had taken a turn for the worse, I immediately got on a plane from Reno to Phoenix. By the time I got to my mother's bedside, she was no longer speaking or opening her eyes, but her head moved slightly when Suzanne said, "Steve's here."

Surrounded by my sister and her grown children, Adam and Meghan, I sat with my hand on my mother and watched over a period of hours as her breathing slowed and her feet turned black as her body shut down. My mind drifted to the last time I saw her.

She'd forgotten I was coming—her mind could not hold new information well anymore. In a frail voice, she had exclaimed, "Steven! My son!" as I entered the dayroom in the extended-care facility she was living in. "He's a famous man," she proudly told a woman sitting next to her in a lowered voice, and then catching her little mom brag, she quickly added, "He's a psychologist," and then, turning to me, as if to remind her beloved son what was *actually* important in life, she concluded quietly but firmly, "He helps people."

My mother exemplified values-based living, and she had worked, to the very end, to guide her children in doing what was *right*, not what was superficially appealing. What had always mattered most to her was what kind of people we were. As her life came to a close, I was so grateful that we could be together, experiencing our sadness and our appreciation and love for one another fully for every precious last moment.

I will go to my own grave savoring that good-bye. We say that the death of a loved one is awful, and it is, but these sacred moments are also full of awe, if we open our hearts to see it. Love and the pain of loss is a sandwich and it does not come any other way.

I hope that as you face the loss of loved ones, the flexibility skills you have will help you experience a sense of peace and the fullness of love that lies within your sadness in their passage.

Chapter Twenty-One

SOCIAL TRANSFORMATION

We are in kind of race against ourselves. If you read between the lines in our communications with each other, everyone is wondering if we can develop psychologically and culturally fast enough to forestall disaster. The particular disaster varies with the tweet, Facebook post, blog, or column, whether about warming the planet beyond repair, fostering a killer epidemic, or simply creating a hellacious world in which our children cannot be happy.

This book helps explain what that race is really about. Can we human beings learn how to be at peace with ourselves and act wisely, even though human language and cognition is seemingly creating an endless series of barriers to doing so? Science and technology, the product of those skills, is wonderful but also mindless. The Internet connects us, but it also overwhelms us with difficult information and challenging judgments. Airplanes connect us, but they also add more greenhouse gases to our atmosphere than any other device. We have the capability to make the world virtually unlivable or even uninhabitable, and in a world like that we can no longer trust in a "me" focus—we need a "we" focus that allows us to cooperate with others to meet such challenges.

What we have been lacking is the development and use of evolution and behavioral science knowledge that can match the needs of the modern world. We see the cost of that absence in the rise of mental health issues, chronic pain, and substance abuse problems, and the miserable mess we have created by trying to medicate our way out of them. But we see it also in our inability to foster healthy behavior, rise to the challenge of physical disease, solve the problem of prejudice and stigma, or soften our politics. We see it in our homes, schools, and work sites.

The theme of this book is that we *do* have a way forward, once we realize the nature of the challenge we face. Using principles of evolution and behavioral science, we can consciously evolve ourselves, becoming better able to contend with life's challenges and to transform our homes and societies. Many of the skills we need are known and can be taught, to children and their parents and teachers, to workers and managers, to medical practitioners and their patients, to social services workers and those seeking services. And I believe that if we develop these skills broadly, they can be helpful in tackling the many social, behavioral, economic, and environmental ills that plague individuals, communities, and whole countries.

This hope may sound grandiose, but I'd like to share a story that inspires me to believe in this potential. It's a story of using ACT training to help people in a devastated community open their hearts and minds to adopting a radical change in behavior in order to save lives.

If any nation on Earth were the least likely to cultivate psychological flexibility it might be Sierra Leone. Nearly three-quarters of the country's population of 6.2 million live on less than $1 per day. The country's healthcare system is weak, and mental healthcare as it is understood in the West is virtually nonexistent. As of a handful of years ago, it was home to a single PhD-level psychologist and one retired psychiatrist. I do not think that sad situation has changed.

On top of all that, the country was riven by a decade-long civil war, which ended in 2002, leaving fifty thousand dead, a ruined infrastructure, and approximately twenty thousand amputees. The future of the country is now in the hands of citizens who as children had been recruited to be soldiers and to kill villagers with machetes, or who had been raped or maimed, sometimes in front of their families.

With so much trauma already to contend with, in 2014 Sierra Leone suffered again. The Ebola virus struck early in the year, and soon more than eight thousand people were infected and almost four thousand had died. The WHO was struggling to contain the outbreak, which had likely spread to Sierra Leone from neighboring Guinea and Liberia.

Hundreds of contagious-disease experts from around the world flocked to the countries, and millions of dollars were sent in from the developed world. Expensive clinics were built (many only to be completed after the crisis was over). Military experts helped contain civil unrest while forcing compliance with epidemiological recommendations to stop the spread of the disease. But mental health experts were *not* sent.

Why would *psychotherapists* be helping in fighting Ebola? Because it's not just the disease that is infectious, it's also the fear of being infected, which makes fighting the virus vastly harder. We saw that in Guinea in a horrifying way, when some of the locals in infected communities were so terrified by healthcare workers arriving in the required protective plastic moon-suits that they killed the intruders with machetes. They also hid sick relatives from the authorities, or allowed them to escape to surrounding villages, where they spread the disease.

We saw the spread of fear in the United States as well. Health workers returning from other parts of Africa (countries without Ebola infection) were put in quarantine for extensive time periods for no logical reason. A single case of Ebola in the United States became national news.

Containing an epidemic always requires behavior change, and in that, psychology ought to have much to offer. In Sierra Leone, the people themselves used ACT and evolutionary principles to forgo their sacred practices of kissing and washing the dying and the dead, which are culturally required to honor family ties and foster passage of the spirits of the deceased to the next world.

The practice had to change because when Ebola claims a life, the virus rises to the surface of the skin as the person sweats. Kissing and washing the bodies of the dead are sure ways to become one of Ebola's next victims. The only safe way to treat patients is to quarantine them, and then the bodies of those who pass away must be immediately zipped into plastic bags and burned.

It is easy for governments to impose such policies, and perhaps, with enough guns, to enforce them. Forcing compliance, however, invites leaving behind a culturally traumatized society. A more humane and effective psychological approach was needed. Fortunately for the district around Bo, the country's second-largest city, locals trained in ACT helped innovate a way for community members to accept the requirements.

A German psychologist named Beate Ebert had established an ACT mental health clinic in Bo to help people cope with the horrors of the war and the crushing poverty of their lives. The country almost completely lacked mental health services. Beate began her work to become an ACT trainer after attending a two-day workshop on ACT I gave in London several years earlier, and from the beginning her main interest was to use ACT to foster social transformation.

She founded a nonprofit organization called Commit and Act whose mission is "to bring psychotherapist support to traumatized people in areas of conflict." In 2010, Beate started traveling to Sierra Leone to offer ACT trainings, and one of those she trained was Hannah Bockarie, an amazing young social worker. Hannah, then twenty-nine, was interested in psychotherapy for both communitarian and personal reasons.

She'd grown up during the war and had seen many children hurt. She had also been a victim. When she was turning thirteen, she was captured by rebels. She escaped and hid in a swamp, but soldiers found her. As they approached, she heard one say, "If we find her, we kill her on the spot." But they did not kill her. Instead, they took her to the camp commandant, who immediately raped her. She again escaped and spent her teenage years in hiding, becoming addicted to drugs "to push down the pain," as she says.

Eventually Hannah was able to get off drugs and channel her pain into helping others. She began volunteering with Doctors Without Borders. With assistance from the United Nations, she then earned her degree in social work. After ACT helped her address her own wounds, Hannah became an invaluable partner to Beate in expanding ACT training in the country. ACBS, the professional society that directs the development of ACT, learned of their work and helped raise the funds to fly Hannah and several other Sierra Leone counselors to the United States for more training, as well as flying ACT trainers to Sierra Leone to train more counselors.

When Beate opened the Commit and Act clinic in Bo, Hannah was appointed its director. Having a resource like this was so special that the people of Bo held a parade in celebration of the opening.

Special programs were established for victims of tribal violence and for women who as children had been sold as indentured servants, frequently ending up as sexual slaves. Several hundred clients were treated individually, in groups, and in workshops. An evaluation by the University of Glasgow showed that attendees became more mindful, less trapped by their thoughts, and happier, even among those who screened positive for PTSD (a common problem in a country that has been war-torn for more than a decade).

Then the Ebola outbreak struck. Within a few weeks, Hannah was appointed the regional director of the Ebola response because the Commit and Act clinic was one of the few well-functioning entities that might be able to help change behavior. Recognizing the need to convince the whole community to accept the need for quarantine and the burning of bodies, Hannah and Beate reached out to me and others in the ACBS community for help.

I had been working with David Sloan Wilson, the evolutionary biologist mentioned earlier, to combine ACT with the work of the late Nobel Prize winner Elinor Ostrom. She had identified eight principles by which the members of communities can come together to solve problems, such as managing limited joint resources like pasture land and fishing grounds. Our goal was to develop a more effective approach for fostering prosocial cooperation and caring in communities. We called the blending of Ostrom's principles and ACT that we developed Prosocial. Hannah and Beate bought in and tried to follow this approach to getting the community to respond to the challenge of Ebola. They began doing Prosocial training with groups of villagers in the Bo district, combining educational information about Ebola with instruction and intervention tools taken from ACT and training in the Ostrom principles.

The ACT training used the tool called the Matrix, introduced in the section on work in Chapter Eighteen, which taught people to look for the inner values they wanted to move toward, see the emotional and cognitive barriers that moved them away, and consider what it would take to make their behavior more values-based. The villages were then asked to reflect on how to apply this values connection, along with Ostrom's insights about group cooperation, to stepping up to the challenge of Ebola. Hannah challenged community members to come up with alternatives for how to honor their loved ones instead of praying over them, washing them, and kissing them. In one of the early trainings, one of the villagers suggested a powerful solution.

Sierra Leone is lush with large banana trees, and this person suggested using them to craft a new ritual: cutting a section of the trunk of a tree, washing it in traditional fashion, wrapping it in a clean white sheet, and placing it on a mat to serve as a sort of totem for the dead. Mourners could carry it, kiss it, pray over it, hug it, and even bury it as a symbol of the person with Ebola.

If this notion strikes you as odd, please consider some traditional Western religious rituals. I was raised a Catholic and taught that communion wafers are transubstantiated through ritual into the *actual body of Christ*. If 1.2 billion people can participate in that practice, why can't the people of Sierra Leone use a banana trunk as a stand-in for their loved ones? As the outbreak spread in Bo, this ritual helped people protect both their community and the essential core of their cultural traditions. As a result, in the critical months during the late spring and summer of 2014, Bo had the lowest rate of increase in Ebola of any of the eight heavily infected districts.

ACT training also helped people with Ebola face their terrible fate. One of these was a man who was refusing to submit to a blood test that would prove whether he had Ebola. He was terrified. "If anybody comes close to me, I will spit on them!" he had shouted to the hospital workers. Armed guards were brought in to keep him in the hospital. For days, no one knew what to do. The man told a guard he would rather be shot than give his blood. The hospital workers were both angry with him and scared of him.

When Hannah heard about the situation, she asked to be allowed to see him. She recalled to me, "In ACT, we say people are 'entangled' with thoughts, and he had this concept firmly in his head: 'I'm not going to let anyone near me. I can't face this. This can't be.'" She donned full protective gear, sat on his bed, introduced herself, and asked "What do you care about? To die here alone?"

He replied that he was suffering because no one was allowed to touch him—that everyone would rather kill him than touch him. "Everybody's against me now," he said. "I'm troublesome. I'm problematic. I'm threatened."

Hannah replied: "So what have you *done* about it?"

The man looked at her as though she didn't understand and said, "If I have it, I will spread it."

She responded, "But what do you want to stand for in your life in the midst of all this?" He paused and broke down, sobbing uncontrollably. In halting words, he said he cared most about his family—he wanted to be with them. He wanted them to know he loved them. He wanted them to respect him.

"Then take some actions," Hannah suggested, very quietly. "Let them take the blood sample. Show your love for your family. Show it."

He gave the sample, and as he had feared, he had the disease and would soon die a horrible death. But Hannah helped him see that he could take the energy of his pain and pivot it toward love of family rather than toward anger and fearsomeness. His family could now visit him, wearing their protective gear, and tell him how much they loved him. They would see that he was accepting his fate with courage and dignity, instead of hearing later about his threats and ravings.

Hannah had been to his village a few weeks earlier to do an ACT/Prosocial training and as a result, when he passed away, his family knew what to do. They allowed his body to be carried away and incinerated and they lovingly sent his spirit on to the afterlife with a proper burial, praying over, washing, kissing, and then burying a banana trunk.

In the aftermath of Ebola, the culture in Sierra Leone has been torn asunder. Across the country, families have fallen apart; sexual and domestic violence is on the rise. But the gentler and more socially transformative path blazed by the Commit and Act clinic in Bo continues to yield dividends. A women's movement to confront the violence, and specifically to rein in domestic violence, has emerged out of Prosocial in Bo. For the first time, men who abuse women are going to jail, and behavioral services are being provided to survivors and perpetrators. The Commit and Act clinic was recently cited by the Sierra Leone government as a major reason that sexual violence toward girls is falling in the city (see http://commitandact.com). Healing continues, using the flexibility processes to promote social transformation.

EPILOGUE

All across the world, psychological flexibility is becoming recognized as a vital life skill, in clinics, workplaces, churches, government agencies, and schools. With each person who learns the skills, the culture evolves just a little bit. Human communication softens; human connection grows.

It's not just ACT, of course. Meditation programs have proliferated; values-based groups are growing; you can hardly open a magazine or turn on your computer without encountering blogs, popular books, television shows, or movies that are focused in some way on psychological flexibility writ large. Readers of this book will recognize what is happening, even if the specific outlet uses other terms. For example, tens of millions of children have seen films or cartoons about the importance of psychological flexibility (go to http://bit.ly/StevenUniverseSong if you want to see an amazing example). It's gratifying to me that over the last thirty-five years, ACT has played a role in fostering this change in cultural focus.

We can do much more to foster healthy evolutionary processes in our lives, homes, and communities. In this area, the readers of this book have an important role. I hope by now you are convinced that I've fulfilled the promise made at the beginning of this book to put forward a small set of scientifically established processes that empower doing what matters in virtually every area. I also hope that you have been inspired to help others learn about flexibility processes and that you've already seen benefits in your life and the lives of those you love from doing so.

If so, think about the fact that social change begins with someone making the simple choice to step forward. If this book has been useful to you, stepping forward is what I am asking of you as this last page is being written. I am asking you to share what you have learned and put it to good use. It does not matter much whether you use the terms in this book. What matters more are the actual things you do or encourage in others. When you open up, you empower others to do likewise. When you take the perspective of others, or make your chosen values clear and step in their direction, you help create human connection and healthy motivation. When you let others know that there is an alternative to mental entanglement and emotional avoidance, you give the gift of hope. And all of that leads to a kinder more nurturing world, reducing the negative experiences that foster inflexibility in the first place.

Life is a misery when we allow ourselves to be dominated by the Dictator Within. When we are freed from its grip, there is another mode of mind just a hair's width away—as the title of this book says, a liberated mind that can help us pivot toward what matters.

We have the seeds within already. If you see a spectacular sunset tonight, you will have the intuitive wisdom just to say "wow" as you open your eyes wide to take in the whole of it. You will not say, "It needs a little more pink." That "wow" mode of mind is not restricted to beauty. If tomorrow you meet a crying child telling a tale of personal horror, you might again say "wow" as you listen intently to take in the whole of that child's pain. You will not say, "Could you talk about something a little less disturbing?"

This book did not teach you anything that you did not, at some deep level, already know in your very soul. All it did was lay out the *principles* you can use to evolve your life in a chosen direction by tapping into the power of psychological flexibility—the power of a liberated mind.

Humanity is in a race, a race to create a kinder, more flexible and values-based world—to say it another way, a more loving world that is better able to face the challenges that our own scientific and technological developments present to us. Either we will learn how to create modern minds for this modern world of ours, or we will loom ever closer to disaster.

None of us knows how it will turn out, but based on human history, I put my bet on the human community evolving to meet the challenge. I put my bet on our capacity to choose love over fear. That can only happen one person, couple, family, business, and community at a time. When each of us learns how to put our *own* mind on a leash, and become more able to open up, show up, and move forward toward what we deeply care about, we shine a light into the darkness that helps others do the same. There is a good word for it: the word is *love*.

We know how important that is. The crying eight-year-olds within us know. Deep down, we all know that love isn't everything, it's the only thing.

Peace, love, and life, my friends.

—S

Hold Out Your Hand

Let's forget the world for a while
fall back and back
into the hush and holy
of now

are you listening? This breath
invites you
to write the first word
of your new story

your new story begins with this:
You matter

you are needed—empty
and naked

willing to say yes
and yes and yes

Do you see
the sun shines, day after day
whether you have faith
or not
the sparrows continue
to sing their song
even when you forget to sing
yours

stop asking: Am I good enough?
Ask only
Am I showing up
with love?

Life is not a straight line
it's a downpour of gifts, please—
hold out your hand

—Julia Fehrenbacher

NOTES

Chapter One: The Need to Pivot

3 **That computer in your pocket**: https://www.quora.com/How-much-more-computing-power-does-an-iPhone-6-have-than-Apollo-11-What-is-another-modern-object-I-can-relate-the-same-computing-power-to.

3 **Leukemia killed**: Centers for Disease Control. "Trends in Childhood Cancer Mortality—United States, 1990–2004." http://www.cdc.gov/mmwr/preview/mmwrhtml/mm5648a1.htm.

3 **Deaths from malaria all declined**: National Cancer Institute, *SEER (Statistics, Epidemiology, and End Results) Cancer Statistics Review 1975–2011*, 2014. https://seer.cancer.gov/archive/csr/1975_2011/

4 **the World Health Organization (WHO) rated it number one**: http://www.who.int/mediacentre/factsheets/fs369/en/. A good summary of the current level of burden worldwide of mental health struggles can be found in Steel, Z., Marnane, C., Iranpour, C., Chey, T., Jackson, J. W., Patel, V., & Silove, D. (2014). The global prevalence of common mental disorders: A systematic review and meta-analysis 1980–2013. *International Journal of Epidemiology, 43*, 476–493. DOI: 10.1093/ije/dyu038.

4 **having an anxiety disorder**: Kessler, R. C., Aguilar-Gaxiola, S., Alonso, J., Chatterji, S., Lee, S., Ormel, J., Ustün, T. B., & Wang, P. S. (2009). The global burden of mental disorders: An update from the WHO World Mental Health (WMH) surveys. *Epidemiology and Psychiatric Sciences, 18*, 23–33.

4 **frequent mental distress**: Moriarty, D. G., Zack, M. M., Holt, J. B., Chapman, D. P., & Safran, M. A. (2009). Geographic patterns of frequent mental distress: U.S. adults, 1993–2001 and 2003–2006. *American Journal of Preventive Medicine, 46*, 497–505.

4 **actually becoming more dangerous**: Pinker, S. (2012). *Better angels of our nature: Why violence has declined.* New York: Penguin.

5 **These skills predict**: These claims will be extensively documented in the chapters to come, so rather than add a long list of studies here, an easy way to assess the general truth of what I am saying is to go to Google Scholar and enter the term ["psychological flexibility" OR "experiential avoidance" OR "acceptance and commitment"]. Leafing through the nearly 18,000 results this search will pull up will quickly link you to hundreds of good examples of this work. If you have access to an academic library, the same search on the Web of Science will pull up around 2,200 scholarly journal articles, and several more are added each week.

6 **books such as this one**: See the preceding note, but for studies showing that just reading an ACT book can be helpful, see, for example, Muto, T., Hayes, S. C., & Jeffcoat, T. (2011). The effectiveness of acceptance and commitment therapy bibliotherapy for enhancing the psychological health of Japanese college students living abroad. *Behavior Therapy*, 42, 323–335. You can find a list of the growing number of such studies at http://www.contextualscience.org (search for "state of the evidence").

7 **affirmations make us both feel and do worse:** Wood, J. V., Perunovic, W. Q. E., & Lee, J. W. (2009). Positive self-statements: Power for some, peril for others. *Psychological Science, 20*, 860–866.

8 **Psychological rigidity predicts**: If you've turned here looking for references to support the bold claims made in this paragraph, congratulations. You have healthy skepticism and that will serve you well in considering the arguments in this book. That being said, it is too early to dump scores of references into the endnotes. So be patient just a little while and all of these claims will be addressed one by one later in the book.

8 **It's the latter:** Farach, F. J., Mennin, D. S., Smith, R. L., et al. (2008). The impact of pretrauma analogue GAD and posttraumatic emotional reactivity following exposure to the

September 11 terrorist attacks: A longitudinal study. *Behavior Therapy*, *39*, 262–276.

8 **you have to avoid joy as well**: Kashdan, T. B., & Steger, M. F. (2006). Expanding the topography of social anxiety: An experience-sampling assessment of positive emotions, positive events, and emotion suppression. *Psychological Science*, *17*, 120–128. DOI: 10.1111/j.1467-9280.2006.01674.x.

9 **horrible outcomes follow**: Panayiotou, G., Leonidou, C., Constantinou, E., et al. (2015). Do alexithymic individuals avoid their feelings? Experiential avoidance mediates the association between alexithymia, psychosomatic, and depressive symptoms in a community and a clinical sample. *Comprehensive Psychiatry*, *56*, 206–216.

9 **I call this aspect of our minds the Dictator Within**: I am a behavioral psychologist so perhaps it may seem odd for me to be talking so much about "minds," but all I mean by that word is the collection of higher relational learning abilities we have that allow the generation and following of symbolic rules. A "mind" is a relational framing repertoire; a "mode of mind" is a way of applying that repertoire. I will explain what relational learning is later in the book.

14 **what they "have" hidden inside**: Frances, A. (2013). Saving normal: An insider's revolt against out-of-control psychiatric diagnosis, DSM-5, big pharma and the medicalization of ordinary life. *Psychotherapy in Australia*, *19*, 14–18.

14 **it has only gotten worse since**: You can piece together these statistics from sources such as Olfson, M., & Marcus, S. C. (2010). National trends in outpatient psychotherapy. *American Journal of Psychiatry*, *167*(12), 1456–1463. DOI: 10.1176/appi.ajp.2010.10040570.

14 **incidence of mental health problems has risen**: Robert Whitaker's website Mad in America has a wealth of information on this issue that I think is fairly responsible. His book of the same name is a bit dated now but is also a good place to start.

14 **Friends and family feel less hopeful**: This is a very large literature now, and without question mental illness diagnoses are stigmatizing even if they provide initial relief. I find the work of Pat Corrigan and colleagues persuasive. For example, see Ben-Zeev, D., Young, M. A., & Corrigan, P. W. (2010). DSM-V and the stigma of mental illness. *Journal of Mental Health*, *19*, 318–327. DOI: 10.3109/09638237.2010.492484. Experimental studies make the same point, not just correlational ones. For example, see Eisma, M. C. (2018). Public stigma of prolonged grief disorder: An experimental study. *Psychiatry Research*, *261*, 173–177. DOI: 10.1016/j.psychres.2017.12.064.

24 **They promote prosperity**: Bohlmeijer, E. T., Lamers, S. M. A., & Fledderus, M. (2015). Flourishing in people with depressive symptomatology increases with Acceptance and Commitment Therapy. Post-hoc analyses of a randomized controlled trial. *Behaviour Research and Therapy*, *65*, 101–106. DOI:10.1016/j.brat.2014.12.014.

25 **turned their recovery from cancer into an asset**: Hawkes, A. L., Chambers, S. K., Pakenham, K. I., Patrao, T. A., Baade, P. D., Lynch, B. M., Aitken, J. F., Meng, X. Q., & Courneya, K. S. (2013). Effects of a telephone-delivered multiple health behavior change intervention (CanChange) on health and behavioral outcomes in survivors of colorectal cancer: A randomized controlled trial. *Journal of Clinical Oncology*, *31*, 2313–2321. See also Hawkes, A. L., Pakenham, K. I., Chambers, S. K., Patrao, T. A., & Courneya, K. S. (2014). Effects of a multiple health behavior change intervention for colorectal cancer survivors on psychosocial outcomes and quality of life: A randomized controlled trial. *Annals of Behavioral Medicine*, *48*, 359–370. DOI: 10.1007/s12160-014-9610-2).

25 **poly-drug users**: Hayes, S. C., Wilson, K. G., Gifford, E. V., Bissett, R., Piasecki, M., Batten, S. V., Byrd, M., & Gregg, J. (2004). A randomized controlled trial of twelve-step facilitation and acceptance and commitment therapy with polysubstance abusing methadone maintained opiate addicts. *Behavior Therapy*, *35*, 667–688.

25 **dozens of studies on substance use**: A recent summary of that area of work can be found in Lee, E. B., An, W., Levin, M. E., & Twohig, M. P. (2015). An initial meta-analysis of Acceptance and Commitment Therapy for treating substance use disorders. *Drug and Alcohol Dependence*, *155*, 1–7. DOI: 10.1016/j.drugalcdep.2015.08.004.

26 **flexibility measures can predict**: Again, I will document this throughout the book. Chapter One is not the time for a detailed dive into findings like this, but a list of ACT meta-analyses (summaries of the ACT literature) can be found at http://bit.ly/ACTmetas (type carefully—capitalization matters). Perhaps the wildest idea in this paragraph deserves documentation: psychologically flexible hockey professionals are more worthwhile to team performance. It's true, they are; see Lundgren, T., Reinebo, G., Löf, P.-O., Näslund, M., Svartvadet, P., & Parling, T. (2018). The Values, Acceptance, and Mindfulness Scale for Ice Hockey: A psychometric evaluation. *Frontiers in Psychology*, *9*, 1794. DOI: 10.3389/fpsyg.2018.01794. Why? If an inflexible player makes a mistake, they get all wrapped up in their emotional response and self-criticism. Guess what? While they are doing that, they are not fully

in the game, supporting their teammates properly. In other words, another mistake! Counterintuitive findings like that are all over this book.

27 **randomized controlled trials**: You can see the current list by going to http://www.contextualscience.org and searching for "randomized trials," or go to http://bit.ly/ACTRCTs.

27 **the level of psychological flexibility overweight people exhibit**: Lillis, J., Hayes, S. C., Bunting, K., & Masuda, A. (2009). Teaching acceptance and mindfulness to improve the lives of the obese: A preliminary test of a theoretical model. *Annals of Behavioral Medicine, 37*, 58–69.

27 **fall a hundred times in a single day**: Adolph, K. et al. (2012). How do you learn to walk? Thousands of steps and dozens of falls per day. *Psychological Science, 23*, 1387–1394.

28 **it has been shown again and again**: Some science skeptics will properly note that this very book has not been tested for its ability to produce such changes. That is fair, but it does not tell the whole story because there are dozens of trials of ACT books, tapes, apps, and websites, and most have shown helpful outcomes. You can find the list here: https://contextualscience.org/act_studies_based_on_computers_phones_smartphones_and_books. Furthermore, readers will be more likely to seek out an ACT therapist once the central importance of flexibility processes are understood. Thus, I do not hold this book out as itself being therapy, but I do hold it out as an accurate science-based story that is likely to open up positive ways forward to help you advance your life if you apply yourself to learning and using the flexibility skills and explore the many free resources available on line to help you deepen your learning and getting over rough spots. I particularly recommend the ACT for the Public discussion list in Yahoo Groups as a good place to begin when you need additional ideas and support.

Chapter Two: The Dictator Within

33 **Automatic Thoughts Questionnaire**: The ATQ was developed by Steve Hollon and Phil Kendall (Hollon, S. D., & Kendall, P. C. [1980]. Cognitive self-statements in depression: Development of an Automatic Thoughts Questionnaire. *Cognitive Therapy and Research, 4*, 383–395.). ACT researchers tweaked the ATQ by asking how believable the thoughts were, rather than how often they occurred. For some purposes that turns out to be a better question. For example, see Zettle, R. D., Rains, J. C., & Hayes, S. C. (2011). Processes of change in Acceptance and Commitment Therapy and Cognitive Therapy for depression: A mediational reanalysis of Zettle and Rains (1989). *Behavior Modification, 35*, 265–283. DOI: 10.1177/0145445511398344.

33 **poor mental and physical outcomes**: For example, they correlate with lower levels of well-being and satisfaction with work. See Judge, T. A., & Locke, E. A. (1993). Effect of dysfunctional thought processes on subjective well-being and job-satisfaction. *Journal of Applied Psychology, 78*, 475–490. DOI: 10.1037/0021-9010.78.3.475; for lower life satisfaction, see Netemeyer, R. G., Williamson, D. A., Burton, S., Biswas, D., Jindal, S., Landreth, S., Mills, G., & Primeaux, S. (2002). Psychometric properties of shortened versions of the Automatic Thoughts Questionnaire. *Educational and Psychological Measurement, 62*, 111–129. DOI: 10.1177/0013164402062001008.

42 **These discoveries**: I cover all of these matters later in the book, where I will provide extensive references to document these claims.

42 **last three pivots**: The linear requirements of a book make this seem more sequential than it really was—it was more a matter of emphasis. For example, committed action was there at the beginning but we assumed it more than studied it. Similarly, flexible attention to the now was implicit in the use of mindfulness exercises but gradually became more an object of research. The same point applies to values.

Chapter Three: Finding a Way Forward

46 **among the most cited scholars**: You can see who is on the top of the list here: http://www.webometrics.info/en/node/58. Freud was number three in December 2018 when I last checked. I am on that list too, but at a lowly 1,740 and sinking fast as so many young people push ahead. My mentor David Barlow is at 695—I doubt if I will ever catch him. That wonderful rascal is one tough act to follow!

47 **subsequent work done by other researchers**: Baumeister, R. F., Dale, K., & Sommer, K. L. (1998). Freudian defense mechanisms and empirical findings in modern social psychology: Reaction formation, projection, displacement, undoing, isolation, sublimation, and denial. *Journal of Personality, 66*, 1081–1124. DOI: 10.1111/1467-6494.00043.

48 **Most of the new methods have emphasized**: You can find these data in resources such as the following: Blagys, M., & Hilsenroth, M. (2000). Distinctive features of short-term psychodynamic interpersonal psychotherapy: A review of the comparative psychotherapy process literature. *Clinical Psychology: Science and Practice, 7*, 167–188; Weissman, M. M., Markowitz, J. C., & Klerman, G. L. (2007). *Clinician's quick guide to interpersonal psychotherapy*. New York: Oxford

University Press; Allen, J. G., Fonagy, P., & Bateman, A. W. (2008). *Mentalizing in clinical practice*. Arlington, VA: American Psychiatric.

48 **Maslow argued that traditional**: Maslow, A. H. (1970). *The psychology of science: A reconnaissance*. Chicago: Henry Regnery.

49 **Rogers argued that research**: Rogers, C. R. (1955). Persons or science? A philosophical question. *American Psychologist, 10*, 267–278. The quote I cite is on page 273.

49 **ACT is sometimes covered in books on humanistic therapy**: For example, see Schneider, K. J., Pierson, J. F., & Bugental, J. F. T. (Eds.). (2014). *The handbook of humanistic psychology: Theory, research, and practice* (2nd ed.). Los Angeles: Sage.

50 **part of the treatment did not matter**: There were scores of studies on the "why" of desensitization, which is one reason it is so important in the history of psychotherapy. Careful research such as that of the late, great Gordon Paul showed that desensitization was not effective because it was a placebo, but as research went ahead it turned out that the hierarchy of scenes to imagine could be done top down versus bottom up—Jon Krapfl and Mike Nawas showed that in the 1970 (DOI: 10.1037/h0029351), and relaxation did not matter provided there was a good rationale. The "why" studies happened because the developer of desensitization, Joseph Wolpe, was so specific about how the method should be done and why it worked. I knew Joe Wolpe, and my undergraduate mentor, Irving Kessler, was a huge fan of his. Joe thought desensitization worked through what he called *reciprocal inhibition*—even doing clever animal studies to test the principle. It turns out he was wrong, but all scientific theories are somewhat wrong if you have enough time, and it is enormously to his credit that he tried to answer the "why" question, not just the "what" question.

51 **this era of behaviorism**: I first used the term in Hayes, S. C. (2004). Acceptance and Commitment Therapy, Relational Frame Theory, and the third wave of behavioral and cognitive therapies. *Behavior Therapy*, 35, 639–665. DOI: 10.1016/S0005-7894(04)80013-3.

52 **the topic of my dissertation**: It was published in Hayes, S. C., & Cone, J. D. (1981). Reduction in residential consumption of electricity through simple monthly feedback. *Journal of Applied Behavior Analysis, 14*, 81–88. DOI: 10.1901/jaba.1981.14-81.

54 **which CBT could not readily explain**: Careful reviews of this issue concluded "that there was "little evidence that specific cognitive interventions significantly increase the effectiveness of the therapy" (p. 173). Longmore, R. J., & Worrell, M. (2007). Do we need to challenge thoughts in cognitive behavior therapy? *Clinical Psychology Review, 27*, 173–187. Large dismantling studies reached the same conclusion; see Dimidjian, S., Hollon, S. D., Dobson, K. S., Schmaling, K. B., Kohlenberg, R. J., Addis, M. E., et al. (2006). Randomized trial of behavioral activation, cognitive therapy, and antidepressant medication in the acute treatment of adults with major depression. *Journal of Consulting and Clinical Psychology*, 74(4), 658–670. DOI: 10.1037/0022-006X.74.4.658.

54 **I can stay in the dark**: Kanfer, F. H., & Karoly, P. (1972). Self-control: A behavioristic excursion into the lion's den. *Behavior Therapy*, 3, 398–416.

56 **CBT generally does not work in the way that was originally postulated**: Chawla, N., & Ostafin, B. D. (2007). Experiential avoidance as a functional dimensional approach to psychopathology: An empirical review. *Journal of Clinical Psychology, 63*, 871–890.

56 **can even *subtract***: Jacobson, N. S., Dobson, K. S., Truax, P. A., Addis, M. E., Koerner, K., Gollan, J. K., Gortner, E., & Prince, S. E. (1996). A component analysis of cognitive-behavioral treatment for depression. *Journal of Consulting and Clinical Psychology, 64*, 295–304. DOI: 10.1037/0022-006X.64.2.295; Dimidjian, S., et al. (2006). Randomized trial of behavioral activation, cognitive therapy, and antidepressant medication in the acute treatment of adults with major depression. *Journal of Consulting and Clinical Psychology, 74*, 658–670. DOI: 10.1037/0022-006X.74.4.658.

56 **a major transition is under way**: You can find the first full presentation of what led to this change in the article that was my presidential address for the Association for Behavioral and Cognitive Therapies (good thing it was my presidential paper because it would have been hellacious to publish it otherwise; even as it was, some reviewers did their best to change it). The reference is in the preceding endnote labeled "this era of behaviorism."

58 **the 1960s and 1970s**: Paul Emmelkamp, a brilliant CBT researcher in Belgium who is about my age, says with good humor that the "third wave" just means that the hippies grew up and the crazies are now driving the bus. I laugh, but there is more than a grain of truth in it.

61 **their epigenome is different**: An excellent and accessible book on epigenetic processes that reviews the Dutch winter cohort findings is *Evolution in Four Dimensions* by Eva Jablonka and Marian Lamb.(2nd ed, 2014, Cambridge, MA: Bradford)

61 **serotonin in the brain**: Caspi, A., et al. (2003). Influence of life stress on depression: Moderation by a polymorphism in the 5-HTT gene. *Science, 301*, 386–389.

61 **After the initial "Eureka!"**: Brown, G. W., & Harris, T. O. (2008). Depression and the serotonin transporter 5-HTTLPR polymorphism: a review and a hypothesis concerning gene-environment interaction. *Journal of Affective Disorders, 111*, 1–12.

61 **several other factors influenced**: This is now a fairly large literature, but examples include Barr, C. S., et al. (2004). Rearing condition and rh5-HTTLPR interact to influence limbic-hypothalamic-pituitary-adrenal axis response to stress in infant macaques. *Biological Psychiatry*, 55, 733–738. Other studies include Neumeister, A., et al. (2002). Association between serotonin transporter gene promoter polymorphism (5HTTLPR) and behavioral responses to tryptophan depletion in healthy women with and without family history of depression. *Archives of General Psychiatry*, 59, 613–620.

62 **changing methylation**: Dusek, J. A., Otu, H. H., Wohlhueter, A. L., Bhasin, M., Zerbini, L. F., Joseph, M. G., Benson, H., & Libermann, T. A. (2008). Genomic counter-stress changes induced by the relaxation response. *PLoS ONE*, 3, 1–8.

62 **hurt is just less central**: This has been shown in a couple studies. An example is Smallwood, R. F., Potter, J. S., & Robin, D. A. (2016). Neurophysiological mechanisms in acceptance and commitment therapy in opioid-addicted patients with chronic pain. *Psychiatry Research: Neuroimaging, 250*, 12–14.

Chapter Four: Why Our Thoughts Are So Automatic and Convincing

68 **my lab was among the first to show this**: Lipkens, G., Hayes, S. C., & Hayes, L. J. (1993). Longitudinal study of derived stimulus relations in an infant. *Journal of Experimental Child Psychology*, 56, 201–239. DOI: 10.1006/jecp.1993.1032.

68 **doing research with a senior colleague**: It was Aaron who first exposed me to the seed from which RFT sprang: a phenomenon known as stimulus equivalence, which was first identified by one of the giants in behavioral psychology and a personal hero, Murray Sidman. If young children learn to pick stimulus B when shown A, and C when shown A, they will pick all of the combinations (A given B, B given C, etc.). That outcome does not make behavioral sense—contingencies move in one direction, not two. The wonderful week that led to RFT was based on contemplating that finding and realizing that it was just an example of a much larger behavioral phenomenon of relational learning. The idea that relating was an operant was just a guess—but it had that "click" of everything fitting. Aaron's approval of the idea was key to me, and he would have been on all of the early RFT work except that he died before the first paper appeared. He was a lovely man and one of the best behavioral psychologists I ever met. Behavior analysts in general did not warm to RFT as quickly as Aaron—he took just a few minutes but the field of behavior analysis took four decades. Thankfully as this is being written in 2018, that tipping point has been reached. RFT is fast becoming the most studied behavioral theory of cognition in history.

73 **Children usually learn them in that order**: McHugh, L., Barnes-Holmes, Y., & Barnes-Holmes, D. (2004). Perspective-taking as relational responding: A developmental profile. *Psychological Record, 54*, 115–144.

74 **we lived in small groups, in which cooperation paid off**: Wilson, D. S., & Wilson, E. O. (2008). Evolution "for the good of the group." *American Scientist*, 96, 380–389.

75 **the baby will put the toy in the cleanup box**: Liebal, K., Behne, T., Carpenter, M., & Tomasello, M. (2009). Infants use shared experience to interpret a pointing gesture. *Developmental Science*, 12, 264–271.

76 **Most people are not prolific liars**: For examples of the literature that back up the claims made in this paragraph and the next, see Halevy, R., Shalvi, S., & Verschuere, B. (2014), Being honest about dishonesty: Correlating self-reports and actual lying. *Human Communication Research*, 40, 54–72. DOI: 10.1111/hcre.12019; and DePaulo, B., et al. (1996). Lying in everyday life. *Journal of Personality and Social Psychology*, 70, 984. See also Levine, T. R., Serota, K. B., Carey, F., & Messer, D. (2013). Teenagers lie a lot: A further investigation into the prevalence of lying. *Communication Research Reports*, 30, 211–220. DOI: 10.1080/08824096.2013.806254. And see Panasiti, M. S., et al. (2014). The motor cost of telling lies: Electrocortical signatures and personality foundations of spontaneous deception. *Social Neuroscience*, 9, 573–589. DOI: 10.1080/17470919.2014.934394.

77 **As an expert in this area points out**: Bouton, M. E. (2004). Context and behavioural processes in extinction. *Learning and Memory, 11*, 485–494. DOI: 10.1101/lm.78804. The quote can be found on page 485.

78 **A classic study done years ago**: Nisbett, R. E., & Wilson, T. D. (1977). Telling more than we can know: Verbal reports on mental processes. *Psychological Review*, 84(3), 231–259. DOI: 10.1037/0033-295X.84.3.231.

79 **Research using IRAP tests**: There are studies showing that the IRAP version of measuring experiential avoidance with statements like "anxiety is bad" predicts how arousal impacts behavior better

than overt measures. Levin, M. E., Haeger, J., & Smith, G. S. (2017). Examining the role of implicit emotional judgments in social anxiety and experiential avoidance. *Journal of Psychopathology and Behavioral Assessment*, 39, 264–278. DOI: 10.1007/s10862-016-9583-5. The best-known example of traditional implicit measures is Tony Greenwald's Implicit Association Test (IAT). In head-to-head competition, the data show that the IRAP is a far better test than the IAT, as it should be if RFT is correct. The IRAP does very well as an implicit measure; see Carpenter, K. M., et al. (2012). Measures of attentional bias and relational responding are associated with behavioral treatment outcome for cocaine dependence. *American Journal of Drug and Alcohol Abuse*, 38, 146–154.

79 **people struggling with drug problems**: It turns out, however, that people who are more defused and mindful show a psychological weaker impact of implicit cognition; see Ostafin, B. D., Kassman, K. T, & Wessel, I. (2013). Breaking the cycle of desire: Mindfulness and executive control weaken the relation between an implicit measure of alcohol valence and preoccupation with alcohol-related thoughts. *Psychology of Addictive Behaviors*, 27, 1153–1158. DOI: 10.1037/a0032621.

80 **introduced about a century ago by Edward Titchener**: Titchener, E. B. (1916). *A text-book of psychology*. New York: Macmillan. The word repetition exercise is on page 425.

81 **Say the word *fish* over and over again**: Tyndall, I., Papworth, R., Roche, B., & Bennett, M. (2017). Differential effects of word-repetition rate on cognitive defusion of believability and discomfort of negative self-referential thoughts postintervention and at one-month follow-up. *Psychological Record*, 67(10), 377–386. DOI: 10.1007/s40732-017-0227-2.

81 **shame at an in-patient unit for substance abusers**: Luoma, J. B., Kohlenberg, B. S., Hayes, S. C., & Fletcher, L. (2012). Slow and steady wins the race: A randomized clinical trial of Acceptance and Commitment Therapy targeting shame in substance use disorders. *Journal of Consulting and Clinical Psychology*, 80, 43–53. DOI: 10.1037/a0026070.

Chapter Five: The Problem with Problem Solving

86 **In these studies**: A book-length review of this entire line of research can be found in Hayes, S. C. (Ed.). (1989). *Rule-governed behavior: Cognition, contingencies, and instructional control*. New York: Plenum Press. I am deliberately changing some of the details of these experiments to make them easier to understand. For example, usually the "consequences" are points on a counter that are worth money or chances for money, not actual coins. The tasks are often more complicated than just pushing a button—for example, in our lab we usually had participants move a light through a maze by pushing buttons. The geek reader can learn all of this by reading the original studies—I am trying to get to the essence here.

87 **Behavioral researchers gradually narrowed down**: An early example of studies like that is Matthews, B. A., Shimoff, E., Catania, A. C., & Sagvolden, T. (1977). Uninstructed human responding: Sensitivity to ratio and interval contingencies. *Journal of the Experimental Analysis of Behavior*, 27, 453–467. DOI: 10.1901/jeab.1977.27-453.

87 **In my lab**: See the book in the preceding endnote labeled "In these studies."

87 **Most people still kept charging ahead**: Hayes, S. C., Brownstein, A. J., Zettle, R. D., Rosenfarb, I., & Korn, Z. (1986). Rule-governed behavior and sensitivity to changing consequences of responding. *Journal of the Experimental Analysis of Behavior*, 45, 237–256. DOI: 10.1901/jeab.1986.45-237.

89 **A wonderful study done over sixty years ago**: Hefferline, R., Keenan, B., & Harford, R. (1959). Escape and avoidance conditioning in human subjects without their observation of the response. *Science*, *130*(3385), 1338–1339. By the way, if you are interested in Gestalt therapy, you might recognize the name. You should since Ralph helped create it and was a co-author of the first major text in the area: Perls, F., Hefferline, R. F., & Goodman, P. (1951). *Gestalt therapy: Excitement and growth in the human personality*. New York: Delta. That is an irony: a behavior analyst actually helped create Gestalt therapy but 99 percent of the Gestalt folks think behaviorists are the enemy.

92 **as an adult, pliance is another issue**: It is not that people with clinical disorders follow rules and others do not. It is more subtle than that. The reason people follow rules is key . . . but the diagnostic label confuses the issue because it gathers different kinds of processes under a loose label. With that caution, here is an example of the kinds of studies that are out there: McAuliffe, D., Hughes, S., & Barnes-Holmes, D. (2014). The dark-side of rule governed behavior: An experimental analysis of problematic rule-following in an adolescent population with depressive symptomatology. *Behavior Modification*, 38, 587–613.

92 **they become so entrenched that we cannot see**: We found that rule-based insensitivity is associated with measures of psychological rigidity that are known to predict psychopathology. Wulfert, E., Greenway, D. E., Farkas, P., Hayes, S. C., & Dougher, M. J. (1994). Correlation between a personality test for rigidity and rule-governed

insensitivity to operant contingencies. *Journal of Applied Behavior Analysis, 27,* 659–671. DOI: 10.1901/jaba.1994.27-659.

94 **One was a brief exercise**: Hayes, S. C., Bissett, R., Korn, Z., Zettle, R. D., Rosenfarb, I., Cooper, L., & Grundt, A. (1999). The impact of acceptance versus control rationales on pain tolerance. *Psychological Record, 49,* 33–47.

95 **the more people believed in their own mental reasons**: Addis, M. E., & Carpenter, K. M. (1999). Why, why, why?: Reason-giving and rumination as predictors of response to activation- and insight-oriented treatment rationales. *Journal of Clinical Psychology, 55,* 881–894.

Chapter Six: Turning Toward the Dinosaur

97 **the brain activates the same areas**: For an example of a study of that kind, see Kim, H., Shimojo, S., & O'Doherty, J. P. (2006). Is avoiding an aversive outcome rewarding? Neural substrates of avoidance learning in the human brain. *PLoS Biology* 4(8): e233. DOI: 10.1371/journal.pbio.0040233.

106 **willing to go through the experience again**: Eifert, G. H., & Heffner, M. (2003). The effects of acceptance versus control contexts on avoidance of panic-related symptoms. *Journal of Behavior Therapy and Experimental Psychiatry, 34,* 293–312. DOI: 10.1016/j.jbtep.2003.11.001.

106 **David Barlow's student Jill Levitt**: Levitt, J. T., Brown, T. A., Orsillo, S. M., & Barlow, D. H. (2004). The effects of acceptance versus suppression of emotion on subjective and psychophysiological response to carbon dioxide challenge in patients with panic disorder. *Behavior Therapy, 35,* 747–766. DOI: 10.1016/S0005-7894(04)80018-2.

106 **The findings were confirmed**: For example, see Arch, J. J., Eifert, G. H., Davies, C., Vilardaga, J., Rose, R. D., & Craske, M. G. (2012). Randomized clinical trial of cognitive behavioral therapy (CBT) versus acceptance and commitment therapy (ACT) for mixed anxiety disorders. *Journal of Consulting and Clinical Psychology, 80,* 750–765. DOI: 10.1037/a0028310.

Chapter Seven: Committing to a New Course

112 **our thinking often wanders**: Research shows that our mind is wandering about a third of the time, but in these studies some participants are off somewhere else mentally over 95 percent of the time. See McVay, J. C., Kane, M. J., & Kwapil, T. R. (2009). Tracking the train of thought from the laboratory into everyday life: An experience-sampling study of mind wandering across controlled and ecological contexts. *Psychonomic Bulletin & Review, 16,* 857–863. Another similar study is Poerio, G. L., Totterdell, P., & Miles, R. (2013). Mind-wandering and negative mood: Does one thing really lead to another? *Consciousness and Cognition,* 22, 1412–1421. DOI: 10.1016/j.concog.2013.09.012.

113 **contemplative practice has good effects**: For a recent review, see Khoury, B., et al. (2013). Mindfulness-based therapy: A comprehensive meta-analysis. *Clinical Psychology Review, 33,* 763–771.

113 **Changes in brain structure and reactivity**: Fletcher, L. B., Schoendorff, B., & Hayes, S. C. (2010). Searching for mindfulness in the brain: A process-oriented approach to examining the neural correlates of mindfulness. *Mindfulness, 1,* 41–63. DOI: 10.1007/s12671-010-0006-5.

113 **epigenetic changes that up- and down-regulate**: Dusek, J. A., Otu, H. H., Wohlhueter, A. L., Bhasin M., Zerbini L. F., Joseph, M. G., Benson, H., & Libermann, T. A. (2008). Genomic counterstress changes induced by the relaxation response. *PLoS ONE,* 3, 1–8.

113 **I thought we could adapt some other classic mindfulness processes**: My students and I have written extensively about ways to approach mindfulness as a process instead of just mindfulness as a method of meditation and contemplation. We provided a working RFT-based definition of mindfulness in Fletcher, L., & Hayes, S. C. (2005). Relational Frame Theory, Acceptance and Commitment Therapy, and a functional analytic definition of mindfulness. *Journal of Rational Emotive and Cognitive Behavioral Therapy, 23,* 315–336; and Hayes, S. C., & Plumb, J. C. (2007). Mindfulness from the bottom up: Providing an inductive framework for understanding mindfulness processes and their application to human suffering. *Psychological Inquiry, 18,* 242–248. We worked out some of the details of our process-based approach in these articles: Hayes, S. C., & Shenk, C. (2004). Operationalizing mindfulness without unnecessary attachments. *Clinical Psychology: Science and Practice, 11,* 249–254; Hayes, S. C., & Wilson, K. G. (2003). Mindfulness: Method and process. *Clinical Psychology: Science and Practice, 10,* 161–165; Hayes, S. C. (2002). Acceptance, mindfulness, and science. *Clinical Psychology: Science and Practice,* 9, 101–106; and Hayes, S. C. (2002). Buddhism and Acceptance and Commitment Therapy. *Cognitive and Behavioral Practice,* 9, 58–66.

114 **This exercise and others like it have been studied**: Examples of some studies are Takahashi, M., Muto, T., Tada, M., & Sugiyama, M. (2002). Acceptance rationale and increasing pain

tolerance: Acceptance-based and FEAR-based practice. *Japanese Journal of Behavior Therapy, 28*, 35–46; Marcks, B. A., & Woods, D. W. (2005). A comparison of thought suppression to an acceptance-based technique in the management of personal intrusive thoughts: A controlled evaluation. *Behaviour Research and Therapy, 43*, 433–445; Marcks, B. A., & Woods, D. W. (2007). Role of thought-related beliefs and coping strategies in the escalation of intrusive thoughts: An analog to obsessive-compulsive disorder. *Behaviour Research and Therapy, 45*, 2640–2651; Forman, E. M., Hoffman, K. L., McGrath, K. B., Herbert, J. D., Brandsma, L. L., & Lowe, M. R. (2007). A comparison of acceptance- and control-based strategies for coping with food cravings: An analog study. *Behaviour Research and Therapy, 45*, 2372–2386. It is not enough to give a rationale for this kind of exercise—people have to practice using it to benefit. It appears to help manage intrusive thoughts, to increase pain tolerance, and to reduce the impact of urges, among other benefits.

115 **reconstructed—in the present:** Loftus, E. F. (2004). Memories of things unseen. *Current Directions in Psychological Science, 13*(4), 145–147. DOI: 10.1111/j.0963-7214.2004.00294.x.

122 **But the group with the short ACT-based values training**: Chase, J. A., Houmanfar, R., Hayes, S. C., Ward, T. A., Vilardaga, J. P., & Follette, V. M. (2013). Values are not just goals: Online ACT-based values training adds to goal-setting in improving undergraduate college student performance. *Journal of Contextual Behavioral Science, 2*, 79–84. DOI: 10.1016/j.jcbs. 2013.08.002.

124 **incomplete versions of ACT therapy**: Villatte, J. L., Vilardaga, R., Villatte, M., Vilardaga, J. C. P., Atkins, D. A., & Hayes, S. C. (2016). Acceptance and Commitment Therapy modules: Differential impact on treatment processes and outcomes. *Behaviour Research & Therapy, 77*, 52–61. DOI: 10.1016/j.brat.2015.12.001.

124 **We have done over seventy studies**: Levin, M. E., Hildebrandt, M. J., Lillis, J., & Hayes, S. C. (2012). The impact of treatment components suggested by the psychological flexibility model: A meta-analysis of laboratory-based component studies. *Behavior Therapy, 43*, 741–756. DOI: 10.1016/j.beth.2012.05.003.

Chapter Eight: We All Have the Ability to Pivot

129 **evolutionary scientist David Sloan Wilson agrees**: You can explore some of this in Wilson, D. S., & Hayes, S. C. (Eds.). (2018). *Evolution and contextual behavioral science: An integrated framework for understanding, predicting, and influencing human behavior.* Oakland, CA: Context Press.

131 **The process of evolution can be guided**: Hersh, M. N., Ponder, R. G., Hastings, P. J., & Rosenberg, S. M. (2004). Adaptive mutation and amplification in Escherichia coli: Two pathways of genome adaptation under stress. *Research in Microbiology, 155*, 353–359. DOI: 10.1016/j.resmic.2004.01.020.

132 **This is where flexibility skills come in**: If you put my name in quotes ("Steven C. Hayes") and the word evolution into Google Scholar you will find the kinds of things I'm talking about. The following endnotes also contain some references.

132 **The average public health worker**: Dahl, J., Wilson, K. G., & Nilsson, A. (2004). Acceptance and Commitment Therapy and the treatment of persons at risk for long-term disability resulting from stress and pain symptoms: A preliminary randomized trial. *Behavior Therapy, 35*, 785–802.

134 **copies of this figure to fill in**: This figure is a modified and expanded version.

135 **look more closely at the self-story they've been weaving**: Studies have been done on the values revealed in obituaries and on tombstones. See, for example, Alfano, M., Higgins, A., & Levernier, J. (2018). Identifying virtues and values through obituary data-mining. *Journal of Value Inquiry, 52*, 59–79. DOI: 10.1007/s10790-017-9602-0. Not surprisingly, issues such as family and character are very dominant.

136 **Three years later the figure was nearly identical**: Vowles, K. E., McCracken, L. M., & O'Brien, J. Z. (2011). Acceptance and values-based action in chronic pain: A three-year follow-up analysis of treatment effectiveness and process. *Behaviour Research and Therapy, 49*, 748–755. DOI: 10.1016/j.brat.2011.08.002. Some of the other measures showed some falloff at three years, but the gains were dominantly still significant and clinically meaningful. Across all measures, reliable change was seen in 46.2 percent of the patients (range: 45.0–46.9 percent) at the three-month follow-up and 35.8 percent (range: 29.1–38.0 percent) at the three-year follow-up.

136 **Another study followed fifty-seven people**: Kohtala, A., Muotka, J., & Lappalainen, R. (2017). What happens after five years? The long-term effects of a four-session Acceptance and Commitment Therapy delivered by student therapists for depressive symptoms. *Journal of Contextual Behavioral Science, 6*, 230–238. DOI: 10.1016/j.jcbs.2017.03.003.

136 **These results may seem startling**: There are ACT pain studies with similar outcomes to other treatments, but usually other features need to be looked at more carefully. For example, in this

study the outcomes were similar at follow up but ACT treatment stopped and medication treatment continued through follow-up: Wicksell, R. K., Melin, L., Lekander, M., & Olsson, G. L. (2009). Evaluating the effectiveness of exposure and acceptance strategies to improve functioning and quality of life in longstanding pediatric pain—A randomized controlled trial. *Pain, 141*, 248–257. Other studies have shown similar outcomes but at lower cost. It's not in chronic pain per se, but one recent study seemed to show that on a few measures ACT was not as good as a more elaborate model to help reduce absence from work due to mental health issues: Finnes, A., Ghaderi, A., Dahl, J., Nager, A., & Enebrink, P. (in press). Randomized controlled trial of Acceptance and Commitment Therapy and a workplace intervention for sickness absence due to mental disorders. *Journal of Occupational Health Psychology*. DOI: 10.1037/ocp0000097. However, when cost effectiveness was considered later, ACT was declared the clear winner: Finnes, A., Enebrink, P., Sampaio, F., Sorjonen, K., Dahl, J., Ghaderi, A., Nager, A., & Feldman, I. (2017). Cost-effectiveness of Acceptance and Commitment Therapy and a workplace intervention for employees on sickness absence due to mental disorders. *Journal of Occupational and Environmental Medicine*, 59, 1211–1220. DOI: 10.1097/JOM.0000000000001156. In the chronic pain area especially, the ACT model is emerging as a psychosocial model with vigorous overall support. I mention these cautions because while it is still early and we have a lot to learn, I do believe that the central theme of this book—that psychological flexibility is a key to healthy change—is well supported. That does not mean that study by study things won't vary a bit. Science is never that simple.

Chapter Nine: The First Pivot Defusion—Putting the Mind on a Leash

149 **The defusion methods the ACT community has developed**: The need to consider cognitive flexibility as involving defusion is supported by findings that traditional measures of more flexible thinking, such as Martin, M. M., & Rubin, R. B. (1995). A new measure of cognitive flexibility. *Psychological Reports, 76*, 623–626, is helpful primarily when that is in the service of psychological flexibility more generally. For example, see Palm, K. M., & Follette, V. M. (2011). The roles of cognitive flexibility and experiential avoidance in explaining psychological distress in survivors of interpersonal victimization. *Journal of Psychopathology and Behavioral Assessment*, 33, 79–86.

153 **The parts of the brain involved in mind wandering**: These findings can all be seen in Christoff, K., Gordon, A. M., Smallwood, J., Smith, R., & Schooler, J. W. (2009). Experience sampling during fMRI reveals default network and executive system contributions to mind wandering. *Proceedings of the National Academy of Sciences, 106*, 8719–8724. DOI: 10.1073/pnas.0900234106.

154 **defusion exercises weaken the link**: Those data are summarized in a review article: Levin, M. E., Luoma, J. B., & Haeger, J. A. (2015). Decoupling as a mechanism of change in mindfulness and acceptance: A literature review. *Behavior Modification*, 39, 870–911. DOI: 10.1177/0145445515603707.

155 **Sue and Liz target cognitive fusion with mindfulness**: An example of their research in the area is Roemer, L., Orsillo, S. M., & Salters-Pedneault, K. (2008). Efficacy of an acceptance-based behavior therapy for generalized anxiety disorder: Evaluation in a randomized controlled trial. *Journal of Consulting and Clinical Psychology, 76*, 1083–1089.

157 **She described how it helped this way**: This link should take you to her column: https://www.nbcnews.com/better/health/mental-trick-helped-me-claw-way-back-debilitating-anxiety-ncna834751.

157 **Cognitive Fusion Questionnaire**: Gillanders, D. T., et al. (2014). The development and initial validation of the Cognitive Fusion Questionnaire. *Behavior Therapy, 45*, 83–101. DOI: 10.1016/j.beth.2013.09.001.

160 **one of the most common measures of cognitive flexibility**: Guilford, J. P. (1967). Creativity: Yesterday, today and tomorrow. *Journal of Creative Behavior, 1*, 3–14. DOI: 10.1002/j.2162-6057.1967.tb00002.x.

163 **saying one thing while doing the opposite**: McMullen, J., Barnes-Holmes, D., Barnes-Holmes, Y., Stewart, I., Luciano, C., & Cochrane, A. (2008). Acceptance versus distraction: Brief instructions, metaphors, and exercises in increasing tolerance for self-delivered electric shocks. *Behaviour Research and Therapy*, 46, 122–129.

Chapter Ten: The Second Pivot Self—The Art of Perspective-Taking

172 **High self-esteem is a worthy goal**: Baumeister, R. F., Campbell, J. D., Krueger, J. I., & Vohs, K. D. (2003). Does high self-esteem cause better performance, interpersonal success, happiness, or healthier lifestyles? *Psychological Science in the Public Interest, 4*, 1–44. For more on this issue, see Leary, M. R., & Baumeister, R. F. (2000). The nature and function of self-esteem: Sociometer theory. In M. P. Zanna (Ed.), *Advances*

in experimental social psychology (Vol. 32, pp. 1–62). San Diego, CA: Academic Press.

172 **Research shows that when people focus**: A vast amount of research by researchers in self-determination theory shows this, including Deci, E. L., & Ryan, R. M. (1995). Human autonomy: The basis for true self-esteem. In M. H. Kernis (Ed.), *Efficacy, agency, and self-esteem* (pp. 31–49). New York: Plenum Press; and Deci, E. L., & Ryan, R. M. (2000). The "what" and "why" of goal pursuits: Human needs and the self-determination of behavior. *Psychological Inquiry, 11*, 227–268. For other matters in this section, see Crocker, J., Karpinski, A., Quinn, D. M., & Chase, S. K. (2003). When grades determine self-worth: Consequences of contingent self-worth for male and female engineering and psychology majors. *Journal of Personality and Social Psychology, 85*, 507–516; and Brown, J. D. (1986). Evaluations of self and others: Self-enhancement biases in social judgments. *Social Cognition, 4*, 353–376.

172 **Advertisers happily sell goods**: Escalas, J. E., & Bettman, J. R. (2005). Self-construal, reference groups, and brand meaning. *Journal of Consumer Research*, 32, 378–389. DOI: 10.1086/497549.

172 **We may also try to prove our worth**: Baumeister, R. F., Heatherton, T. F., & Tice, D. M. (1993). When ego threats lead to self-regulation failure—negative consequences of high self-esteem. *Journal of Personality and Social Psychology, 64*, 141–156. DOI: 10.1037/0022-3514.64.1.141. See also Crocker, J., & Park, L. E. (2004). The costly pursuit of self-esteem. *Psychological Bulletin, 130*, 392–414. DOI: 10.1037/0033-2909.130.3.392.

175 **Entire programs are now being established**: If you want to see an example of such programs, enter "PEAK autism" into Google to find Mark Dixon's version. He also has solid books on ACT and RFT with autistic children. See Belisle, J., Dixon, M. R., Stanley, C. R., Munoz, B., & Daar, J. H. (2016). Teaching foundational perspective-taking skills to children with autism using the PEAK-T curriculum: Single-reversal "I-you" deictic frames. *Journal of Applied Behavior Analysis, 49*, 965–969. DOI: 10.1002/jaba.324.

176 **You will notice an old woman**: I have written about a moment exactly like that in this short piece: Hayes, S. C. (2012). The women pushing the grocery cart. In R. Fields (Ed.), *Fifty-two quotes and weekly mindfulness practices: A year of living mindfully* (pp. 18–20). Tucson, AZ: FACES Conferences.

178 **Now read each sentence again, slowly**: Some of these ideas come from my work with Matthieu and Jennifer Villatte in Villatte, M. (2016). *Mastering the clinical conversation*. New York: Guilford Press.

185 **Then restate the experience in three forms**: This exercise used to include only the first two steps, but RFT research has clearly shown that it is important to include containment or hierarchical relations, not just distinction relations. For example, see Foody, M., Barnes-Holmes, Y., Barnes-Holmes, D., & Luciano, C. (2013). An empirical investigation of hierarchical versus distinction relations in a self-based ACT exercise. *International Journal of Psychology and Psychological Therapy, 13*(3), 373–388. I like the fact that basic research keeps modifying ACT methods. It is how it should be.

Chapter Eleven: The Third Pivot Acceptance—Learning from Pain

193 **Genetics research has revealed that**: This literature is growing rapidly. The study showed that the epigenetic impact of abuse was even involved in who would later commit suicide: McGowan, P. O. et al. (2009). Epigenetic regulation of the glucocorticoid receptor in human brain associates with childhood abuse. *Nature Neuroscience, 12*, 342–348. This study shows how it was related to physical disease: Yanh, B.-Z., et al. (2013). Child abuse and epigenetic mechanisms of disease risk. *American Journal of Preventive Medicine, 44*, 101–107. DOI: 10.1016/j.amepre.2012.10.012.

193 **We can also experience emotional instability**: Biglan, A. (2015). *The nurture effect*. Oakland, CA: New Harbinger.

195 **One of the horrible outcomes for sexually abused children**: Messman-Moore, T. L., Walsh, K. L., & DiLillo, D. (2010). Emotion dysregulation and risky sexual behavior in revictimization. *Child Abuse & Neglect, 34*, 967–976. DOI: 10.1016/j.chiabu.2010.06.004.

196 **What is especially sad**: Fiorillo, D., Papa, A., & Follette, V. M. (2013). The relationship between child physical abuse and victimization in dating relationships: The role of experiential avoidance. *Psychological Trauma: Theory, Research, Practice, and Policy*, 5(6), 562–569. DOI: 10.1037/a0030968.

196 **When good things happened**: Todd and his team have done a whole series of studies like this. This one is a good example: Machell, K. A., Goodman, F. R., & Kashdan, T. B. (2015). Experiential avoidance and well-being: A daily diary analysis. *Cognition and Emotion, 29*, 351–359. DOI: 10.1080/02699931.2014.911143.

199 **The mainstream CBT community has now come around**: You can find my claim in my first major write-up about ACT: Hayes, S. C. (1987). A contextual approach to therapeutic change. In Jacobson, N. (Ed.), *Psychotherapists in clinical practice: Cognitive and behavioral perspectives* (pp. 327–387). New York: Guilford Press. Mainstream

CBT arrived at a similar view around 2008. See, for example, the dialogue with Michelle Craske on this point in Hayes, S. C. (2008). Climbing our hills: A beginning conversation on the comparison of ACT and traditional CBT. *Clinical Psychology: Science and Practice, 15,* 286–295.

Chapter Twelve: The Fourth Pivot Presence—Living in the Now

213 **higher levels of emotional acceptance**: Teper, R., & Inzlicht, M. (2013). Meditation, mindfulness and executive control: The importance of emotional acceptance and brain-based performance monitoring. *Social Cognitive and Affective Neuroscience, 8,* 85–92. DOI: 10.1093/scan/nss045. There are other examples of studies of this kind, such as Riley, B. (2014). Experiential avoidance mediates the association between thought suppression and mindfulness with problem gambling. *Journal of Gambling Studies, 30,* 163–171. DOI: 10.1007/s10899-012-9342-9.

214 **observing what is present can lead to *more* rumination**: Royuela-Colomer, E., & Calvete, E. (2016). Mindfulness facets and depression in adolescents: Rumination as a mediator. *Mindfulness, 7,* 1092–1102. DOI: 10.1007/s12671-016-0547-3.

216 **The research on meditation**: Parsons, C. E., Crane, C., Parsons, L. J., Fjorback, L. O., & Kuyken, W. (2017). Home practice in Mindfulness-Based Cognitive Therapy and Mindfulness-Based Stress Reduction: A systematic review and meta-analysis of participants' mindfulness practice and its association with outcomes. *Behaviour Research and Therapy, 95,* 29–41. DOI: 10.1016/j.brat.2017.05.004.

216 **The *quality* of the practice is more important**: Hafenbrack, A. C., Kinias, Z., & Barsade, S. G. (2013). Debiasing the mind through meditation. *Psychological Science, 25,* 369–376. DOI: 10.1177/0956797613503853. The researcher being quoted in this paragraph is Zoe Kinias, an assistant professor of organizational behavior at INSEAD. The quote can be found here: https://www.sciencedaily.com/releases/2014/02/140212112745.htm.

217 **A wonderfully simple method of meditating**: Hardy, R. R. (2001). *Zen master: Practical Zen by an American for Americans.* Tucson, AZ: Hats Off Books.

219 **This is a version of one of the most effective and yet simplest mindfulness exercises**: A good description can be found in Singh, N. N., Lancioni, G. E., Manikam, R., Winton, A. W., Singh, A. A., Singh, J., & Singh, A. A. (2011). A mindfulness-based strategy for self-management of aggressive behavior in adolescents with autism. *Research in Autism Spectrum Disorders, 5,* 1153–1158. DOI: 10.1016/j.rasd.2010.12.012. Examples of studies showing the effects I mention here include Singh, N. N., Lancioni, G. E., Winton, A. W., Adkins, A. D., Wahler, R. G., Sabaawi, M., & Singh, J. (2007). Individuals with mental illness can control their aggressive behavior through mindfulness training. *Behavior Modification, 31,* 313–328. DOI: 10.1177/0145445506293585; Singh, N. N., Lancioni, G. E., Myers, R. E., Karazsia, B. T., Winton, A. W., & Singh, J. (2014). A randomized controlled trial of a mindfulness-based smoking cessation program for individuals with mild intellectual disability. *International Journal of Mental Health and Addiction, 12,* 153–168. DOI: 10.1007/s11469-013-9471-0; and Singh, N. N., Lancioni, G. E., Singh, A. N., Winton, A. W., Singh, J., McAleavey, K. M., & Adkins, A. D. (2008). A mindfulness-based health wellness program for an adolescent with Prader-Willi syndrome. *Behavior Modification, 32,* 167–181. DOI: 10.1177/0145445507308582. As I mention in the next paragraph, attentional training like this is a core of Adrian Wells's Meta-Cognitive Therapy (MCT). I love his work and suggest MCT as a worthwhile set of methods to explore. There is a growing base of support for MCT. See Wells, A. (2011). *Metacognitive therapy for anxiety and depression.* New York: Guilford Press.

220 **it's just as important to broaden your attention**: This approach was developed by Les Fehmi. I have never met Les, but he is why I am a psychologist. I had a bad letter from the chair of my department at Loyola-Marymount—the late Father Ciklic. I was one of the first hippies on campus and the good Father Ciklic was not pleased. Unknown to me, he put in his letter of recommendation for entry to graduate school that I was a drug addict (I wasn't by the way . . . just a normal hippie). Needless to say, I did not get in anywhere. After two years of this, I decided to try one last time. A friend of my brother asked a new faculty member at the State University of New York at Stony Brook (where I had applied for graduate training), to look in my file. He kindly did and passed along the information about the bad letter. I did not ask Father Ciklic for a letter that third time out, and I got into several doctoral programs. Finally, my education could start. The name of the psychologist at Stony Brook who did that favor? You can guess it by now: Les Fehmi. I wrote him a thank-you letter a few years ago. He did not remember the incident, but it changed my life. Think of it: tiny kindnesses you do today can profoundly alter people's lives, but you may never know it, or remember it if you eventually do! That's cool, no?

221 **my boss told me I would never amount to anything**: In fact, that did happen—to me! In the

mid-1980s the late Gilbert Gottlieb (a brilliant man who did foundational work on evolution and early experience) told me that. He looked at the breadth of my interests and said point-blank that I was a dilettante. It hurt—a lot—but I did not change course. To be honest in hindsight I was a handful . . . and I *was* all over the place with my interests. Ironically, were that not the case I never would have amounted to much because that breadth eventually all interlinked, helping to create contextual behavioral science. I did not stay at the University of North Carolina at Greensboro much longer after that conversation. Aaron Brownstein died and I secretly (and somewhat unfairly) blamed Gottlieb because he did something similar to Aaron, which put him under tremendous stress. I left a year later for the University of Nevada, Reno, where I have been ever since. It is ironic because Gottlieb's work is now an important part of my thinking. I have a book of his in my briefcase as I write this endnote! I wish I could have another conversation with him just to explore interests. At the time, however, all he could see in me was a crazy young man who he thought would never make a difference.

Chapter Thirteen: The Fifth Pivot Values—Caring by Choice

225 **we escape from the freedom life gives us**: It may seem strange for a behaviorist to be speaking of "escape from freedom," but we can use such words without turning them into things that exist as objects—that is, into ontology. Even words like *spirit* have behaviorally sensible meanings; see Hayes, S. C. (1984). Making sense of spirituality. *Behaviorism, 12*, 99–110. Realizing that is part of how ACT research started (I tell the story of this paper later in the book in the chapter on spirituality). But coming back to freedom, I did research long ago that showed that even nonhuman animals will escape from freedom (normally they greatly prefer choice) if you provide them with experiences that lead them to fear their own choices, *even if they did not make the wrong choice*: Hayes, S. C., Kapust, J., Leonard, S. R., & Rosenfarb, I. (1981). Escape from freedom: Choosing not to choose in pigeons. *Journal of the Experimental Analysis of Behavior, 36*, 1–7. DOI: 10.1901/jeab.1981.36-1. Human beings have enormously amplified reasons to fear choices that reside in symbolic language and the cognitive networks it produces.

225 **Consider the effects of materialism**: Richins, M. L. (2004). The Material Values Scale: Measurement properties and development of a short form. *Journal of Consumer Research, 31*, 209–219. DOI: 10.1086/383436.

226 **Fame, power, sensory gratification**: A good summary of that work is in Ryan, R. M., Huta, V., & Deci, E. L. (2008). Living well: A self-determination theory perspective on eudaimonia. *Journal of Happiness Studies, 9*, 139–170. DOI: 10.1007/s10902-006-9023-4.

226 **what it will take to have enough money**: John Paul Getty is said to have answered a similar question in exactly that way, despite having more wealth than almost anyone alive.

230 **because I *choose* to**: I'm not arguing for or against "free will" in a literal sense. I'm a behaviorist, and sitting atop Mt. Olympus I presume there are "reasons" we do everything. But we don't live there and the language of freedom puts the ability to respond (in other words, responsibility) back where it belongs. We do what we do, and based on that we get what we get. That's the knowledge we really need and it is here, inside our experience. If the language of freedom helps us see that, I'm all for it.

231 **Our thirst for chosen meaning and purpose will be unquenched**: One study that shows that clearly is Kashdan, T. B., & Breen, W. E. (2007). Materialism and diminished well-being: Experiential avoidance as a mediating mechanism. *Journal of Social and Clinical Psychology, 26*, 521–539. DOI: 10.1521/jscp.2007.26.5.521.

234 **Valued Living Questionnaire**: Wilson, K. G., Sandoz, E. K., Kitchens, J., & Roberts, M. (2010). The Valued Living Questionnaire: Defining and measuring valued action within a behavioral framework. *Psychological Record, 60*, 249–272. The version I'm using includes aesthetics and the environment, which were added later.

239 **values writing has more impact**: Sandoz, E., & Hebert, E. R. (2016). Meaningful, reminiscent, and evocative: An initial examination of four methods of selecting idiographic values-relevant stimuli. *Journal of Contextual Behavioral Science, 4*, 277–280. DOI: 10.1016/j.jcbs.2015.09.001.

239 **making us more receptive to information**: Crocker, J., Niiya, Y., & Mischkowski, D. (2008). Why does writing about important values reduce defensiveness? Self-affirmation and the role of positive other-directed feelings. *Psychological Science, 19*, 740–747. DOI: 10.1111/j.1467-9280.2008.02150.x.

Chapter Fourteen: The Sixth Pivot Action—Committing to Change

246 **they combine into the one skill**: One reason I say that is that it is very hard to break them apart in assessment. If you force them apart, statistically there is what is called a *latent variable* (a deep underlying structure) that goes across all of them. I have used the metaphor of six sides of a box to explain it. The sides of a box are aspects of a whole. You would not look at a square piece of

wood and say, "That is a side of a box," but once you saw it assembled and then disassembled, that is exactly what you would say, and rightly so. The six pivots are like that.

246 **all of that work begins to come to fruition**: There are data in support of that idea. For example, a recent study showed that acceptance of pain predicted positive outcomes for chronic pain patients, but primarily if it was linked to actual behavior change: Jeong, S., & Cho, S. (2017). Acceptance and patient functioning in chronic pain: The mediating role of physical activity. *Quality of Life Research, 26*, 903–911. DOI: 10.1007/s11136-016-1404-5. See also Villatte, J. L., Vilardaga, R., Villatte, M., Vilardaga, J. C. P., Atkins, D. A., & Hayes, S. C. (2016). Acceptance and Commitment Therapy modules: Differential impact on treatment processes and outcomes. *Behaviour Research and Therapy, 77*, 52–61. DOI: 10.1016/j.brat.2015.12.001, which found that with flexibility skills left out, behavior change methods alone sometimes took people into distressing areas without needed tools.

249 **sit with a marshmallow in close reach**: The original study was done in the mid-1970s. It and a long string of subsequent studies that confirmed the effect are summarized in the late Walter Mischel's book: Mischel, M. (2015). *The marshmallow test: Why self-control is the engine of success.* New York: Back Bay Books. I knew Mischel but not well—he was a giant in the field.

250 **some forms of persistence are actually forms of avoidance**: Many studies show this. For example, see Shimazu, A., Schaufeli, W. B., & Taris, T. W. (2010). How does workaholism affect worker health and performance? The mediating role of coping. *International Journal of Behavioral Medicine, 17*, 154. DOI: 10.1007/s12529-010-9077-x.

259 **habit reversal is even more powerful**: My former student Mike Twohig and Douglas Woods have done a lot of the research work on habit reversal and how to combine it and related behavioral methods with ACT. They have written a book for the public on these methods as applied to hair pulling, for example: Woods, D., & Twohig, M. P. (2008). *Trichotillomania: An ACT-enhanced behavior therapy approach workbook.* New York: Oxford University Press. An example of their research in this area is Twohig, M. P., Woods, D. W., Marcks, B. A., & Teng, E. J. (2003). Evaluating the efficacy of habit reversal: Comparison with a placebo control. *Journal of Clinical Psychiatry, 64*, 40–48.

260 **public commitments are more likely to be maintained**: For example, see Lyman, R. D. (1984). The effect of private and public goal setting on classroom on-task behavior of emotionally-disturbed children. *Behavior Therapy, 15*, 395–402.

260 **a similar behavior change is now more likely in your friends**: Christakis, N., & Fowler, J. H. (2009). *Connected: The surprising power of our social networks and how they shape our lives.* New York: Little, Brown.

Part Three: Introduction

265 **Give Difficult Feelings a Color, Weight, Speed, Shape**: That one is in a book I co-wrote with Spencer Smith: Hayes, S. C., with Smith, S. (2005). *Get out of your mind and into your life: The new acceptance and commitment therapy.* Oakland, CA: New Harbinger.

265 **Do a Values Card Sort**: There are commercially available ACT values card decks and websites to sort your values. You can easily Google them, but I have a list of resources for them at http://www.stevenchayes.com.

266 **There is no need for you ever to get bored**: I borrowed the toolkit idea from Kirk Strosahl (an ACT for the Public list serve member named Bill helped me see how useful it was: thanks Bill). For more help, go to http://www.stevenchayes.com or to other ACT books I've cited, or just follow the resource guidance I gave right before Chapter One.

273 **We're *Homo prosocialis***: I think this is why Elinor Ostrom won the Nobel Prize in 2009. She showed that there was a "middle path" between command economies and the "invisible hand" of *Homo economicus*—namely the evolution of prosocial groups that protected their common pool resources by cooperation. It takes specific principles to do this. If you want to see how we are combining Ostrom's design principles and ACT, see http://www.prosocial.world. I will cover some of this work in the last chapter, but I also have a book that explains it: Atkins, P., Wilson, D. S., & Hayes, S. C. (2019). *Prosocial: Using evolutionary science to build productive, equitable, and collaborative groups.* Oakland, CA: Context Press.

274 **WHO has created an ACT self-help program**: The name of the program is "self-help plus." It is described here in an open access format you can download: Epping-Jordan, J. E., Harris, R., Brown, F. L., Carswell, K., Foley, C., García-Moreno, C. , Kogan, C., & van Ommeren, M. (2016). Self-Help Plus (SH+): A new WHO stress management package. *World Psychiatry, 15*, 295–296. DOI: 10.1002/wps.20355. It is now being tested around the world, especially with refugees. The European Union has a large grant to do so called RE-DEFINE (http://re-defineproject.eu) and WHO is testing it with South Sudanese refugees in Uganda: Brown, F., Carswell, K., Augustinavicius, J., Adaku, A., Leku, M., White, R., . . . Tol, W. (2018). Self Help Plus: Study protocol for a cluster-randomised controlled trial

of guided self-help with South Sudanese refugee women in Uganda. *Global Mental Health*, 5, E27. DOI: 10.1017/gmh.2018.17.

Chapter Fifteen: Adopting Healthy Behaviors

275 **Nearly two-thirds of all poor health is due to behavior**: You can find those data in Forouzanfar, M. H., et al. (2013). Global, regional, and national comparative risk assessment of 79 behavioural, environmental and occupational, and metabolic risks or clusters of risks in 188 countries, 1990–2013: A systematic analysis for the Global Burden of Disease Study. *Lancet*, 386, 2287–2323. In some ways, this analysis—impressive as it is—actually underestimates how important behavior is to health because such things as exposure to environmental toxins is often due to our behavior as well. For example, air pollution comes from our excessive energy use and policies that encourage it. I started my career as an environmental activist, showing how to change environmentally relevant behavior: Cone, J. D., & Hayes, S. C. (1980). *Environmental problems/ behavioral solutions*. Monterey, CA: Brooks/Cole. (Republished in 1986 by Cambridge University Press; Reprinted in 2011.) I moved out of that area when I realized the data I produced would be ignored unless I became a member of large industrial organizations and worked from the inside. My goals were too broad for that to make sense for me.

275 **just to name a few**: There are ACT trials in all of these areas. Yes, even teeth cleaning (in fact there are two!). One I like was done with young adults: Wide, U., Hagman, J., Werner, H., & Hakeberg, M. (2018). Can a brief psychological intervention improve oral health behavior? A randomized controlled trial. *BCM Oral Health, 18(163)*, 1-8. DOI: 10.1186/s12903-018-0627-y and the ACT group took far better care of their teeth. I think values work is especially important in areas like this, although perspective taking and emotional openness helps too. I have a very progressive dentist, Todd Sala, who tries to help careless adolescent and young adults by asking them ("usually young males need this more" he says) to imagine what it is like to be interested in a person who has body odor or teeth that are not being cleaned. Yipes. A bit of health perspective-taking, that.

276 **this is almost cruel**: Of course, the researchers also secretly marked the chocolates to make sure no one cheated, ate one, and then replaced it. The study can be found in Moffitt, R., Brinkworth, G., Noakes, M., & Mohr, P. (2012). A comparison of cognitive restructuring and cognitive defusion as strategies for resisting a craved food. *Psychology & Health*, 27, 77–94. DOI: 10.1080/08870446.2012.694436.

277 **Even the best and most extensive science-based programs**: MacLean, P. S., Wing, R. R., Davidson, T., et al. (2015). NIH working group report: Innovative research to improve maintenance of weight loss. *Obesity*, 23, 7–15.

277 **Consider one of the most effective programs**: Brownell, K. D. (2000). *The LEARN program for weight management*. Dallas, TX: American Health.

277 **Shame is also a common problem**: Our measure of inflexibility in this area is discussed in Lillis, J., & Hayes, S. C. (2008). Measuring avoidance and inflexibility in weight related problems. *International Journal of Behavioral Consultation and Therapy*, 4, 348–354; our measure of weight-related shame and self-stigma is discussed in Lillis, J., Luoma, J. B., Levin, M. E., & Hayes, S. C. (2010). Measuring weight self-stigma: The weight self-stigma questionnaire. *Obesity*, 18, 971–976. DOI: 10.1038/oby.2009.353. Data on body dissatisfaction can be found in Fallon, E. A., Harris, B. S., & Johnson, P. (2014). Prevalence of body dissatisfaction among a United States adult sample. *Eating Behaviors*, 15, 151–158. DOI: 10.1016/j.eatbeh.2013.11.007. Data on physicians shaming overweight clients is in Harris, C. R., & Darby, R. S. (2009). Shame in physician-patient interactions: Patient perspectives. *Basic and Applied Social Psychology*, 31, 325–334. DOI: 10.1080/01973530903316922.

278 **To precisely measure the role of shame**: see the immediately preceding endnote for the reference.

278 **Our research team conducted a study**: Decreasing distress and shame itself is a physical benefit, since they tend to lead to physical distress and health problems: Mereish, E. H., & Poteat, V. P. (2015). A relational model of sexual minority mental and physical health: The negative effects of shame on relationships, loneliness, and health. *Journal of Counseling Psychology*, 62, 425–437.

279 **athletes can do better work by focusing on their willingness**: Emily Leeming found this in her 2016 dissertation on mental toughness, which I describe in Chapter Eighteen: Leeming, E. (2016). *Mental toughness: An investigation of verbal processes on athletic performance*. Unpublished doctoral dissertation. University of Nevada, Reno. I hope it is out in publication form soon. The data on exercise addiction are presented in Alcaraz-Ibanez, M., Aguilar-Parra, J., & Alvarez-Hernandez, J. F. (2018). Exercise addiction: Preliminary evidence on the role of psychological inflexibility. *International Journal of Mental Health and Addiction*, 16, 199–206. DOI: 10.1007/s11469-018-9875-y.

279 **Values work also helps with shame**: Vartanian, L. R., & Shaprow, J. G. (2008). Effects of weight stigma on exercise motivation and behavior: A preliminary investigation among college-aged females. *Journal of Health Psychology, 13*, 131–138. DOI: 10.1177/1359105307084318.

281 **books devoted to applying ACT to eating and exercise**: Some of those books are cited in the following endnote labeled "You can do all of this without acting on the craving."

282 ***what I've seen with my own body***: Both of these things I mention are now reasonably well supported empirically, but I did them initially more out of trial and error. To find those specific data, search online for studies on "time-restricted eating" as well as "avoiding flour." I never do risky things by trial and error, however. You need a smart research-oriented physician who is willing to talk to you, or an ability to research the medical literature before venturing out into trial and error. My internist, Dr. Shaheen Ali, is awesome and I can indeed read much of the medical literature—but if you do not have that kind of support, be cautious and do trial-and-error learning within more normal ranges. This is not the place for dumb moves (long, unsupervised fasts; eating nothing but carrots; you name it).

282 **ACT plus (wait for it) walnuts**: Tapsell, L. C., Lonergan, M., Batterham, M. J., Neale, E. P., Martin, A., Thorne, R., Deane, F., & Peoples, G. (2017). Effect of interdisciplinary care on weight loss: a randomised controlled trial. *BMJ Open*, 7:e014533.. DOI: 10.1136/bmjopen-2016-014533.

283 **You can do all of this without acting on the craving**: There are solid ACT books for help with diet, although I know of none that have been evaluated in book form, so while the theory is known to be helpful you do need to keep your eye on how it plays out more specifically (this book is like that too, as I said earlier). Two good ones are Lillis, J., Dahl, J., & Weineland, S. M. (2014). *The diet trap: Feed your psychological needs and end the weight loss struggle using Acceptance and Commitment Therapy*. Oakland, CA: New Harbinger; and Bailey, A., Ciarrochi, J., & Harris, R. (2014). *The weight escape: How to stop dieting and start living*. Boulder, CO: Shambala.

283 ***slowly* do curls or triceps presses**: I love the work of Rick Winett, who is a psychologist of my era (and still going strong) who does work on exercise sort of on the side. A reference that explains why a couple of short, properly done sessions of resistance training has great health benefits is Winett, R. A., & Carpinelli, R. N. (2001). Potential health-related benefits of resistance training. *Preventive Medicine*, 33, 503–513. DOI: 10.1006/pmed.2001.0909.

285 **pioneering research on applying ACT to work**: A book of his that I like in this area is Flaxman, P. E., Bond, F. W., & Livheim, F. (2013). *The mindful and effective employee: An acceptance and commitment therapy training manual for improving well-being and performance*. Oakland, CA: New Harbinger.

285 **the first ACT study done on worksite stress**: Bond, F. W., & Bunce, D. (2000). Mediators of change in emotion-focused and problem-focused worksite stress management interventions. *Journal of Occupational Health Psychology, 5*, 156–163.

289 **worry about getting to sleep**: Nota, J. A., & Coles, M. E. (2015). Duration and timing of sleep are associated with repetitive negative thinking. *Cognitive Therapy and Research*, 39, 253–261. DOI: 10.1007/s10608-014-9651-7.

289 **People with poor sleep patterns**: Kapur, V. K., Redline, S., Nieto, F., Young, T. B., Newman, A. B., & Henderson, J. A. (2002). The relationship between chronically disrupted sleep and healthcare use. *Sleep, 25*, 289–296.

289 **ACT studies in chronic pain and depression**: There are several examples of ACT studies with side benefits in sleep, including McCracken, L. M., Williams, J. L., & Tang, N. K. Y. (2011). Psychological flexibility may reduce insomnia in persons with chronic pain: A preliminary retrospective study. *Pain Medicine, 12*, 904–912. DOI: 10.1111/j.1526-4637.2011.01115.x; Westin, V. Z., et al. (2011). Acceptance and Commitment Therapy versus Tinnitus Retraining Therapy in the treatment of tinnitus: A randomised controlled trial. *Behaviour Research and Therapy*, 49, 737–747. DOI: 10.1016/j.brat.2011.08.001; and Kato, T. (2016). Impact of psychological inflexibility on depressive symptoms and sleep difficulty in a Japanese sample. *Springerplus, 5*, 712. DOI: 10.1186/s40064-016-2393-0. An ACT study in this area that directly targeted insomnia (successfully) is Zetterqvist, V., Grudina, R., Rickardsson, J., Wicksell, R. K., & Holmström, L. (in press). Acceptance-based behavioural treatment for insomnia in chronic pain: A clinical pilot study. *Journal of Contextual Behavioral Science*. DOI: 10.1016/j.jcbs.2018.07.003.

290 **a combination of ACT training and a modified form of CBTi**: Dalrymple, K. L., Fiorentino, L., Politi, M. C., & Posner, D. (2010). Incorporating principles from Acceptance and Commitment Therapy into Cognitive-Behavioral Therapy for insomnia: A case example. *Journal of Contemporary Psychotherapy, 40*, 209–217. DOI: 10.1007/s10879-010-9145-1.

Chapter Sixteen: Mental Health

292 **The group of psychiatrists and psychologists tasked**: These quotes come from the work group

that developed the strategy for the new *Diagnostic and Statistical Manual of the American Psychiatric Association*: Kupfer, D. J., et al. (2002). *A research agenda for DSM-V.* Washington, DC: American Psychiatric Association.

292 a **shift to a more process-oriented approach**: See my text on process-based CBT with my colleague Stefan Hofmann: Hayes, S. C., & Hofmann, S. (2018). *Process-based CBT: The science and core clinical competencies of cognitive behavioral therapy.* Oakland, CA: Context Press / New Harbinger..

293 **genetically primed to react to negative events**: Many studies show that genetics interact with environment in ways that can take the same genetic factor in a positive or negative direction. I like this study as a good example: Gloster, A. T., Gerlach, A. L., Hamm, A., Höfler, M., Alpers, G. W., Kircher, T., et al. (2015). 5HTT is associated with the phenotype psychological flexibility: Results from a randomized clinical trial. *European Archives of Psychiatry and Clinical Neuroscience, 265*(5), 399–406.

293 **behavior that may be adaptive in some contexts**: The DSM-V workgroup (see Kupfer et al. 2002, cited in the preceding endnote labeled "The group of psychiatrists and psychologists tasked") said that clearly as well: "many, if not most, conditions and symptoms represent a somewhat arbitrarily defined pathological excess of normal behaviors and cognitive processes." I agree.

294 **one in five people will experience a common mental health condition**: One reason I have some patience with researchers who call these conditions "brain diseases" is that although they may know they are fibbing, they hope that doing do will reduce stigma. Sadly, over the long haul it appears as though it actually *increases* some aspects of stigma. That research has taken a while to get out, but now that it is, I hope this begins to change. Corrigan, P. W. & Watson, A. C. (2004). At issue: Stop the stigma: Call mental illness a brain disease. *Schizophrenia Bulletin, 30*, 477–479.

294 **People with mental illness are tagged**: See Corrigan, P. W., & Watson, A. C. (2002). Understanding the impact of stigma on people with mental illness. *World Psychiatry 1*(1), 16–20. https://www.ncbi.nlm.nih.gov/pmc/articles/PMC1489832/; and Corrigan, P. W., Larson, J. E., & Rusch, N. (2009). Self-stigma and the "why try" effect: impact on life goals and evidence-based practices. *World Psychiatry* 8(2), 75–81. https://www.ncbi.nlm.nih.gov/pmc/articles/PMC2694098/.

294 **about one in five will seek assistance**: Centers for Disease Control and Prevention et al. (2012). *Attitudes toward mental illness: results from the Behavioral Risk Factor Surveillance System.* Atlanta: Centers for Disease Control and Prevention. https://www.cdc.gov/hrqol/Mental_Health_Reports/pdf/BRFSS_Full%20Report.pdf.

295 **350 million people around the globe**: MacGill, M. (2017). What is depression and what can I do about it?? *Medical News Today* (last updated November 30). https://www.medicalnewstoday.com/kc/depression-causes-symptoms-treatments-8933; see also https://www.cdc.gov/nchs/fastats/depression.htm.

296 **long-term or high-dose use carries the risk**: A meta-analysis of sexual side effects can be found here: Serretti, A., & Chiesa, A. (2009). Treatment-emergent sexual dysfunction related to antidepressants: A meta-analysis. *Journal of Clinical Psychopharmacology, 29*, 259–266. DOI: 10.1097/JCP.0b013e3181a5233f. Long-term relapse data are shown in many studies and are significantly higher for medications than for psychotherapy. See, for example, Hollon, S. D., et al. (2005). Prevention of relapse following cognitive therapy vs medications in moderate to severe depression. *Archives of General Psychiatry, 62*, 417–422. DOI: 10.1001/archpsyc.62.4.417. Both of these are serious problems that the pharmaceutical industry has failed to acknowledge adequately.

296 **the combination for lesser depression is not significantly more effective**: Khan, A., Faucett, J., Lichtenberg, P., Kirsch, I., & Brown, W. A. (2012) A systematic review of comparative efficacy of treatments and controls for depression. *PLoS ONE, 7*(7): e41778. DOI: 10.1371/journal.pone.0041778. See also the previous endnote for this broader body of work.

296 **the benefits of CBT are largely due to the behavioral elements**: I cited these studies in earlier footnotes. For example, see Chawla, N., & Ostafin, B. D. (2007). Experiential avoidance as a functional dimensional approach to psychopathology: An empirical review. *Journal of Clinical Psychology, 63*, 871–890.

296 **we know more about why it works**: There are many successful mediational studies on ACT. A list is available at https://contextualscience.org/act_studies_with_mediational_data. See also the summary article at http://bit.ly/ACTmediation2018.

296 **ruminating to avoid difficult emotions**: Eisma, M. C., et al. (2013). Avoidance processes mediate the relationship between rumination and symptoms of complicated grief and depression following loss. *Journal of Abnormal Psychology, 122*, 961–970. DOI: 10.1037/a0034051.

297 **one of the best types of therapy for depression, Behavioral Activation**: Carlbring, P., et al. (2013). Internet-based behavioral activation and acceptance-based treatment for depression: A randomized controlled trial. *Journal of Affective*

Disorders, 148, 331–337. DOI: 10.1016/j.jad.2012.12.020.

298 **an anxiety condition during the course of our lives**: Craske, M. G., & Stein, M. B. (2016). Anxiety. *Lancet, 388* (10063), 3048–3059. DOI: 10.1016/S0140-6736(16)30381-6.

298 **the ACT group showed much greater improvement**: Arch, J. J., Eifert, G. H., Davies, C., Vilardaga, J., Rose, R. D., & Craske, M. G. (2012). Randomized clinical trial of cognitive behavioral therapy (CBT) versus acceptance and commitment therapy (ACT) for mixed anxiety disorders. *Journal of Consulting and Clinical Psychology, 80,* 750–765. DOI: 10.1037/a0028310.

300 **over a dozen decent quality studies**: Lee, E. B., An, W., Levin, M. E., & Twohig, M. P. (2015). An initial meta-analysis of Acceptance and Commitment Therapy for treating substance use disorders. *Drug and Alcohol Dependence, 155,* 1–7. DOI: 10.1016/j.drugalcdep.2015.08.004.

301 **That internalization is pushed deeper by psychological inflexibility**: My colleagues and I have explored this in several studies. See, for example, Luoma, J. B., Rye, A., Kohlenberg, B. S., & Hayes, S. C. (2013). Self-stigma in substance abuse: Development of a new measure. *Journal of Psychopathology and Behavioral Assessment, 35,* 223–234. DOI: 10.1007/s10862-012-9323-4; and Luoma, J. B., Kohlenberg, B. S., Hayes, S. C., Bunting, K., & Rye, A. K. (2008). Reducing the self stigma of substance abuse through acceptance and commitment therapy: Model, manual development, and pilot outcomes. *Addiction Research & Therapy, 16,* 149–165. DOI: 10.1080/16066350701850295.

301 **Acceptance can help stay the course**: Hayes, S. C., Wilson, K. G., Gifford, E. V., Bissett, R., Piasecki, M., Batten, S. V., Byrd, M., & Gregg, J. (2004). A randomized controlled trial of twelve-step facilitation and acceptance and commitment therapy with polysubstance abusing methadone maintained opiate addicts. *Behavior Therapy, 35,* 667–688. DOI: 10.1016/S0005-7894(04)80014-5.

302 **a release of dopamine into their brains**: Volkow, N. D., Fowler, J. S., Wang, G. J., Baler, R., & Telang, F. (2009). Imaging dopamine's role in drug abuse and addiction. *Neuropharmacology, 56* (Suppl. 1), 3–8. DOI: 10.1016/j.neuropharm.2008.05.022.

303 **twice as likely to be substance abusers**: Recovery First. "The Connection between Depression and Substance Abuse." https://www.recoveryfirst.org/co-occuring-disorders/depression-and-substance-abuse/.

303 **applying ACT training specifically to shame**: Luoma, J. B., Kohlenberg, B. S., Hayes, S. C., & Fletcher, L. (2012). Slow and steady wins the race: A randomized clinical trial of Acceptance and Commitment Therapy targeting shame in substance use disorders. *Journal of Consulting and Clinical Psychology, 80,* 43–53. DOI: 10.1037/a0026070.

304 **the ACT message for addiction**: That quote is on page 13 of Kelly Wilson and Troy Dufrene's ACT book on addiction: Wilson, K., & Dufrene, T. (2012). *The wisdom to know the difference.* Oakland, CA: New Harbinger.

304 **About twenty million women**: Wade, T. D., Keski-Rahkonen, A., & Hudson J. (2011). Epidemiology of eating disorders. In M. Tsuang and M. Tohen (Eds.), *Textbook in psychiatric epidemiology* (3rd ed., pp. 343–360). New York: Wiley. For data on the increase in ED, see Sweeting, H., Walker, L., MacLean, A., Patterson, C., Räisänen, U., & Hunt, K. (2015). Prevalence of eating disorders in males: A review of rates reported in academic research and UK mass media. *International Journal of Men's Health 14*(2). https://www.ncbi.nlm.nih.gov/pmc/articles/PMC4538851/. For data on etiology, see National Eating Disorders Association. "What Are Eating Disorders? Risk Factors." https://www.nationaleatingdisorders.org/factors-may-contribute-eating-disorders.

305 **the desire to avoid difficult thoughts and feelings**: A large number of studies support that point and the other points made in this paragraph. As a beginning, you can consult Juarascio, A., Shaw, J., Forman, E., Timko, C. A., Herbert, J., Butryn, M., . . . Lowe, M. (2013). Acceptance and commitment therapy as a novel treatment for eating disorders: An initial test of efficacy and mediation. *Behavior Modification, 37,* 459–489. DOI: 10.1177/0145445513478633; and Bluett, E. J., et al. (2016). The role of body image psychological flexibility on the treatment of eating disorders in a residential facility. *Eating Behaviors, 23,* 150–155. DOI: 10.1016/j.eatbeh.2016.10.002. See also Ferreira, C., Palmeira, L., Trindade, I. A., & Catarino, F. (2015). When thought suppression backfires: Its moderator effect on eating psychopathology. *Eating and Weight Disorders—Studies on Anorexia Bulimia and Obesity, 20,* 355–362. DOI: 10.1007/s40519-015-0180-5; and Cowdrey, F. A., & Park, R. J. (2012). The role of experiential avoidance, rumination and mindfulness in eating disorders. *Eating Behavior, 13,* 100–105. DOI: 10.1016/j.eatbeh.2012.01.001. Finally, look at Pearson, A. N., Follette, V. M., & Hayes, S. C. (2012). A pilot study of Acceptance and Commitment Therapy (ACT) as a workshop intervention for body dissatisfaction and disordered eating attitudes. *Cognitive and Behavioral Practice, 19,* 181–197. DOI: 0.1016/j.cbpra.2011.03.001.

305 **two-thirds of people with EDs also have an anxiety disorder**: Kaye, W. H., Bulik, C. M.,

Thornton, L., Barbarich, N., & Masters, K. (204). Comorbidity of anxiety disorders with anorexia and bulimia nervosa. *American Journal of Psychiatry, 161*, 2215–2221.

306 **ACT values work was added**: Strandskov, S. W., Ghaderi, A., Andersson, H., Parmskog, N., Hjort, E., Warn, A. S., Jannert, M., & Andersson, G. (2017). Effects of tailored and ACT-influenced Internet-based CBT for eating disorders and the relation between knowledge acquisition and outcome: A randomized controlled trial. *Behavior Therapy, 48*, 624–637.

306 **results from six hundred of his patients**: Walden, K., Manwaring, J., Blalock, D. V., Bishop, E., Duffy, A., & Johnson, C. (2018). Acceptance and psychological change at the higher levels of care: A naturalistic outcome study. *Eating Disorders, 26*, 311–325. DOI: 10.1080/10640266.2017.1400862.

307 **determine your own degree of flexibility**: Manwaring, J., Hilbert, A., Walden, K., Bishop, E. R. & Johnson, C. (2018). Validation of the acceptance and action questionnaire for weight-related difficulties in an eating disorder population. *Journal of Contextual Behavioral Science, 7*, 1–7. The original scale we developed was Lillis, J., & Hayes, S. C. (2008). Measuring avoidance and inflexibility in weight related problems. *International Journal of Behavioral Consultation and Therapy, 4*, 348–354.

308 **a significant reduction in rehospitalization**: Bach, P., Gaudiano, B. A., Hayes, S. C., & Herbert, J. D. (2013). Acceptance and Commitment Therapy for psychosis: Intent to treat hospitalization outcome and mediation by believability. *Psychosis, 5*, 166–174. You can predict who is likely to struggle by how they deal with their hallucinations. We created a measure to do this and it works reasonably well: Shawyer, F., Ratcliff, K., Mackinnon, A., Farhall, J., Hayes, S. C., & Copolov, D. (2007). The Voices Acceptance and Action Scale: Pilot data. *Journal of Clinical Psychology, 63*, 593–606. DOI: 10.1002/jclp.20366. ACT interventions can also deflect the depression that often follows psychotic breaks, especially the first one: Gumley, A., White, R., Briggs, A., Ford, I., Barry, S., Stewart, C., Beedie, S., McTaggart, J., Clarke, C., MacLeod, R., Lidstone, E., Salgado Riveros, B., Young, R., & McLeod, H. (2017). A parallel group randomised open blinded evaluation of acceptance and commitment therapy for depression after psychosis: Pilot trial outcomes (ADAPT). *Schizophrenia Research, 183*, 143–150.

Chapter Seventeen: Nurturing Relationships

311 **thoughtful, caring communication**: Sprecher, S., & Regan, P. C. (2002). Liking some things (in some people) more than others: Partner preferences in romantic relationships and friendships. *Journal of Social and Personal Relationships, 19*, 463–481. DOI: 10.1177/0265407502019004048.

311 **articulate those feelings to others**: Uysal, A., Lin, H. L., Knee, C. R., & Bush, A. L. (2012). The association between self-concealment from one's partner and relationship well-being. *Personality and Social Psychology Bulletin, 38*, 39–51. DOI: 10.1177/0146167211429331.

312 **the capacity for healthy attachment**: La Guardia, J. G., Ryan, R. M., Couchman, C. E., Deci, E. L. (2000). Within-person variation in security of attachment: A self-determination theory perspective on attachment, need fulfillment, and well-being. *Journal of Personality and Social Psychology, 79*, 367–384. DOI: 10.1037//0022-3514.79.3.367.

312 **actions that nurture relationships**: The bottom line for all of this literature on ACT for couples is small but growing. ACT also has many similarities to integrative behavioral couple therapy and emotional-focused therapy, which are both evidence-based intervention methods. A recent review of IBCT is Christensen, A., & Doss, B. D. (2017). Integrative behavioral couple therapy. *Current Opinion in Psychology, 13*, 111–114. DOI: 10.1016/j.copsyc.2016.04.022. The EFT literature is reviewed in Johnson, S. (2019). *Attachment theory in practice*. New York: Guilford Press. There are several randomized trials of ACT for marital difficulties, but most are small and most have been done in Iran (oddly enough).

312 **Commitment practice helps with these actions**: Vohs, K. D., Finkenauer, C., & Baumeister, R. F. (2011). The sum of friends' and lovers' self-control scores predicts relationship quality. *Social Psychological and Personality Science, 2*, 138–145. DOI: 10.1177/1948550610385710.

317 **By the time little Stevie goes off to college**: Not that I didn't have massive help raising these rascals from my three wives, Angle, Linda, and Jacque; Stevie's loving nanny and honorary grandmother, Inge Skeans; and others who have loved and cared for them.

317 **psychological inflexibility makes it hard to interact with our children**: There are quite a number of studies of this kind. See Brockman, C., et al. (2016). Relationship of service members' deployment trauma, PTSD symptoms, and experiential avoidance to post-deployment family reengagement. *Journal of Family Psychology, 30*, 52–62. DOI: 10.1037/fam0000152; and Shea, S. E., & Coyne, L. W. (2011). Maternal dysphoric mood, stress, and parenting practices in mothers of head start preschoolers: The role of experiential

avoidance. *Child and Family Behavior Therapy, 33,* 231–247. DOI: 10.1080/07317107.2011.596004. Also see these three studies: Brassell, A. A., Rosenberg, E., Parent, J., Rough, J. N., Fondacaro, K., & Seehuus, M. (2016). Parent's psychological flexibility: Associations with parenting and child psychosocial well-being. *Journal of Contextual Behavioral Science, 5,* 111–120. DOI: 10.1016/j.jcbs.2016.03.001; Whittingham, K., Sanders, M., McKinlay, L., & Boyd, R. N. (2014). Interventions to reduce behavioral problems in children with cerebral palsy: An RCT. *Pediatrics, 133,* E1249–E1257. DOI: 10.1542/peds.2013-3620; and Brown, F. L., Whittingham, K., Boyd, R. N., McKinlay, L., & Sofronoff, K. (2014). Improving child and parenting outcomes following paediatric acquired brain injury: A randomised controlled trial of Stepping Stones Triple P plus Acceptance and Commitment Therapy. *Journal of Child Psychology and Psychiatry, 55,* 1172–1183. DOI: 10.1111/jcpp.12227.

318 **those with especially inflexible parents**: Polusny, M. A., et al. (2011). Effects of parents' experiential avoidance and PTSD on adolescent disaster-related posttraumatic stress symptomatology. *Journal of Family Psychology, 25,* 220–229; Cheron, D. M., Ehrenreich, J. T., & Pincus, D. B. (2009). Assessment of parental experiential avoidance in a clinical sample of children with anxiety disorders. *Child Psychiatry and Human Development, 40,* 383–403. DOI: 10.1007/s10578-009-0135-z.

318 **ACT researchers in Australia followed 750 children**: Williams, K. E., Ciarrochi, J., & Heaven, P. C. L. (2012). Inflexible parents, inflexible kids: A 6-year longitudinal study of parenting style and the development of psychological flexibility in adolescents. *Journal of Youth and Adolescence, 41,* 1053–1066. DOI: 10.1007/s10964-012-9744-0.

319 **most high school students**: The data are a bit old now, but a well-known study is Friedman, J. M. H., Asnis, G. M., Boeck, M., & DiFiore, J. (1987). Prevalence of specific suicidal behaviors in a high school sample. *American Journal of Psychiatry, 144,* 1203–1206. You have to ask the question in a pretty open way to get rates this high, but still it shows that our kids are thinking about it to a degree. Why not? Have you ever had such a thought?

320 **how best to address suicidality**: A good summary of those data and guidance about how best to address suicidality based on the evidence is in a book by psychiatrist John Chiles and ACT co-developer Kirk Strosahl: Chiles, J. A., & Strosahl, K. (2005). *Clinical manual for assessment and treatment of suicidal patients.* Washington, DC: American Psychiatric Association. The second edition is now out and has well-known Stanford professor Laura Weiss Roberts as the third author. I consider it the most authoritative book currently available on suicidality, and it is completely compatible with an ACT model. Multiple studies show that ACT helps with suicidality—a good example is Ducasse, D., et al. (2018). Acceptance and Commitment Therapy for the management of suicidal patients: A randomized controlled trial. *Psychotherapy and Psychosomatics, 87,* 211–222. DOI: 10.1159/000488715.

322 **our partners are more satisfied when we are more accepting**: Lenger, K. A., Gordon, C. L., & Nguyen, S. P. (2017). Intra-individual and cross-partner associations between the five facets of mindfulness and relationship satisfaction. *Mindfulness, 8,* 171–180. DOI: 10.1007/s12671-016-0590-0.

322 **communicating their own emotions and values**: Wachs, K., & Cordova, J. V. (2007). Mindful relating: Exploring mindfulness and emotion repertoires in intimate relationships. *Journal of Marital and Family Therapy, 33,* 464–481. DOI: 10.1111/j.1752-0606.2007.00032.x.

324 **Across the planet, 30 percent of women**: Devries, K. M., et al. (2013). The global prevalence of intimate partner violence against women. *Science, 340,* 1527–1528. DOI: 10.1126/science.1240937. See also Ellsberg, M., et al. (2008). Intimate partner violence and women's physical and mental health in the WHO multi-country study on women's health and domestic violence: An observational study. *Lancet, 371,* 1165–1172. DOI: 10.1016/S0140-6736(08)60522-X.

324 **using an online program based on a book**: The study that evaluated the book was Fiorillo, D., McLean, C., Pistorello, J., Hayes, S. C., & Follette, V. M. (2017). Evaluation of a web-based Acceptance and Commitment Therapy program for women with trauma related problems: A pilot study. *Journal of Contextual Behavioral Science, 6,* 104–113. DOI: 10.1016/j.jcbs.2016.11.003. The book itself is Follette, V. M., & Pistorello, J. (2007). *Finding life after trauma.* Oakland, CA: New Harbinger. The website for the online version of the book is at https://elearning.newharbinger.com.

325 **WHO concluded**: Harvey, A., Garcia-Moreno, C., & Butchart, A. (2007). *Primary prevention of intimate-partner violence and sexual violence.* Geneva: World Health Organization.

325 **both have shown only a minor reduction**: Babcock, J. C., Green, C. E., & Robie, C. (2004). Does batterers' treatment work? A meta-analytic review of domestic violence treatment. *Clinical Psychology Review, 23,* 1023–1053. DOI: 10.1016/j.cpr.2002.07.001.

326 **The first study testing this approach**: Zarling, A., Lawrence, E., & Marchman, J. (2015). A randomized controlled trial of acceptance and

commitment therapy for aggressive behavior. *Journal of Consulting and Clinical Psychology*, 83, 199–212. DOI: 10.1037/a0037946.

326 **In the next study Zarling conducted**: Zarling, A., Bannon, S., & Berta, M. (2017). Evaluation of Acceptance and Commitment Therapy for domestic violence offenders. *Psychology of Violence*. DOI: 10.1037/vio0000097. The study was not fully randomized because the men picked their groups based on schedule, not knowing the kind of group they would get. Future research will need to test this finding in a bit more tightly controlled study.

327 **how deeply and completely the same**: Posth, C., et al. (2016). Pleistocene mitochondrial genomes suggest a single major dispersal of non-Africans and a late glacial population turnover in Europe. *Current Biology*, *26*, 827–833. DOI: 10.1016/j.cub.2016.01.037.

328 **a major study of the impact of diversity**: Putnam, R. (2007). E pluribus unum: Diversity and community in the twenty-first century—the 2006 Johan Skytte Prize Lecture. *Scandinavian Political Studies*, *30*, 137–174. DOI: 10.1111/j.1467-9477.2007.00176.x.

328 **the world's best tests of people's implicit biases**: There are other and more popular measures of implicit cognition but the RFT-based measure, the Implicit Relational Assessment Procedure (IRAP), has been shown empirically to be the best available measure. See, for example, Barnes-Holmes, D., Waldron, D., Barnes-Holmes, Y., & Stewart, I. (2009). Testing the validity of the Implicit Relational Assessment Procedure and the Implicit Association Test: Measuring attitudes toward Dublin and country life in Ireland. *Psychological Record*, *59*, 389–406. DOI: 10.1007/BF03395671. That superiority is why I'm referring to RFT almost as if it's the only measure of implicit bias. It's not, and other methods are more popular, but empirically speaking it is the best. An example of how the IRAP is used is Power, P. M., Harte, C., Barnes-Holmes, D., & Barnes-Holmes, Y. (2017). Exploring racial bias in a European country with a recent history of immigration of black Africans. *Psychological Record*, *67*, 365–375. DOI: 10.1007/s40732-017-0223-6.

329 **it was the telltale Ruth Esther:** My middle daughter's name is Esther Marlena. She is an artist like her grandmother; her names are the middle names of my mother and my maternal grandmother. My mother, Ruth, said a tear came to her eye when she first heard the baby's name—it was a kind of closing of a painful circle that spanned generations.

331 **if you try to suppress prejudiced thoughts**: Hooper, N., Villatte, M., Neofotistou, E., & McHugh, L. (2010). The effects of mindfulness versus thought suppression on implicit and explicit measures of experiential avoidance. *International Journal of Behavioral Consultation and Therapy*, 6(3), 233–244. DOI: 10.1037/h0100910.

331 **what psychological factors lead some people to settle into authoritarian distancing**: Levin, M. E., Luoma, J. B., Vilardaga, R., Lillis, J., Nobles, R., & Hayes, S. C. (2016). Examining the role of psychological inflexibility, perspective taking and empathic concern in generalized prejudice. *Journal of Applied Social Psychology*, *46*, 180–191. DOI: 10.1111/jasp.12355.

Chapter Eighteen: Bringing Flexibility to Performance

338 **procrastination is predicted by psychological inflexibility**: Gagnon, J., Dionne, F., & Pychyl, T. A. (2016). Committed action: An initial study on its association to procrastination in academic settings. *Journal of Contextual Behavioral Science*, *5*, 97–102. DOI: 10.1016/j.jcbs.2016.04.002. See also Glick, D. M., Millstein, D. J., & Orsillo, S. M. (2014). A preliminary investigation of the role of psychological inflexibility in academic procrastination. *Journal of Contextual Behavioral Science*, *3*, 81–88. DOI: 10.1016/j.jcbs.2014.04.002.

338 **ACT programs for procrastination**: Scent, C. L., & Boes, S. R. (2014). Acceptance and Commitment Training: A brief intervention to reduce procrastination among college students. *Journal of College Student Psychotherapy*, *28*, 144–156. DOI: 10.1080/87568225.2014.883887.

340 **this cognitive skill correlates greatly with traditional IQ scores**: An example, one of several, is O'Hora, D., et al. (2008). Temporal relations and intelligence: Correlating relational performance with performance on the WAIS-III. *Psychological Record*, *58*, 569–583. DOI: 10.1007/BF03395638 . A more recent and elaborate study is Colbert, D., Dobutowitsch, M., Roche, B., & Brophy, C. (2017). The proxy-measurement of intelligence quotients using a relational skills abilities index. *Learning and Individual Differences*, *57*, 114–122. DOI: 10.1016/j.lindif.2017.03.010. Still another is O'Toole, C., & Barnes-Holmes, D. (2009). Three chronometric indices of relational responding as predictors of performance on a brief intelligence test: The importance of relational flexibility. *Psychological Record*, *59*, 119–132.

340 **a rise over several months**: This work began with a humble pilot study: Cassidy, S., Roche, B., & Hayes, S. C. (2011). A relational frame training intervention to raise intelligence quotients: A pilot study. *Psychological Record*, *61*, 173–198. More elaborate and controlled studies have since

appeared, including Hayes, J., & Stewart, I. (2016). Comparing the effects of derived relational training and computer coding on intellectual potential in school-age children. *British Journal of Educational Psychology, 86*, 397–411. DOI: 10.1111/bjep.12114.

340 **cognitive functioning improved moderately**: Presti, G., Torregrosssa, S., Migliore, D., Roche, B., & Cumbo, E. (2017). Relational Training Intervention as add-on therapy to current specific treatments in patients with mild-to-moderate Alzheimer's disease. *International Journal of Psychology and Neuroscience*, 3(2), 89–97.

343 **Gallup polls show**: Examples include Mann, A., & Harter, J. (2016). The worldwide employee engagement crisis. Gallup. http://news.gallup.com/businessjournal/188033/worldwide-employee-engagement-crisis.aspx; Zenger, J., & Folkman, J. (2012). How damaging is a bad boss, exactly? *Harvard Business Review.* https://hbr.org/2012/07/how-damaging-is-a-bad-boss-exa.

343 **the term job sculpting**: A recent online discussion of their work is here: Butler, T., & Waldroop, J. "Job Sculpting: The Art of Retaining Your Best People." Harvard Business School. https://hbswk.hbs.edu/archive/job-sculpting-the-art-of-retaining-your-best-people.

345 **leaders who manage with psychological flexibility**: Peng, J., Chen, Y. S., Xia, Y., & Ran, Y. X. (2017). Workplace loneliness, leader-member exchange and creativity: The cross-level moderating role of leader compassion. *Personality and Individual Differences, 104*, 510–515. DOI: 10.1016/j.paid.2016.09.020. Many studies show these kinds of results. See Reb, J., Narayanan, J., & Chaturvedi, S. (2014). Leading mindfully: Two studies on the influence of supervisor trait mindfulness on employee well-being and performance. *Mindfulness*, 5, 36–45. DOI: 10.1007/s12671-012-0144-z. Also see Leroy, H., Anseel, F., Dimitrova, N. G., & Sels, L. (2013). Mindfulness, authentic functioning, and work engagement: A growth modeling approach. *Journal of Vocational Behavior*, 82, 238–247. DOI: 10.1016/j.jvb.2013.01.012; Park, R., & Jang, S. J. (2017). Mediating role of perceived supervisor support in the relationship between job autonomy and mental health: moderating role of value-means fit. *International Journal of Human Resource Management*, 28, 703–723. DOI: 10.1080/09585192.2015.1109536.

345 **When leaders use individual rewards as incentives**: A meta-analysis of that kind is provided by Judge, T. A., & Piccolo, R. F. (2004). Transformational and transactional leadership: A meta-analytic test of their relative validity. *Journal of Applied Psychology*, 89, 755–768. A later and larger meta-analysis found the same thing but added that contingent reward especially helped at the level or the person and transformational leadership at the level of the team: Wang, G., Oh, I. S., Courtright, S. H., & Colbert, A. E. (2011). Transformational leadership and performance across criteria and levels: A meta-analytic review of 25 years of research. *Group and Organization Management*, 36, 223–270. DOI: 10.1177/1059601111401017. See also King, E., and Haar, J. M. (2017). Mindfulness and job performance: A study of Australian leaders. *Asia Pacific Journal of Human Resources*, 55, 298–319. DOI: 10.1111/1744-7941.12143.

346 **the Matrix**: This is a well-known ACT tool. My version is upside down but Kevin approved it—doing so allows me to use the easy to understand metaphor of head and heart versus hands and feet. I would like to thank Crissa Levin, Mike Levin, and Jacque Pistorello for the thinking behind this change.

348 **being in the flow of the game**: Zhang, C. Q., et al. (2016). The effects of mindfulness training on beginners' skill acquisition in dart throwing: A randomized controlled trial. *Psychology of Sport and Exercise*, 22, 279–285. DOI: 10.1016/j.psychsport.2015.09.005. See also Gross, M., et al. (2016) An empirical examination comparing the Mindfulness-Acceptance-Commitment approach and Psychological Skills Training for the mental health and sport performance of female student athletes. *International Journal of Sport and Exercise Psychology, 16*, 431-451. DOI: 10.1080/1612197X.2016.1250802.

348 **not only for physical sports, but other types of sporting competition or performance situations**: Some examples are Salazar, M. C. R., & Ballesteros, A. P. V. (2015). Effect of an ACT intervention on aerobic endurance and experiential avoidance in walkers. *Revista Costarricense de Psicologia*, 34, 97–111. Also look at Ruiz, F. J., & Luciano, C. (2012). Improving international-level chess players' performance with an acceptance-based protocol: Preliminary findings. *Psychological Record*, 62, 447–461. DOI: 10.1007/BF03395813; and Ruiz, F. J., & Luciano, C. (2009). Acceptance and commitment therapy (ACT) and improving chess performance in promising young chess-players. *Psicothema*, 21, 347–352. There are also now beginning studies on ACT for musical performances: Juncos, D. G., & Markman, E. J. (2017). Acceptance and Commitment Therapy for the treatment of music performance anxiety: A single subject design with a university student. *Psychology of Music*, 44, 935–952.

349 **competitive CrossFit athletes**: Leeming, E. (2016). *Mental toughness: An investigation of verbal processes on athletic performance.* Unpublished doctoral dissertation. University of Nevada, Reno.

349 **Otherwise they are at risk of injury**: Timpka, T., Jacobsson, J., Dahlström, Ö., et al. (2015). The psychological factor "self-blame" predicts overuse injury among top-level Swedish track and field athletes: A 12-month cohort study. *British Journal of Sports Medicine, 49,* 1472–1477. DOI: 10.1136/bjsports-2015-094622. See also Nicholls, A. R., Polman, R. C. J., Levy, A. R., & Backhouse, S. H. (2008). Mental toughness, optimism, pessimism, and coping among athletes. *Personality and Individual Differences, 44,* 1182–1192. DOI: 10.1016/j.paid.2007.11.011.

349 **go through rehabilitation successfully**: DeGaetano, J. J., Wolanin, A. T., Marks, D. R., & Eastin, S. M. (2016). The role of psychological flexibility in injury rehabilitation. *Journal of Clinical Sport Psychology, 10,* 192–205. DOI: 10.1123/jcsp.2014-0023.

Chapter Nineteen: Cultivating Spiritual Well-Being

351 **Spiritual well-being is an important contributor**: This highly cited study is one of many such examples: McClain, C. S., Rosenfeld, B., & Breitbart, W. (2003). Effect of spiritual well-being on end-of-life despair in terminally-ill cancer patients. *Lancet, 361,* 1603–1607. DOI: 10.1016/S0140-6736(03)13310-7. An example in actual physical health is Carmody, J., Reed, G., Kristeller, J., & Merriam, P. (2008). Mindfulness, spirituality, and health-related symptoms. *Journal of Psychosomatic Research, 64,* 393–403. DOI: 10.1016/j.jpsychores.2007.06.015.

351 **no one universally agreed upon definition of spiritual wellness**: An example of a measure in this area that fits with this broad definition is the Spiritual Well-Being Scale: Ellison, C. W. (1983). Spiritual well-being: Conceptualization and measurement. *Journal of Psychology and Theology, 11,* 330–340).; Another example is the Functional Assessment of Chronic Illness Therapy-Spiritual Well-Being (FACIT-Sp): Peterman, A. H., Fitchett, G., Brady, M. J., Hernandez, L., & Cella, D. (2002). *Annals of Behavioral Medicine, 24,* 49–58. DOI: 10.1207/S15324796ABM2401_06.

353 **between a third and four-fifths of all adults**: An example of a whole series of studies like that is Thomas, L. E., Cooper, P. E., & Suscovich, D. J. (1983). Incidence of near-death and intense spiritual experiences in an intergenerational sample: An interpretation. *OMEGA—Journal of Death and Dying, 13,* 35–41. DOI: 10.2190/G260-EWY3-6V4H-EJU3.

353 **it almost seems wrong**: Davis, J., Lockwood, L., & Wright, C. (1991). Reasons for not reporting peak experiences. *Journal of Humanistic Psychology, 31,* 86–94. DOI: 10.1177/0022167891311008.

353 **the first article I wrote**: Hayes, S. C. (1984). Making sense of spirituality. *Behaviorism, 12,* 99–110.

353 **a more enduring sense of connection to this place of transcendence**: There is today an active exploration of psychedelics as a way of achieving such experiences, not in the chaotic way in which that form of self-exploration spread across the world in the 1960s and 1970s, but in a way that fits more with their use as part of a spiritual journey. Michael Poolan's book summarizes this new area of study: Poolan, M. (2018). *How to change your mind: What the new science of psychedelics teaches us about consciousness, dying, addiction, depression, and transcendence.* New York: Penguin. Properly used, psychedelics may indeed open the "doors of perception" (as Aldous Huxley famously titled his book on the topic), but even here repeated use does not mean repeated transformational experiences. The ACT community has established a special interest group to examine the use of ACT and psychedelics, and a special issue on the topic in the *Journal of Contextual Behavioral Science* is being planned for 2019 under the guidance of Jason Luoma.

354 **divergent *both/and* thinking is central to these experiences**: The interest in psychedelics is making empirical study of profound spiritual experiences more possible, so that we can see if the relationship of thinking style to spiritual experience is more than a mere correlation. An example that supports the claim I am making here is Kuypers, K., Riba, J., de la Fuente Revenga, M., Barker, S., Theunissen, E., and Ramaekers, J. (2016). Ayahuasca enhances creative divergent thinking while decreasing conventional convergent thinking. *Psychopharmacology* 233, 3395–3403. DOI: 10.1007/s00213-016-4377-8.

361 **ACT has been embraced by many religious leaders**: The program referred to in the paragraph began in 2013 and has spread across the world. The other specific interventions chaplains are trained in are motivational interviewing, and problem-solving therapy: "Mental Health Integration for Chaplain Services (MHICS)." https://www.mirecc.va.gov/mentalhealthandchaplaincy/docs/MHICS%20Brochure%20(2017-18).pdf. You can find a description of the training in the website for the U.S. Department of Veterans Affairs program in Mental Health Integration for Chaplain Services: https://www.mirecc.va.gov/mentalhealthandchaplaincy/MHICS.asp.

361 **a book on ACT for use by clergy and pastoral counselors**: For a review of this whole area of ACT work, see Nieuwsma, J. A., Walser, R. D., & Hayes, S. C. (Eds.). (2016). *ACT for clergy and pastoral counselors: Using Acceptance and Commitment Therapy to bridge psychological and spiritual care.* Oakland, CA: Context Press.

361 **combine your ACT learning with your religious practice**: I have edited a book for clergy and pastoral counselors. It is cited in the preceding endnote. Books on ACT for Christians have appeared, such as Knabb, J. (2016). *Faith-based ACT for Christian clients: An integrative treatment approach.* New York: Routledge; the workbook that goes with it is *Acceptance and commitment therapy for Christian clients: A faith-based workbook*. Another book of that kind is Ord, I. (2014). *ACT with faith. D.F. Mexico: Compass Publishing.* Several others are coming—searching online will find them.

361 **A devotedly Christian Greek-Cypriot woman**: Karekla, M., & Constantinou, M. (2010). Religious coping and cancer: Proposing an Acceptance and Commitment Therapy approach. *Cognitive and Behavioral Practice, 17,* 371–381. DOI: 10.1016/j.cbpra.2009.08.003.

Chapter Twenty: Coping with Illness and Disability

363 **Even in expert hands**: I'm part of the CBT community, broadly speaking, but ACT comes out of concern for challenging thoughts. Meta-analyses (summaries of entire sets of studies) conclude that it is not very helpful; see Longmore, R. J., & Worrell, M. (2007). Do we need to challenge thoughts in cognitive behavior therapy? *Clinical Psychology Review, 27,* 173–187. Also, when you take out these elements of CBT and leave in only the behavioral elements, outcomes are the same or better. The classic study of that kind was Dimidjian, S., et al. (2006). Randomized trial of behavioral activation, cognitive therapy, and antidepressant medication in the acute treatment of adults with major depression. *Journal of Consulting and Clinical Psychology, 74*(4), 658–670. DOI: 10.1037/0022-006X.74.4.658.

364 **But that is not *nearly* enough**: The literature varies, but a meta-analysis of the impact of education on glycated hemoglobin has called the improvement "modest"; see Ellis, S. E., Speroff, T., Dittus, R. S., Brown, A., Pichert, J. W., & Elasy, T. A. (2004). Diabetes patient education: A meta-analysis and meta-regression. *Patient Education and Counseling,* 52, 97–105. DOI: 10.1016/S0738-3991(03)00016-8. The benefits of such educational efforts do outweigh the costs of their implementation, however; see Boren, S. A., Fitzner, K. A., Panhalkar, P. S., & Specker, J. E. (2009). Costs and benefits associated with diabetes education: A review of the literature. *Diabetes Educator,* 35, 72–96. DOI: 10.1177/014572170 8326774.

364 **My good friend Kirk Strosahl**: Kirk and Patti have numerous books and articles on this topic. See, for example, Robinson, P. J., Gould, D. A., & Strosahl, K. D. (2011). *Real behavior change in primary care: Improving patient outcomes and increasing job satisfaction.* Oakland, CA: New Harbinger.

365 **survivors of colorectal cancer**: This study showed the main outcomes: Hawkes, A. L., Chambers, S. K., Pakenham, K. I., Patrao, T. A., Baade, P. D., Lynch, B. M., Aitken, J. F., Meng, X. Q., & Courneya, K. S. (2013). Effects of a telephone-delivered multiple health behavior change intervention (CanChange) on health and behavioral outcomes in survivors of colorectal cancer: A randomized controlled trial. *Journal of Clinical Oncology, 31,* 2313–2321. A second study reported psychosocial outcomes such as quality of life: Hawkes, A. L., Pakenham, K. I., Chambers, S. K., et al. (2014). Effects of a multiple health behavior change intervention for colorectal cancer survivors on psychosocial outcomes and quality of life: A randomized controlled trial. *Annals of Behavioral Medicine, 48,* 359–370.

365 **Studies have shown similarly promising results**: This literature is voluminous. Anyone can test the veracity of my claim by searching for "psychology flexibility" or "psychological inflexibility" and [enter physical health areas here] in Google Scholar. For a recent review, see Graham, C. D., Gouick, J., Krahé, C., & Gillanders, D. (2016). A systematic review of the use of Acceptance and Commitment Therapy (ACT) in chronic disease and long-term conditions. *Clinical Psychology Review, 46,* 46–58.

365 **a rare *representative sample***: Gloster, A. T., Meyer, A. H., & Lieb, R. (2017). Psychological flexibility as a malleable public health target: Evidence from a representative sample. *Journal of Contextual Behavioral Science, 6,* 166–171. DOI: 10.1016/j.jcbs.2017.02.003.

366 **Research has shown that elderly people**: Davis, E. L., Deane, F. P., Lyons, G. C. B., & Barclay, G. D. (2017). Is higher acceptance associated with less anticipatory grief among patients in palliative care? *Journal of Pain and Symptom Management, 54,* 120–125. DOI: 10.1016/j.jpainsymman.2017.03.012; Romero-Moreno, R., Losada, A., Marquez-Gonzalez, M., & Mausbach, B. T. (2016). Stressors and anxiety in dementia caregiving: Multiple mediation analysis of rumination, experiential avoidance, and leisure. *International Psychogeriatrics,* 28, 1835–1844. DOI: 10.1017/S1041610216001009; and Losada, A., Márquez-González, M., Romero-Moreno, R., & López, J. (2014). Development and validation of the Experiential Avoidance in Caregiving Questionnaire (EACQ). *Aging & Mental Health, 18,* 293.

367 **Scandinavian countries spent**: Organisation for Economic Co-operation and Development. "Public Spending on Incapacity." https://data.oecd.org/socialexp/public-spending-on-incapacity.htm.

367 **The medical cost of chronic pain**: Reuben, D. B., et al. (2015). National Institutes of Health pathways to prevention workshop: The role of opioids in the treatment of chronic pain. *Annals of Internal Medicine, 162*, 295–300.

367 **over half of the U.S. population experienced pain**: Nahin, R. L. (2015). Estimates of pain prevalence and severity in adults: United States, 2012. *Journal of Pain, 16*, 769–780. DOI: 10.1016/j.jpain.2015.05.002.

367 **the fifth vital sign**: In January 2018 the Joint Commission, which accredits hospitals, claimed they said no such thing (http://www.jointcommission.org/joint_commission_statement_on_pain_management/)—but that is not correct. A careful reading shows that they *did* use the term and they *did* suggest that all patients be given a pain assessment, and when combined with the marketing of pharmaceutical companies, that was enough for the problematic use of opiate medications to get traction. Everyone wants to run from responsibility for the opiate crisis, but many hands by many players are not clean and the Joint Commission played a key role, even if inadvertently.

367 ***persisting aversive memory network***: De Ridder, D., Elgoyhen, A. B., Romo, R., & Langguth, B. (2011). Phantom percepts: Tinnitus and pain as persisting aversive memory networks. *Proceedings of the National Academy of Sciences of the United States of America, 108*, 8075–8080. DOI: 10.1073/pnas.1018466108. The case of phantom limb is a powerful demonstration of that network. See Nikolajsen, L., & Christensen, K. F. (2015). Phantom limb pain. In R. S. Tubbs et al. (Eds.), *Nerves and nerve injuries. Vol. 2: Pain, treatment, injury, disease and future directions* (pp. 23–34). London: Academic Press. DOI: 10.1016/B978-0-12-802653-3.00051-8; and Flor, H. (2008). Maladaptive plasticity, memory for pain and phantom limb pain: Review and suggestions for new therapies. *Expert Review of Neurotherapeutics*, 8.

368 **an 80 percent chance it will persist**: Elliott, A. M., Smith, B. H., Hannaford, P. C., Smith, W. C., & Chambers, W. A. (2002). The course of chronic pain in the community: Results of a 4-year follow-up study. *Pain*, 99, 299–307. DOI: 10.1016/S0304-3959(02)00138-0.

368 **Several world-class pain centers**: Wicksell, R. K., et al. (2009). Evaluating the effectiveness of exposure and acceptance strategies to improve functioning and quality of life in longstanding pediatric pain–a randomized controlled trial. *Pain, 141*, 248–257. See also Thorsell, J., et al. (2011). A comparative study of 2 manual-based self-help interventions, Acceptance and Commitment Therapy and applied relaxation, for persons with chronic pain. *Clinical Journal of Pain, 27*, 716–723.

368 **deploy ACT at the right time**: Dindo, L., Zimmerman, M. B., Hadlandsmyth, K., St. Marie, B., Embree, J., Marchman, J., Tripp-Reimer, B., & Rakel, B. (2018). Acceptance and Commitment Therapy for prevention of chronic post-surgical pain and opioid use in at-risk veterans: A pilot randomized controlled study. *Journal of Pain, 19*, 1211–1221. DOI: 10.1016/j.jpain.2018.04.016.

369 **The limits of the standard approach**: Rates of diabetes are shown in Guariguata, L. et al. (2014). Global estimates of diabetes prevalence for 2013 and projections for 2035. *Diabetes Research and Clinical Practice, 103*, 137–149. DOI: 10.1016/j.diabres.2013.11.002. Rates of undiagnosed diabetes are in Beagley, J., Guariguata, L., Weil, C., & Motalab, A. A. (2014). Global estimates of undiagnosed diabetes in adults. *Diabetes Research and Clinical Practice, 103*, 150–160. DOI: 10.1016/j.diabres.2013.11.001. See also Shi, Y., & Hu, F. B. (2014). The global implications of diabetes and cancer. *Lancet* 383(9933): 1947–1948. DOI: 10.1016/S0140-6736(14)60886-2. For estimates of expenditures, see Zhang, P., Zhang, X., Brown, J., et al. (2010). Global healthcare expenditure on diabetes for 2010 and 2030. *Diabetes Research and Clinical Practice, 87*, 293–301.

370 **patients do not stick rigorously to the appropriate regimes**: Diabetes is a disease with one of the lowest rates of patient adherence to medical recommendations. DiMatteo, M. R. (2004). Variations in patients' adherence to medical recommendations: A quantitative review of 50 years of research. *Medical Care*, 42, 200–209.

370 **help patients manage their disease**: Gregg, J. A., Callaghan, G. M., Hayes, S. C., & Glenn-Lawson, J. L. (2007). Improving diabetes self-management through acceptance, mindfulness, and values: A randomized controlled trial. *Journal of Consulting and Clinical Psychology*, 75(2), 336–343. The protocol is available in book form: Gregg, J., Callaghan, G., & Hayes, S. C. (2007). *The diabetes lifestyle book: Facing your fears and making changes for a long and healthy life*. Oakland, CA: New Harbinger.

370 **Jennifer and I developed an assessment of psychological flexibility**: If you're interested in taking it, you can find it at http://www.stevenchayes.com.

371 **the results were fully replicated**: Shayeghian, Z., Hassanabadi, H., Aguilar-Vafaie,

M. E., Amiri, P., & Besharat, M. A. (2016). A randomized controlled trial of Acceptance and Commitment Therapy for Type 2 diabetes management: The moderating role of coping styles. *PLoS ONE, 11*(12), e0166599. DOI: 10.1371/ journal.pone.0166599.

371 **40 percent of the population will be diagnosed with cancer**: Adler, N. E., & Page, A. E. K. (Eds.). (2008). *Cancer care for the whole patient: Meeting psychosocial health needs.* Washington, DC: National Academies Press.

372 **Training in the ACT skills**: Evidence can be found in Páez, M. B., Luciano, C., & Gutiérrez, O. (2007). Tratamiento psicológico para el afrontamiento del cáncer de mama. Estudio comparativo entre estrategias de aceptación y de control cognitivo. *Psicooncología, 4,* 75–95; and Arch, J. J., & Mitchell, J. L. (2016). An Acceptance and Commitment Therapy (ACT) group intervention for cancer survivors experiencing anxiety at re-entry. *Psycho-Oncology, 25,* 610–615. DOI: 10.1002/pon.3890.

373 **The counselor began by asking**: Angiola, J. E., & Bowen, A. M. (2013). Quality of life in advanced cancer: An Acceptance and Commitment Therapy approach. *Counseling Psychologist, 41,* 313–335. DOI: 10.1177/0011000012461955.

374 **psychological inflexibility turns the loudness of the ringing:** The questionnaire was published in Westin, V., Hayes, S. C., & Andersson, G. (2008). Is it the sound or your relationship to it? The role of acceptance in predicting tinnitus impact. *Behaviour Research and Therapy, 46,* 1259–1265. DOI: 10.1016/j.brat.2008.08.008. Additional data on its role in tinnitus distress can be found in Hesser, H., Bankestad, E., & Andersson, G. (2015). Acceptance of tinnitus as an independent correlate of tinnitus severity. *Ear and Hearing, 36,* e176–e182. DOI: 10.1097/AUD.0000000000000148. You can find the measure of tinnitus acceptance at http://www.stevenchayes.com.

374 **Gerhard and his team then conducted a trial:** Westin, V. Z., Schulin, M., Hesser, H., Karlsson, M., Noe, R. Z., Olofsson, U., Stalby, M., Wisung, G., & Andersson, G. (2011). Acceptance and Commitment Therapy versus Tinnitus Retraining Therapy in the treatment of tinnitus distress: A randomized controlled trial. *Behaviour Research and Therapy, 49,* 737–747.

375 **We tracked the frequency with which patients made statements**: Hesser, H., Westin, V., Hayes, S. C., & Andersson, G. (2009). Clients' in-session acceptance and cognitive defusion behaviors in acceptance-based treatment of tinnitus distress. *Behaviour Research and Therapy, 47,* 523–528. DOI: 10.1016/j.brat.2009.02.002.

375 **help people with a diagnosis of terminal illness:** Rost, A. D., Wilson, K. G., Buchanan, E., Hildebrandt, M. J., & Mutch, D. (2012). Improving psychological adjustment among late-stage ovarian cancer patients: Examining the role of avoidance in treatment. *Cognitive and Behavioral Practice, 19,* 508–517.

Chapter Twenty-One: Social Transformation

379 **Nearly three-quarters of the country's population:** U.S. Department of State, Bureau of Economic and Business Affairs. "2013 Investment Climate Statement–Sierra Leone." March 2013.

382 **An evaluation by the University of Glasgow:** Stewart, C., White, R. G., Ebert, B., Mays, I., Nardozzi, J., & Bockarie, H. (2016). A preliminary evaluation of Acceptance and Commitment Therapy (ACT) training in Sierra Leone. *Journal of Contextual Behavioral Science, 5,* 16–22. DOI: 10.1016/j.jcbs.2016.01.001.

382 **the blending of Ostrom's principles and ACT:** You can explore this protocol for free and if it applies to groups you care about you can get help in applying it. Visit http://www.prosocial.world.

Epilogue

388 **Hold Out Your Hand:** This beautiful poem is published by permission of the author. Julia has a book of her poems available called (fittingly for me and for the last page of this book) *On the Other Side of Fear* (Balboa Press, 2012), and you can find her e-books at http://www.etsy.com/shop/juliafeh.

INDEX